Social Indicators Research Series

Volume 67

This series aims to provide a public forum for single treatises and collections of papers on social indicators research that are too long to be published in our journal *Social Indicators Research*. Like the journal, the book series deals with statistical assessments of the quality of life from a broad perspective. It welcomes the research on a wide variety of substantive areas, including health, crime, housing, education, family life, leisure activities, transportation, mobility, economics, work, religion and environmental issues. These areas of research will focus on the impact of key issues such as health on the overall quality of life and vice versa. An international review board, consisting of Ruut Veenhoven, Joachim Vogel, Ed Diener, Torbjorn Moum, Mirjam A.G. Sprangers and Wolfgang Glatzer, will ensure the high quality of the series as a whole.

More information about this series at http://www.springer.com/series/6548

Ronald E. Anderson
Editor

Alleviating World Suffering

The Challenge of Negative Quality of Life

Springer

Editor
Ronald E. Anderson
Faculty of Sociology, Department of Sociology
University of Minnesota
Minneapolis, MN, USA

ISSN 1387-6570 ISSN 2215-0099 (electronic)
Social Indicators Research Series
ISBN 978-3-319-51390-4 ISBN 978-3-319-51391-1 (eBook)
DOI 10.1007/978-3-319-51391-1

Library of Congress Control Number: 2017934073

Printed on acid-free paper

This Springer imprint is published by Springer Nature
The registered company is Springer International Publishing AG
The registered company address is: Gewerbestrasse 11, 6330 Cham, Switzerland

Preface

This book project serves as a companion volume to *World Suffering and Quality of Life* (*http://www.springer.com/us/book/9789401796699*), which I edited and Springer published in early 2015. That volume introduced an agenda for studying global quality of life, including both negative and positive aspects of daily life. Since then the concepts of negative quality of life and ill-being have gained greater attention among researchers.

In this new book, my vision, and that of the other authors, has been to understand and heal the roots of suffering, in other words, to more effectively alleviate suffering. Our chapters could reinvigorate policies related to global well-being by providing new approaches and more thorough evaluation of these approaches. We hope that a side effect of this project will be to add sufficient clarity to public understanding, such that both humanitarian institutions and individuals take additional steps to relieve more suffering.

This follow-up volume of 27 chapters written by experts around the world is clearly distinguished from the first volume by concentrating upon the *alleviation* of world suffering rather than world suffering itself. We also take on the challenge of integrating suffering and its relief into the research on negative quality of life. Importantly, alleviation will be defined to include prevention of suffering as well as relief actions and institutions. Most chapters evaluate aspects of the ways that relief, development, health, and other social programs ultimately attempt to reduce suffering. The scope of these chapters encompasses analyses of social policies and programs on relief work, economic development, environmental policies, human rights promotion, caregiving, and compassion. The resulting book serves as an example of quality work that addresses such major sources of suffering as violence, inequity, cruelty, poverty, and climate change, focusing on how these conditions can be more effectively contained.

Removing or reducing extreme suffering symbolizes kindness, compassion, humanitarianism, empathy, and, most importantly, altruism. Some would even say it springs from the better angels of our nature. Yet some moral traditions punish specific types of alleviation, for example, taking illegal drugs for severe pain, aborting a deformed fetus, or performing mercy suicides. These controversial topics are not discussed in this book, with the exception of abortion, which is discussed in two chapters as a topic related to global health.

In a society where self-interest is valued more highly than solidarity, giving alms or providing welfare for the poor could become taboo and even declared immoral by some. Such cultural ambivalence about suffering may explain why the alleviation of suffering often goes unrewarded, even though it has been offered empathetically, sincerely, and generously.

Alleviation of large, complex sources of suffering such as poverty or discrimination poses another problem: that the path to alleviation has not been mapped. This problem can be addressed by researching the roots of social suffering and studying forms of intervention intended to relieve suffering.

It is apparent that the alleviation of suffering is not always perceived as a uniformly desirable trait or social activity. However, for the most part, it remains a humane, caring action that can provide scaffolding for solidarity, trust, and mutual caring. Therefore, it appears to be a solid place to start in the mobilization of civil society and programs to improve mutuality and, ultimately, human betterment.

Audience

This work primarily targets researchers, academics, and students in the social sciences, international studies, psychology, health sciences, and health professions. It is also aimed at nonacademic readers with a personal interest in the relief of suffering, whether intellectual, policy oriented, or practical. As I assembled the chapters, I divided them in many different ways, including by study methods used and key themes. From this process, the principal audience communities became more apparent. Anticipated audiences include:

- Those supporting or participating in humanitarian activities, including human rights and development
- Those trying to understand suffering and how to ameliorate its effects
- Researchers wanting to assess the quality of life of different groups
- Those studying communities, including online community, and the impact social suffering has on these
- Health-care providers and informal caregivers, especially those who struggle with someone's suffering

Project Development

Over the past two years, in preparation for writing this book, I digested hundreds of articles and books about suffering and its alleviation. I found the diversity of approaches and opinions startling. Such divergence made the mission for this book even more compelling.

To develop the chapters for this volume, I emailed invitations to about 100 authors of academic books or articles related to suffering and its relief. Each was charged with writing something important pertaining to the *alleviation of world suffering* in 5000 to 9000 words. I received about 50 good abstracts and asked for the authors to write chapter drafts.

Over a 9-month period, I worked with these authors and obtained reviews in order to create high-quality, in-depth but succinct reports for this volume. Together, the 27 chapters assembled here represent the best of contemporary thought and cutting-edge research on world suffering and its alleviation. The authors live in many different countries and represent each major continent except Antarctica. The authors don't necessarily agree on precisely how to define suffering, but their work contributes to a cumulative body of knowledge about suffering that ultimately will be enormous. By bringing a more precise and complete vocabulary of suffering into every day and humanitarian discourse, we have the basic tools to collaborate to alleviate suffering and reduce its future occurrences.

Challenges

In today's world, it is nearly impossible to escape images showing violence, famine, disease, and other calamities. As noted in Chap. 3, media scholars tend to agree that social media and other new technologies, combined with narcissist marketing of humanitarian aid, produce half-hearted concern for global suffering. Thus, the public sees secondhand a barrage of disasters, epidemics, wars, and terrorism. Existing institutions such as human rights organizations and humanitarian relief agencies rally support for relief from these calamities. But often their appeals fall flat because the giving public has not been socialized in the humane values that demand social responsibility for all tragically suffering human beings. Working against full support for alleviation of suffering is public indifference from growing weary of so many appeals for help.

Avoiding preventable suffering is an ultimate human concern. This means that human beings must come to terms with it and understand it as a central social responsibility in exchange for being human. Research on suffering will help us identify and evaluate how best to act responsibly.

In contrast, unpreventable suffering, such as natural death, can be a tragedy that we learn to approach with serenity and accept as part of life. Toward that end, some of the chapters here offer enlightenment on how suffering can become a source of greater meaning and an aid to making peace in a cruel world.

Acknowledgments

A book this size—with 34 authors and 27 chapters—requires an extended "family" to conceive, produce, and deliver a new, literary life. The book's production had its moments of excitement and suspense as well as hard, tedious—but challenging—work. The book project began in Buenos Aires at an ISQOLS (International Society for Quality of Life Studies) conference in July 2012, when I met Esther Otten, editor of health, well-being, and sociology publications at Springer Science + Business Media (commonly known as Springer) in Dordrecht, the Netherlands. She expressed interest in my work on the topic of suffering, and by the end of the year, I had presented two successful book proposals to Springer. After finishing the first book in June 2013, I immediately started an edited book, *World Suffering and the Quality of Life*, which was completed a year later. After the book's publication, it became clear that many people were buying or reading it, so I proposed another volume, this time emphasizing alleviation, not just suffering.

During the writing and preparation of this book, I sent dozens of email requests for help to the Springer staff, namely, Esther Otten, editor; Tuerlings Hendrikje and Miranda Dijksman, both editorial assistants; and Joseph Daniel, project coordinator, all at Springer in Dordrecht, the Netherlands. I am very grateful for their support throughout.

Here in Minnesota, I began the project doing everything myself, but as the draft chapters started arriving, I hired Sherri Hildebrandt to help with the copy editing of the documents. Kathryn Albrecht served as the project's expert on citations and references, as well as working with statistics and making charts. Some authors helped by reviewing papers and finding additional prospective authors. This writing project benefited greatly from a small grant to me from the University of Minnesota Office of the Vice President for Research and the University of Minnesota Retirees Association (UMRA).

Finally, the contribution of my wife, Nancy Kehmeier, was the most important of all. Not once did she claim to suffer from social rejection due to my preoccupation every day, from sunup to sundown, with this intense and time-consuming project.

Minneapolis, MN, USA Ronald E. Anderson

Contents

Contributors

Cawo Mohamed Abdi Associate Professor, Department of Sociology, University of Minnesota, USA

Ronald E. Anderson Faculty of Sociology, Department of Sociology, University of Minnesota, Minneapolis, MN, USA

Muhammad Faress Bhuiyan Faculty of Economics, Carleton College, Northfield, MN, USA

Elizabeth Heger Boyle Faculty of Sociology, University of Minnesota, Minneapolis, MN, USA

Lilie Chouliaraki Faculty of Media and Communications, London School of Economics and Political Science, London, UK

Mick Cooper Department of Psychology, University of Roehampton, London, UK

Richard J. Estes School of Social Policy & Practice, University of Pennsylvania, Philadelphia, PA, USA

Élise Féron Tampere Peace Research Institute, University of Tampere, Tampere, Finland

Rengin B. Firat Global Studies Institute, Department of Sociology and Neuroscience Institute, Georgia State University, Atlanta, GA, USA

Lea Hagoel The Department of Community Medicine and Epidemioogy, Carmel Medical Center and the Faculty of Medicine, Technion, Haifa, Israel

Laura M. Harder Faculty of Psychology, Metropolitan State University, St. Paul, MN, USA

Jason Hickel Faculty of Anthropology, London School of Economics and Political Science, London, UK

Ryan T. Kaminski United Nations Foundation, Washington, DC, USA

Meg Wilkes Karraker University of St. Thomas, St. Paul, MN, USA

Ellen J. Kennedy World Without Genocide, Mitchell Hamline School of Law, St Paul, MN, USA

Mehmet Kocaoğlu Department of Political Science, Purdue University, Beering Hall of Liberal Arts and Education, West Lafayette, IN, USA

Andrzej Kulczycki Deptartment of Health Care Organization & Policy, University of Alabama at Birmingham (UAB), Birmingham, AL, USA

Hye Won Kwon Department of Sociology, University of Iowa, Iowa City, IA, USA

Mark P. Lagon Walsh School of Foreign Service, Georgetown University, Washington, DC, USA

Caitlin O. Mahoney Faculty of Psychology, Metropolitan State University, St. Paul, MN, USA

Adam Muller Department of English, Film and Theatre, University of Manitoba, Winnipeg, MB, Canada

Robert A. Neimeyer Faculty of Psychology, University of Memphis, Memphis, TN, USA

Samuel P. Oliner Emeritus Professor of Sociology, Humboldt State University, Arcata, CA, USA

Rhonda Phillips Purdue University, West Lafayette, IN, USA

Poul Poder Centre for Resolution of International Conflict, Department of Political Science, University of Copenhagen, Copenhagen, Denmark

Paul C. Rosenblatt Department of Family Social Science, University of Minnesota, Saint Paul, MN, USA

Daniel Rothbart School for Conflict Analysis and Resolution (S-CAR), George Mason University, Fairfax, VA, USA

Joachim J. Savelsberg Department of Sociology, University of Minnesota, Minneapolis, MN, USA

Struan Sinclair Department of English, Film, and Theatre, University of Manitoba, Winnipeg, MB, Canada

M. Joseph Sirgy Virginia Tech Real Estate Professor of Marketing, Virginia Polytechnic Institute & State University, Blacksburg, VA, USA

J. Joseph Speidel Bixby Center for Global Reproductive Health, University of California, San Francisco, San Francisco, CA, USA

Joseph Svec Department of Sociology, University of Minnesota, Minneapolis, MN, USA

Iain Wilkinson School of Social Policy, Sociology, University of Kent, North East Canterbury, UK

Andrew Woolford Department of Sociology, University of Manitoba, Winnipeg, MB, Canada

About the Editor

Ronald (Ron) E. Anderson is Professor Emeritus at the University of Minnesota. He received his PhD in sociology from Stanford University in 1970. From 1968 until retiring in 2005, he served on the faculty of sociology at the University of Minnesota. From 1990 to 2005, he coordinated several international studies of the social and learning effects of information technology within primary and secondary education in 20 or more countries in each study. From that and earlier work, he wrote or edited seven books and over 100 articles. Since retirement, his research interests have shifted to suffering and caring. In 2014, Springer published his book *Human Suffering and Quality of Life: Conceptualizing Stories and Statistics*, as a 105-page Springer Brief. In 2015, Springer published a contributed book of 32 chapters and 46 authors, entitled *World Suffering and Quality of Life*. This 439-page book, which was edited by Anderson, is a "companion book" to this one. Both that book and this one are part of the Social Indicators Research Series of Springer's Science+Business Media Publishing Company.

Abbreviations

AIDS	acquired immune deficiency syndrome
CRC	colorectal cancer
DfID	Department for International Development (Britain)
DHS	Demographic and Health Surveys
DRC	Danish Refugee Council
FGC	female genital cutting
FOA	UN Food and Agriculture Organization
FP	family planning
GDP	gross domestic product
GHG	greenhouse gas
GPI	genuine progress indicator
HDI	human development index
HIV	human immunodeficiency virus
ICC	International Criminal Court
ICCESCR	International Covenant on Economic, Social and Cultural Rights
ICCPR	International Covenant on Civil and Political Rights
ICPD	International Conference on Population and Development
ICTR	International Criminal Tribunal for Rwanda
ICTY	International Criminal Tribunal for the Former Yugoslavia
INGO	international nongovernmental organization
IPCC	Intergovernmental Panel on Climate Change
IPPF	International Planned Parenthood Federation
IPV	intimate partner violence
IRS	Indian residential school
ISQOLS	International Society for Quality of Life Studies
IUD	intrauterine device
LGBTQ	lesbian, gay, bisexual, transgender, queer or questioning
LMIC	low- and middle-income countries
MDG	Millennium Development Goals
MENA	Middle East and North Africa
MMR	maternal mortality rate

MSF	Medecins Sans Frontieres (Doctors Without Borders)
NCANDS	National Child Abuse and Neglect Data System
NCVC	National Center for Victims of Crime
NGO	nongovernmental organization
ODA	official development assistance
PAC	postabortion care
PAFP	postabortion family planning
PP	positive psychology
ppm	parts per million
PPP	purchasing power parity
QOL	quality of life
SDG	Sustainability Development Goals
SIDS	Small Island Developing States
SSA	sub-Saharan Africa
STI	sexually transmitted infections
TAN	transnational advocacy network
TFR	total fertility rate
TRC	truth and reconciliation commission
UN	United Nations
UNDP	United Nations Development Programme
UNEP	United Nations Environment Programme
UNFCCC	United Nations Framework Convention on Climate Change
UNFPA	United Nations Fund for Population Activities
UNHCR	United Nations High Commissioner for Refugees
UNICEF	United Nations Children's Fund
UNOCHA	United Nations Office for the Coordination of Humanitarian Affairs
USAID	US Agency for International Development
WB	World Bank
WFP	World Food Programme
WHO	World Health Organization
WMO	World Meteorological Organization
WTO	World Trade Organization

Part I
Humanitarian and Social Perspectives on Suffering Alleviation

Chapter 1
A Worldview of the Alleviation of Suffering

Ronald E. Anderson

Introduction

Alleviation of suffering lies at the core of caring for others, humanitarian relief, civil society, social solidarity, and social welfare policy. For many people and some societies, it is the essence of human purpose, and for some it is the source of greatest meaning in their lives. And yet this is the first book to have addressed this topic from the perspective of not only individuals but societies and global society in particular.

Strangely, the one book that has a title anything like *Alleviation of World Suffering* is the name of a report from a U.S. Congressional hearing in 1921, almost 100 years ago (U.S. Congress 1921). Named as the hearing on "Relief of Suffering Populations of the World," the event passed a resolution to endorse a private philanthropic organization's contribution to provide relief for the "deplorable conditions that exist in Central and Eastern Europe." Not only did the initiative avoid spending any government money, but the target of concern covered only a tiny portion of the world.

Perhaps the neglect of suffering-alleviation in the published literature can be traced back to cultural aversions to negative words and events (Baumeister et al. 2011). A variety of studies of words have found that negative words have much greater staying power than positive words. And a number of studies have found that negative events have more influence than positive events in predicting future success in whatever task individuals or groups are working (Tugend 2012). This probably explains the aversion within academic disciplines to deal with the negative rather than the positive. In particular, studies on human progress use terms like well-being and quality of life, but "ill-being" and "negative quality of life" have been almost totally neglected. Furthermore, it is not just the words that have been

R.E. Anderson (✉)
Faculty of Sociology, Department of Sociology, University of Minnesota,
Minneapolis, MN 55455, USA
e-mail: rea@umn.edu

R.E. Anderson (ed.), *Alleviating World Suffering*, Social Indicators Research
Series 67, DOI 10.1007/978-3-319-51391-1_1

ignored, but researchers have ignored the possibilities to be gained by doing research on negative aspects of these dimensions of human experience.

As the absolute number of persons forced into extreme suffering continues to rise by the millions, if not billions, the need to study and help these persons is becoming much more compelling and urgent. Joseph Sirgy's chapter in this volume proposes that the word "ill-being" not only be widely used in conversations and theories of wellbeing, but that ill-being actually be measured in studies of wellbeing, both locally and globally. I propose that researchers invest in measuring negative quality of life as well as positive quality of life. Measuring negative quality of life must necessarily include suffering, which adds complexity to the research, but the results would be much more comprehensive and true to the actual experiences of all individuals from the top to the bottom of social hierarchies.

Better measurement of suffering will boost research on the alleviation of suffering. Now, we often do not have any idea whether suffering relief efforts actually reduce suffering. While this obviously applies to quantitative measurement, it also applies to qualitative research where the main tools are interviews and social observations. Knowing whether alleviation of suffering is occurring necessarily depends on valid qualitative judgments about peoples' responses to the world around them.

This volume has such a variety of topics and chapters that it necessarily will add to our understanding of both suffering and its alleviation or reduction. After an overview of the concepts of suffering and social suffering, I describe six useful frames for thinking about and conceptualizing suffering-alleviation. These frames include suffering-alleviation as moral and social responsibility; as undesirable or even harmful; as a central human purpose; as civil society; as quality of life; and as the future. Following this are characterizations of four different sectors of society that reveal how cultures are structured to accommodate different approaches to relieving suffering. Additional topics include (1) philosophical approaches for thinking about how to set practice priorities for the work of suffering-alleviation, (2) suggestions for how to alleviate extreme suffering, (3) data on global trends in suffering, and (4) a final section overviewing each chapter.

The Definition and Concept of Suffering

In the companion book, *World Suffering and the Quality of Life,* as editor I spent considerable time defining suffering (Anderson 2015: 3–12). The essence of the definition is severe distress that damages one's body, mind or interpersonal relationships and also damages one's self-identify. Thus, it encompasses not only physical hurt but mental and emotional trauma and destruction of the dignity of individuals, social groups, and even entire societies. The latter divisiveness occurs when the cruelty of one group of people humiliates or bullies another group as in racism, sexism, or even entrapment in poverty. As noted in the companion book (Anderson 2015: 5–6), this type of collective suffering is called *social suffering.* A common, recent form of social suffering has been neglect of and aggression toward refugees.

This rejection has had not only physical manifestations such as blocked border closings, but social stigmas that humiliate refugees, which without intervention can end in violent conflict.

The World Health Organization (WHO 1995) has asserted that poverty is the world's greatest killer. And Farmer (1996) built upon that assumption in describing social suffering by pointing to the intimate relationship between social suffering and structural violence. The essential notion of structural violence is that not only does deep poverty increase one's chances of dying of illnesses and injuries but it creates susceptibility to "hunger, torture, and rape" (Farmer 1996; p. 262). Farmer said that "the poor are not only more likely to suffer but they also are more likely to have their suffering silenced."

"Structural violence" also is a social arrangement (social structure) of conditions that unfairly disadvantage a category of people and puts them at risk. Social suffering and structural violence go hand in hand in that they co-occur and mutually reinforce each other. "In the most recent, comprehensive treatise on social suffering, Wilkinson and Kleinman (2016) capture in words the catastrophic burden of those trapped by the human plight of tormenting trauma. They also argue that "implicitly if not explicitly, social suffering has come to represent a call to moral responsibility and humanitarian care."

Wilkinson and Kleinman (2016) conclude that most "terrible and disabling events of suffering tend to involve us in the experience of losing our roles and identities as husbands, wives, children, friends, and citizens; and thus we are made lost to ourselves." Viewed from the perspective of civil society, social suffering rips apart the social fabric of one's world, leaving it potentially beyond repair.

Basic Principles of Alleviating Suffering

Almost all books and articles on the topic of suffering focus on suffering itself, whereas in this volume we emphasize alleviating it, which includes ameliorating, relieving, reducing, easing, erasing or preventing suffering. Those who seek to provide relief for suffering in the world usually adopt one of two general approaches. One is to offer and provide care for close others feeling trapped by suffering. The other approach is to become an advocate or activist for organizations and/or institutional change to bring suffering relief to large communities of people, sometimes even around the world. Of course, one can attempt to do both, but unless explicit priorities are set and followed, those distant from us physically or socially tend to be neglected.

The decision to reduce suffering, whether at the individual, community, or global levels, arises from a variety of sources such as a sense of social or moral responsibility. Charitable behavior does not necessarily take suffering into account. In fact, a large share of charity does not appear to be guided by suffering. Instead, it seems to be driven by the desire to improve general well-being or even by the desire to get something in return, such as recognition, payment, power, or prestige. Such types of charitable giving should be labeled as self-centered rather than other-centered.

Actions to alleviate suffering may also simultaneously reduce poverty, hunger, homelessness, illness, chemical dependence and so on. Such contributions to welfare or well-being generally benefit the giver as well as the recipient. The degree of observable suffering can serve as a guide to social priorities. A suffering-based policy decision process necessarily takes into account factors such as the severity or degree of hurt and whether or not the hurt has become chronic, that is, lasting 6 months or more. For social suffering, a suffering-based policy decision process would take into account other considerations such as justice and human rights.

Because suffering has many underlying roots, actions to alleviate severe suffering almost certainly need to include the alleviation of basic structural problems of society in order to keep the suffering from re-occurring. Here is a list of goals (which could also be called sub-goals) intended to eliminate the structural problems underlying suffering. Primarily they are goals required for the alleviation of widespread, severe suffering.

Ending violent conflict
Ending ongoing hunger
Ending persistent poverty
Providing disaster relief
Providing refugee relief
Eco-system preservation
Caring for the traumatized
Increasing equality
Raising human dignity

These considerations are not equally important in relieving all types of suffering. The complexities of social life and eco-systems need to be taken into account in alleviation strategies for any large-scale suffering. Furthermore, taking action to reduce suffering may yield additional social benefits.

Useful Frames for Thinking About Suffering-Alleviation

To better understand the role of suffering-alleviation across time, it is helpful to identify and trace some major frames (or points of view) that people use to organize their thoughts. Frames are complex perspectives that structure thought and build a rationale for a particular rhetoric, ideology, ethical principle, or social movement. Frame analysis explores how the frame links to social categories and its role in social change.

In the subsections that follow, I identify six frames with the first three frames focusing upon personal points of view and the last three on societal perspectives. The definition of each frame is not fixed or absolute but heuristic (illustrative of the implications of the frames), and the implications of each frame may change over time. Unless otherwise designated, the frames refer to contemporary culture.

Suffering-Alleviation as Moral and Social Responsibility

Some are driven primarily by a feeling of moral responsibility for others' wellbeing (Kleinman and van der Geest 2009; Mayerfeld 2005; Tronto 1993; Williams 2008). The most common literary metaphor of such commitment to others is the parable of the Good Samaritan as told by Jesus Christ. Now people with humanitarian commitments to helping others, no matter their race or stature, are sometimes called good Samaritans. A similar sentiment motivated hundreds of thousands of people (regardless of faith) to commit themselves to following the principles of the Charter for Compassion (Armstrong 2011). One of charges of the Charter is "to alleviate the suffering of our fellow creatures" and another is "to cultivate an informed empathy with the suffering of all human beings."

A long tradition of research on bystander intervention points to the many ways that people who encounter others in extreme suffering need assistance with delivering relief of suffering. When people are exposed to either a contrived or real situation of severe suffering such as sexual violence or domestic violence, the research question is "Under what conditions does a bystander offer assistance?" The implicit assumption underlying this social situation is that the well-being of such victims of violence depends upon whether or not an observer (bystander) engages in any attempts to relieve the victim's suffering. Darley and Latane (1970) found what has come to be known as the "bystander effect:" that the more people who concurrently observe the suffering, the less likely any one person will attempt to relieve it, presumably because responsibility for helping has been defused across all bystanders.

The large body of research on this situation reveals that accepting moral responsibility typically cannot be reduced to a simple choice of right and wrong (Darley and Latane 1970). Instead, responsible choices inevitably must take into account the array of considerations embedded in the decision situation itself as well as the cultural understanding of how to treat different types of strangers. Because of this complexity, the person who seeks to act with compassion and alleviate the suffering at hand should reflect on whether or not the reasons for not helping a stranger are valid or convenient excuses. In summary, this frame for suffering-alleviation is an important one, in part because moral responsibility is often forgotten.

Suffering-Alleviation as Unnecessary If Not Harmful

Literature of many genres claim that suffering builds character. Larson (2012) embellishes this notion with the additional claim that suffering makes great artists, religious leaders, and social reformers, and she wrote that: "The problem is not suffering per se, but rather our identification with our own ego: our divided, dualistic, cramped view of things."

Psychologist McGonigal (2015) brought together a host of academic research studies that provide evidence that stress and suffering do not necessarily have a negative effect on one's life. She concludes that it is possible to learn to act with resilience to stress and suffering and thus benefit from the experience of suffering. She argues that learning to respond resiliently to stress and certain types of suffering is essential to maintaining personal and social well-being.

Extreme suffering, on the other hand, often cannot be resolved by an individual's training or will power alone. Extreme sufferers often require support and assistance from others in the face of major injury, persecution, torture and equivalent sources of extreme suffering.

The question of this frame's usefulness probably is best answered in terms consistent with some spiritual approaches. Specifically, upon taking a personal path to greater resilience to suffering, there will be a reduced need to rely upon suffering-alleviation. But this does not give one an excuse to withhold suffering-alleviation from others who suffer. These "others" in your life may not have the personal tools yet to learn the resilience necessary to make them immune to events that trigger suffering. Developing this immunity or resilience poses a challenge to everyone because a clear dividing line does not exist between mild and extreme suffering. Thus resilience typically involves a long process of learning the tools to transform painful hardships into strengths of character.

Suffering-Alleviation as Human Purpose and Meaning

The principle purpose of many humans is self-promotion, hoping to obtain (or maintain) comfort, power, popularity, and wealth. At the opposite extreme are those with a purpose to love, care for, or help others. Suffering provides a basis by which to prioritize limited time and attention in doing things for others (Johnson and Schollar-Jaquish 2007). Helping those who truly suffer severely is generally viewed as more fulfilling. Since the traditional definition of compassion is a desire to relieve another's suffering, the work of suffering-alleviation becomes the yardstick by which to measure an authentic life. Contributing to humanity in this sense could mean helping a few close friends or all 7 billion people alive today.

The mission to relieve suffering does not require one-to-one contact. It can be accomplished by providing time and resources to global relief organizations. By giving to varied causes or helping a variety of different types of people in need, you increase the likelihood that your pro-social actions will truly have benefited one or more people. While positive feedback is not mandatory for gaining purpose and satisfaction from compassionate actions, it does help prop up and support the energy put into reducing the suffering of others.

Research on the role of media communications in the humanitarian sector reveals that marketing strategies such as celebrity contacts or rock concerts to raise money for major disasters have undercut the desire to contribute to human well-being and the alleviation of suffering (Chouliaraki 2013). Giving money to disaster relief has because a matter of entertainment and celebrity watching rather than taking steps to aid another human being in dire straits. On the surface the mix of entertainment and humanitarianism seems like a happy marriage but in fact the transition to trivialized benevolence almost totally undermines the meaning of donation as suffering-alleviation and replaces it with the meaning of donation as fun and privilege.

Suffering-Alleviation as Key to Community and Civil Society

The phrase *Civil Society*, while a very important concept, creates confusion and misunderstanding. Across hundreds of definitions, the essential meaning of the phrase is that of a public space between the state and the market (government and business) where people and their representative organizations can debate and tackle action. Therefore, actions and organizations of civil society will be voluntary and intended to advance society and its core values. In addition, the concept looks very much like community and the promotion of community, which is known as communitarianism (Etzioni 2009).

The latter notion of civil society is consistent with the shared ideal of alleviating the suffering of others. Human interdependency combined with concern for others justifies ameliorating the suffering of others whenever possible and appropriate.

Korten (2016) defined "global civil society" as "rejoicing in love of all beings," and actions that are rooted in "a sense of who we are, who we want to be, and how we relate to each other and the living body of Earth." Korten's notion of civil society tends to be future oriented and optimistic about peoples' ability to avoid self-destruction.

Suffering-Alleviation as Improving Quality of Life

The process of meaningful relief of others' suffering, as discussed in the preceding frames, applies to this frame as well. When you are relieving another's suffering, you are also improving their quality of life. This frame is uniquely justified by its emphasis on quality of life as a human need and its emphasis on *social* suffering as a qualitatively different type of suffering.

As a common phrase, "quality of life" (QOL) goes back only a few decades (Mukherjee 1989). However, in the twenty-first century, the concept has become well known, especially within research on health and economics (Land et al. 2012). There is even a professional group called the International Society for Quality of Life Studies, and it publishes several academic journals with "quality of life" in their titles. Many national and international policy reports also use the phrase, sometimes equating it with general well-being and/or happiness (Jordan 2012). The governments of several nations are now using the concept in attempting to construct new measures of national and human progress.

The second wave of Positive Psychology (sometimes called PP 2.0) reflects an attempt to engage in suffering-alleviation and improve quality of life (Ivtzan et al. 2015). Traditional positive psychology (Seligman 2011) presumed that the negatives would disappear if one focused on the positives of life. The second wave of positive psychology emerged to address the limitations of this approach. Ivtzan et al. (2015) assume that it is necessary to engage with the "dark side," recognizing suffering of all kinds. "Engage" means to experience and develop the skills to address suffering such that positive growth becomes the outcome. The weakness of this approach is that positive outcomes may not always be possible.

Present-day approaches to suffering-alleviation framed as improvements in the quality of life can occur in many arenas including public health, human rights projects, humanitarian disaster relief, social services, security, safety precautions, and environmental preservation.

Suffering-Prevention as a Perspective on the Future

Many natural systems, biological and otherwise, depend upon balancing mechanisms for survival. Human societies depend upon these and other social systems to function over time. Suffering is an outward manifestation of threats to individual and social functioning. In addition, suffering serves as a warning sign for persons and civil society to engage in actions that help avoid chaos or social collapse. Actions taken to protect future conditions and future generations should be called "suffering prevention."

Some suffering-producing calamities perpetuate suffering long after it begins. In such circumstances it is more a matter for the future rather than the present. Climate change and global warming are cases in point. Under the assumption that greenhouse gases will continue to be emitted at high rates, suffering-prevention cannot be taken lightly. Strategies primarily for future survival include ecosystem health maintenance, sustainable development reforms, global security systems, and structural economic reforms. Just as we owe distant strangers relief from disasters, we owe our future generations more suffering-prevention activities in the present day. This theme of the future continues in the last chapter (Chap. 27).

Global Social Sectors of Suffering-Alleviation

English-speaking Western nations have evolved such that most suffering-alleviation that transpires collectively occurs within one of these four social sectors: the humanitarian sector, the social policy sector, the caregiving sector, and the spiritual sector.

This pattern arises from the social institutions that have been constructed within these sectors to facilitate coordinated and individual behavior to reduce suffering.

Each of the four sectors generates a unique frame with which to view the world, so this section in part continues the list of six frames in the previous section. But as you will see, these sectors each play such a special role in the practice of suffering-alleviation that they deserve special consideration. The four sectors overlap because all share a common goal to improve human wellbeing. And many projects have components within each of the four sectors. For example, a civil society program to increase racial and ethnic inclusion almost certainly will be consistent with humanitarian goals, support key social policies, create caregiving organizations and generate ethical projects that promote racial inclusion.

Each of these four sectors has sparked its own discussions and literature related to the mission of the sector. In fact, I identified these sectors by conducting a variety of literature and book searches using the keywords "alleviating suffering" and "relief of suffering." The labels for these four sectors emerged from content analyzing the literature related to suffering and its alleviation.

The caregiving and spiritual sectors have by far the largest representation among books and articles. However, the other two sectors (the humanitarian and the social policy sectors) each were represented by over 10% of the published writing. In the discussions below, each sector will be briefly described because not only do they each reflect a body of literature and live website discussions, but they each reveal very different approaches to suffering-alleviation.

The Humanitarian Sector

This sector usually equates with humanitarianism because it champions charitable causes such as disaster relief, socio-economic development and meeting unmet needs such as food, water, and healthcare. Often this sector appeals to its constituents solely on the basis of moral integrity or the ethics of humanitarian responsibility. The International Red Cross website states its mission is to "prevent and alleviate human suffering in the face of emergencies by mobilizing the power of volunteers and the generosity of donors." Often fund-raising solicitations by humanitarian organizations refer to suffering and their activities to reduce it.

These humanitarian organizations often are called non-governmental organizations (NGOs, or INGOs, if the NGO is truly international in scope). During the twentieth century, the number of NGOs evolved from a few hundred social action agencies to an estimated 10 million organizations with 1.5 billion donors worldwide (OnGood 2016). This sector of global society has become so large and dominant that some equate NGOs with civil society (World Bank 2016).

In addition to NGOs and INGOs, a major share of the humanitarian sector is the United Nations, which is an inter-governments agency that works closely with many private NGOs. The United Nations filled a vacuum for global government at a time when inter-nation cooperation emerged as a critical need. The UN now employs more than 50,000 people and takes a major, if not a primary, lead in such areas as health, labor, and development.

Given that the UN plays such a critical leadership role in the global sphere, it is most significant that the World Humanitarian Summit on May 24, 2016, declared one of its primary goals was the minimization of suffering around the world (UN 2016a). In addition, on September 22, 2016, UN Secretary-General Ban Ki-moon declared the alleviation of suffering as a goal toward which all UN staff worked every day (UN 2016b). The UN routinely calls for alleviation of suffering on special events and days such as International Migrants Day.

In this volume, a number of chapters explore elements of the humanitarian sector and how it has changed over time. (Longer summaries are given of each chapter in the last section of this first chapter.) In separate chapters by Lilie Chouliaraki and Iain Wilkinson, these well-known scholars of social suffering trace how the humanitarian sector has evolved rapidly over the past few decades due to the communications and the technology sectors.

Several chapters in this volume discuss genocide, which perhaps poses the greatest challenge to humanitarianism. Joachim Savelsberg takes the case of Darfur to examine the interrelationship between the media and International Criminal Law. Samuel Oliner focuses upon the holocaust while Ellen Kennedy uses five different genocides to summarize the state of knowledge about sexual violence against women. And Adam Muller and his associates describe their project to educate the public about North American cultural genocide against their indigenous people.

The Social Policy Sector

This sector consists of government agencies and nonprofit organizations relevant to social policy, including social welfare, crime, and justice work; safety and security; education, labor, pensions, and child benefits. Also, included within social policy are social issues that do not fit into these broad policy areas. These social issues include animal treatment, legalizing drugs such as medical cannabis for suffering reduction, allowing for assisted suicide in conditions of extreme suffering, abortion, domestic violence, criminal sentencing policies, and actions to minimize discrimination on the basis of race, gender and other inappropriate bases (Jimeniz et al. 2014).

The breadth of the social policy sector depends largely on the local standards for defining what can be included within social policy and implemented by local governance institutions. For example, if laws regarding unlimited consumption of natural resources do not exist or are not enforced, then natural disasters will likely follow at considerable social and economic cost.

New social policy may become necessary under conditions of extreme inequality if it leads to crippling poverty and new costs from high crime and incarceration rates. Poverty, crime and debilitating illnesses together create intractable social suffering, which may threaten the actual survival of a community or society.

Issues such as legalizing medical cannabis and doctor-assisted suicide remain controversial because, while they may dramatically reduce suffering, they conflict with core values of specific social groups within many societies.

It should be obvious by now that the humanitarian and the social policy sectors often overlap. While disasters and economic development tend to be subsumed under the humanitarian sector, social development tends to be seen as part of social policy. If a community issue deals with social inclusion, social isolation, or civil society, chances are that it is seen as a matter of social policy. The World Bank has been primarily concerned with economics and economic support for development around the world. However, a few years ago it established a Social Development division that concentrates upon social issues such as social exclusion, reducing violence, building cohesive and resilient societies, and making institutions accessible and accountable to citizens (World Bank 2005).

Several chapters in this book address social policy by dissecting major human problems. One is Elise Féron, who describes recovery programs for male survivors of sexual violence in armed conflict situations. Examining female rather than male victimization, Elizabeth Heger Boyle and Joseph Svec summarize research on the slow progress being made around the world in reducing the cultural practice of female genital cutting. They focus upon how practice often overwhelms policy, and how social change often requires education in the negative health consequences of following existing social practice.

Several additional chapters primarily pertain to social policy, but they have important implications for humanitarianism as well. One is Richard Estes' report describing research on sexual exploitation of children in North America. He reviews the impact of various social policy legislation intended to curtail child sexual exploitation including child trafficking across borders.

Another chapter reports on a survey of Bangladesh villagers by Faress Bhuiyan. He found naturally occurring alleviation of mental suffering to be highest among those married, those with the best access to health services, and those with relatively little disparity in income with their neighbors.

Thirdly, Cawo Abdi describes her field work findings in South Africa. She concludes that even though Somali refugees to South Africa suffered greatly from refugee camps and lack of resources, the South African indigenous people living in urban shanty towns (also called squatter camps) suffered even more from the lack of resources that left them without adequate housing, sanitation, healthcare, and steady employment.

The Caregiving Sector

As defined in this volume, the caregiving sector encompasses both institutionalized healthcare practice (Farmer et al. 2013) and informal caregiving, which consists of both situations of care and caring (Glenn 2010). The healthcare community, which includes professional groups and organizations such as hospitals, lacks a single position on the priority of relieving people's suffering. Given the diversity in healthcare needs across nations and regions, an overall strategy on global healthcare poses a major challenge. But thanks to Farmer et al. (2013) and his associates and Kleinman (2010a, b), progress has begun toward defining global priorities and strategies in worldwide healthcare. The alleviation of suffering in the caregiving sector depends upon the nature of the challenge at hand, the personal opinions of individual professionals, healthcare facilities, community culture, and governmental regulations.

The first "code" of medical ethics, the Hippocratic Oath, says nothing directly about suffering or obligations to the suffering. Thus, contemporary codes of ethics for healthcare professionals share little agreement on obligations to relieve client suffering (Aswegan 2007). Up until the twentieth century palliative care and hospice movements, patients undergoing severe pain and suffering could not count on receiving state-of-the art treatment for suffering relief.

Within the past few decades the emergence of hospice and palliative care services has been an important development in suffering relief. Palliative care can begin upon diagnosis of terminal illness, but hospice care begins after treatment of the terminal disease is stopped and when it is clear that the patient is not going to survive the illness more than a few days or weeks before life's ending. A turning point in the United States occurred in 1995 when Medicare started offering free hospice care. Not only does this service cover medications and other care to alleviate the patient's suffering, but it includes grief counseling and assistance to loved ones as well.

Switching to the arena of informal caregiving, in the United States more than 34 million unpaid caregivers provide care to another adult who is ill or disabled (CDC 2016). And an estimated 38 million households are family households with children under 18 (U.S. Census 2013). Thus, more than half of all households in the U.S. deliver care either to other adults or to children or both. Most nations in the world have an even higher proportion of households with children.

Not all informal caregiving serves family members or others who carry the burden of extreme suffering. Many are merely ill or incapacitated in less serious ways. However, the breadth of the burden for both sufferers and caregivers is suggested by the hundreds and hundreds of books published about the needed techniques and competencies for successful caregiving.

Table 1.1 gives a typology of three major types of capabilities that help to alleviate the suffering of others. The typology especially captures the skills and competencies needed in caregiving. The types of knowledge and skill, represented by the rows of the table, were adapted from Ohlen (2002), who identified skill classes, using the language of Aristotle, to analyze how to be an effective caregiver in palliative care.

A useful insight suggested by Table 1.1 is the distinction between knowing and doing or "knowing how." Even more significant is the third type of capability, "practical ability with wisdom." This points to the fact that caregiver decisions sometimes require wisdom as well as knowledge and skills. This framework applies not only to caregiving, but, as shown in the last column, to policy-making as well. This analysis

Table 1.1 Capabilities and competencies for alleviating suffering

Aristotle's categories	General descriptions	Learning to alleviate suffering	Effective caregiving	Effective policy decisions and implementation
Episteme	Knowing principles	Knowing risks, hurts, solutions	Knowing theory of caregiving	Knowing goals and resources
Techne	Knowing how (hands-on)	Knowing action alternatives and their efficacy	Caregiving, alleviating skills	Implementation skills
Phronesis	Practical abilities (wise actions)	Wise, prudent ability to reduce suffering of others	Wise, informed comforting and caring	Long-term resolution of large-scale suffering

also applies to most social policy, especially that which has a direct effect on the degree of suffering of any constituencies involved.

The challenge of alleviating severe suffering through either informal care or professional healthcare is addressed by several chapters in this volume. Several authors of these chapters work as professional psychological counselors, namely Mick Cooper and Robert Neimeyer. Neimeyer's chapter specializes in grief, and he shows how intervening in a sufferer's interpretation of the meanings underlying one's grief can result in major reduction of suffering. Mick Cooper also uses the exploration of personal meanings in his approach to suffering reduction. His chapter presents a model of these personal meanings in terms of synergetic and dysergetic desires and how they can be used in moving toward a reduction in suffering.

Two other chapters provide frameworks for evaluating thoughts and feelings toward reduced suffering. Caitlin Mahoney and Laura Harder focus upon emotions and empathy, and Paul Rosenblatt applies a number of theories to explain why many people may be slow in acting to alleviate the suffering of others.

The Spiritual Sector

In the United States, and probably in most other nations, much of the writing on suffering and its alleviation has a spiritual flavor. In the USA the literature most often takes a Christian or Buddhist perspective (Peerman 2008). A significant portion of this literature avoids religion and promotes the importance of personal meaning and existential concerns. These existential discussions address life and death issues. When anxiety arises about these issues, it is called existential suffering.

People who routinely contemplate the meaning of life are considered spiritual in the broad sense of the word. Many people take a narrow view and equate the spiritual with religion. Here "spiritual" encompasses both of these groups because both support taking action to alleviate suffering out of concern for personal meaning.

Most theistic religious faiths such as Christianity explain suffering by individuals' failure to conform to the presumed will of God (Bowker 1970). In contrast, non-theistic religious traditions like Buddhism explain suffering as a failure to maintain a relaxed or spiritual state of mind (Pruett 1987). Also, Buddhism teaches that one should have compassion and care for others who suffer because such acts will reduce one's own susceptibility to suffering. Some Buddhist traditions teach that pain cannot be reduced, only suffering.

Existential frameworks, as already noted, focus on purposes and meanings in life. Furthermore, they also generally claim that helping others adds significant meaning to one's life. This assumption generally emphasizes the important role of helping to relieve the suffering of others.

You will find in this volume at least two chapters that address topics that have a spiritual component. In her chapter, Meg Wilkes Karraker evaluated the acquisition in knowledge and change in spiritual values of students assigned to a work in a homeless shelter as part of a college class assignment. The students' class assignment was to volunteer at Catholic Charities day centers for the homeless. While Karraker's students did not acquire as much knowledge and change in values as she had hoped, the project was successful and the student learning was in the desired direction.

In a chapter on existential suffering, Lea Hagoel describes her interviews and fieldwork with those advised to undergo testing for cancer without any physical signs of cancer. Some public health experts advise that large groups of people be tested for cancer even though the people have no signs of cancer. The rationale is that mortality can be reduced substantially. However, the mere fact of being tested for a deadly disease produces an existential crisis for many people. Programs of this type should try to anticipate and ameliorate any new existential suffering produced by the interventions.

Philosophical Issues in Prioritizing Suffering-Alleviation

Next we turn to the question of prioritizing actions intended to alleviate suffering. For guidance in this challenge, it makes sense to turn to moral philosophy and ethical systems. For centuries the utilitarian principle of giving highest priority to that which brings the greatest happiness to the most people appealed to those seeking an ethical principle that justified preoccupation with happiness. But in 1952, Karl Popper proposed an improvement, which he called *negative utilitarianism* (Popper 1952). Its essence was to make charitable decisions on the basis of either reducing the worst suffering or reducing the suffering of the largest number of sufferers. Or if viewed together, he proposed trying to achieve the least suffering for all.

An important extension of this philosophy was proposed by Arneson (2000) under the label *prioritarianism*, a negative utilitarianism that weights the value of action higher for those suffering the most. For example, with this approach, poor, developing countries would be given higher priority for more resources or assistance than rich, developed countries.

Table 1.2 Extreme suffering and prevalence statistics in 2014

Extreme suffering	Relevant statistics
Torture	Occurring in 130 out of 160 countries
Violent war crimes	Evidence from 18 countries
Violent homicides	Half million homicides in 2012 (UNODC 2013)
Refugees displaced	4 million refugees fled from Syria alone
Severe Malnutrition	2.1 million (Hickel 2017)

Unless otherwise noted, data are from Amnesty International (2015)

Given that no one can eradicate all suffering, how can we decide which type of suffering to tackle first and how much effort to invest in it? In Table 1.2, some extreme types of suffering are ordered in decreasing severity, with torture producing the greatest suffering for any one person and malnutrition the least. Under the premise of negative utilitarianism, the greatest priority would be to eliminate torture, assuming a policy was to alleviate the most severe suffering. But if the policy was to help the most people, then it would make sense to try to eliminate malnutrition because the elimination of malnutrition would probably represent assisting the most people. *Prioritarianism* over-weights suffering severity, so it might give preference to eliminating torture, even if only a few persons were helped.

Another criterion for choosing which strategy to use in reducing suffering has been called *effective altruism.* This concept was developed by philosopher Peter Singer (2009 and 2015), who also founded the Centre for Effective Altruism (https://www.centreforeffectivealtruism.org/) at the University of Oxford in the UK. Singer proposes that emotion and strategy be blended in order to be most effective in altruistic action such as maximizing charitable giving. Effective altruism is a growing social movement founded on the desire to make the world as good a place as it can be, the use of evidence and reason to find out how to do so, and the audacity to try (MacAskill 2016).

Approaches to Alleviating Extreme Suffering

To clarify how a suffering-alleviation decision process might work, consider first the worst suffering imaginable, which we will call *extreme suffering.* Table 1.3 lists examples of these instances of extreme suffering, with a sample of possible roots and alleviation sources.

The table lists only a fraction of the many ways that people feel extreme suffering. Many more people severely suffer from injury or illness with deep, excruciating pain, especially from the large share of the world where pain-relief medications are not available or are unaffordable. Another large share of the world's population suffers from extreme poverty and associated diseases, loss of family members, and deaths due to contamination of drinking water and unsanitary living conditions.

Table 1.3 Extreme suffering, its roots and its resolutions

Suffering	Roots	Alleviation sources
Torture	Injustice	Human rights law
Violent war crimes	Aggression	Human rights law
Violent homicides	Violent conflict	Emotional regulation
Refugees displaced	Global warming	Peace and justice
Severe malnutrition	Greed	Humanitarian policy

The roots of these extreme conditions are challenging to identify and resolve. Factors underlying world suffering not only cut across many layers of systems, both natural and social, but little consensus exists on their precise nature or what should be done to resolve the problems. Table 1.3 lists some roots to the problems and some potential methods for resolving them.

This is only a beginning attempt to identify and clarify the forces underlying extreme contemporary suffering. The objective is to begin to identify the sources of the suffering and their interacting roles such that solutions can be discussed and explored for their alleviation. A more complete analysis deserves considerable attention.

The next section in this chapter addresses the question of whether global suffering has been declining or rising. By considering both global and selected national trends in suffering it becomes possible to better evaluate the importance of suffering-alleviation at this time in global history.

Global Trends in Suffering and Suffering-Alleviation

Despite many globalizing forces, relatively few non-economic global indicators are available across time for evaluating suffering or suffering-alleviation. Exceptions include damage due to global warming and world refugee counts. The Gallup World Poll (Gallup 2015a, b) now collects dozens of metrics every year using random samples within nearly 150 countries, covering 95% of the world adult population. This new resource represents a powerful opportunity to document how the global system works as a natural home for billions of people.

Gallup's Life Evaluation Index measures subjective suffering based upon respondents' very low satisfaction with their life now and 5 years in the future. Very low was defined as a response of 0–4 on a 0–10 "ladder" scale (Gallup 2015b). Gallup labels these responses as 'suffering.'

The percent suffering, as measured by very low life satisfaction scores, are shown by global region in Fig. 1.1. Asia, which contains more than half the world population in this analysis, experienced a rise of over 5% in suffering, especially between 2007 and 2013. As shown in Fig. 1.1, even Europe and the Americas had small rises in suffering. The really steep rise in suffering occurred during this period for the

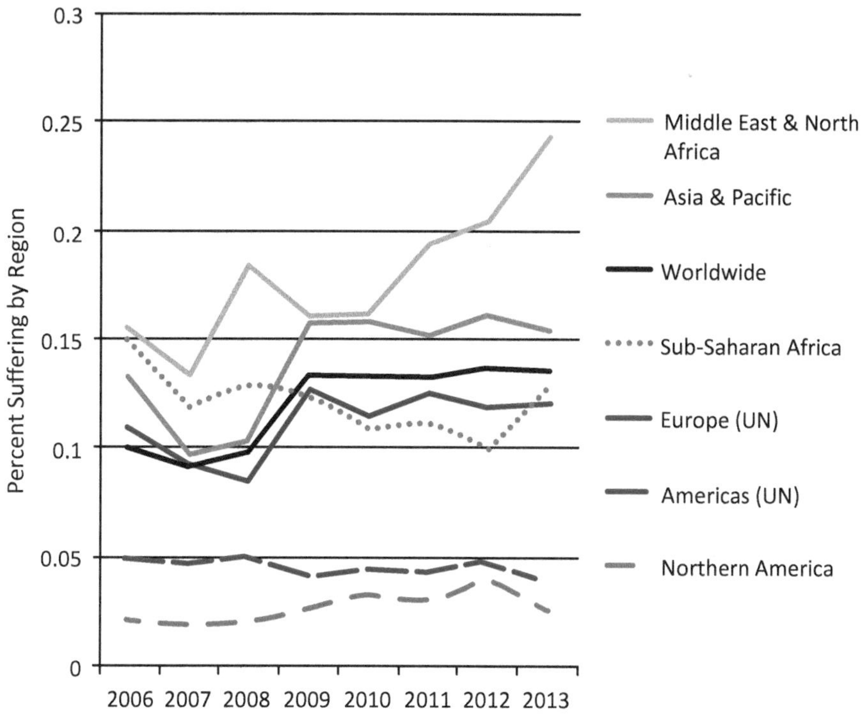

Fig. 1.1 Gallup suffering index by global region

Middle East and North Africa (MENA). Their percent suffering jumped 10% from 14% in 2009 to 24% in 2013. The amount of armed conflict in this region undoubtedly contributed greatly to this tragic rise in suffering.

Worldwide suffering and other negative experiences have been slowly increasing over the past decade, despite positive economic global growth. One way to characterize these findings is that the benefits of global economic growth have been overwhelmed by harmful forces such as ethnic conflicts, widespread armed conflict, and the resulting refugee crisis. Another likely culprit is the rising inequality of income and wealth. In a world where those trapped in poverty produce the highest population growth, any forces such as inequality of power and income contribute to increasing suffering.

Claims of huge poverty reduction have been made by the reports such as MDG 2015. These claims, when placed in the context of evidence of rising global suffering, suggest that the statistical improvements can easily be exaggerated and misleading. An increase in earnings may move one across the poverty line, but not change the risks of pain and suffering that accrue from depending upon negligible income.

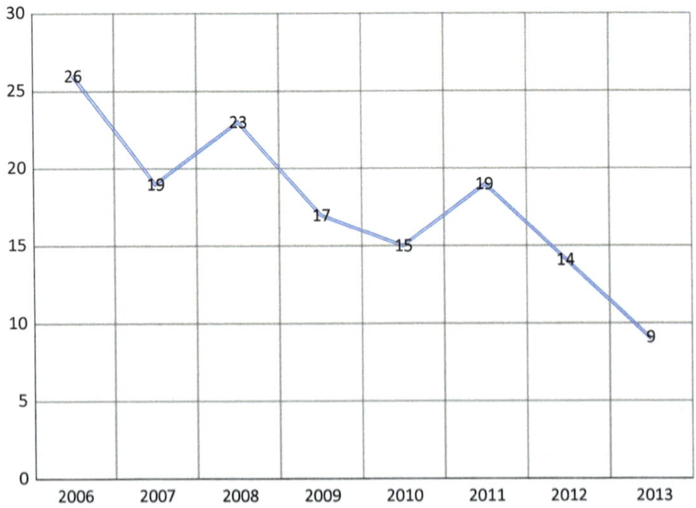

Fig. 1.2 Percent adults in Nicaragua reporting suffering, 2006–2013

Nations with Dramatic Declines in Suffering

Using the same measure of suffering, it is possible to examine countries with dramatic changes in suffering between 2006 and 2013. The countries with large drops in suffering reveal conditions that alleviated suffering substantially over the course of nearly a decade. The largest drop in suffering occurred in Zimbabwe, but before the decline began, it had the highest subjective suffering of all nations. Zimbabwe had been ruled for decades by a dictator, and the people had been living with hyperinflation and starvation. Over the course of only 4 years, suffering dropped from 44% to 6%. The country's leader, Robert Mugabe, implemented a variety of new policies and self-reported suffering plunged.

Another country with high suffering in 2006 was Nicaragua with 26% of the adult population suffering. Figure 1.2 reveals how the percent suffering dropped by 17% to 9% over the seven-year period. During this time, political events in Nicaragua helped spur a variety of improvements in health care and economic opportunity. Thus, Nicaragua is a good example of incremental socio-economic structural improvements and how they alleviate suffering.

Nicaragua was among the top ten countries in terms of declining suffering during this period. This rapid decline in suffering should give nations hope that subjective suffering can be alleviated without a campaign or policy to explicitly relieve suffering. Because severe suffering is so closely interwoven with the structural conditions of a society, by improving these structural conditions, suffering can be reduced indirectly but significantly, improving many lives.

Overview of the Chapters

This last section of this first chapter provides a brief summary of each of the chapters that follow. The book has been divided into five parts in the interest of pointing out the different approaches taken by the authors in addressing the alleviation of suffering. At the same time, the discussions in these sections will reveal how many of the chapters flow together to bring continuity despite different authorship and goals in each of the 27 chapters in this volume.

Part I contains chapters that primarily lay a foundation for understanding the remaining sections. A common theme is that of humanitarianism and its role in alleviating suffering. Part II moves to two major topics for this volume and any other discussion of suffering: the topic of quality of life (QOL) and the topic of care and caregiving. QOL, which is closely allied with human wellbeing, is a research tradition that should embrace suffering because suffering offers a major approach to studying negative qualities of life. Care and caregiving, on the other hand are the principal approaches of personal strategies to try to alleviate individual suffering.

Part III tackles the topic of development head-on and from a global perspective. The authors not only deal with the economics of development, but the topics of health and population growth take up a lot of their attention. Of course, the challenge of poverty arises and the Sustainable Development Goals (SDG) are given attention by a number of authors. Part IV raises the role of human rights from several standpoints, but the primary focus is violent conflict. Not surprisingly several of the papers in this section deal with a facet of one or more major genocides.

Part V centers around the future, applying several different themes. One is the most obvious question of how to prevent future suffering. Another is how to balance a combination of immediate needs with needs of future generations. These challenging questions emerge within discussions of education, economics, and climate change.

Part I. Humanitarian and Social Perspectives on Suffering-Alleviation

All the chapters in the first section, Part I, relate to a core topic: humanitarianism, although some do not even mention the word. At least two of the chapters discuss humanitarianism with the help of historical lenses. And the other two chapters take a perspective more consistent with that of individuals or groups doing humanitarian work. What is important to note is that all the authors in this section analyze their topics sociologically, even though they are not necessarily sociologists. At least part of each chapter analyzes the world from the standpoint of institutions and large sectors of society. And even more significantly, they all ask the rhetorical question, how does one or more aspects of society contribute toward a better understanding of large-scale and extreme suffering.

As editor, I began this first chapter with suffering-related definitions, including social suffering and its alleviation, followed by six frames for thinking about suffering-alleviation. These frames portray suffering-alleviation as a moral responsibility; as undesirable or even harmful; as a central human purpose; as civil society; as quality of life; and as a major future concern. Following this are characterizations of four different sectors of society that reveal how cultures are structured to accommodate different approaches to relieving suffering. Additional topics include philosophical approaches for thinking about how to set priorities for the work of suffering-alleviation; suggestions for how to alleviate extreme suffering; data on a global trend in rising suffering; and a final section overviewing each chapter.

Daniel Rothbart and Poul Poder creatively weave together themes of inequality, social exclusion, and humiliation with the harsh reality of social suffering. The result is a powerful description of highly intractable societies trapped by inequality and discrimination. Rather than leave us with pessimism about alleviating rigid social suffering, they detail some "instruments" that are used by elites to subjugate those of lower status. These instruments include laws favoring elites; an ideology of supremacy; using demeaning labels; using images that demean those on lower rungs of the ladder; and erasing the accomplishments of the degraded people. The proposed mechanism for deactivation of ruthless inequality is increased awareness of the devastating role that humiliation plays in separating hierarchical groupings. The authors argue that dominant elites deploy instruments that control disadvantaged group members through propaganda, by diminishing their self-worth. Rothbart and Poder detail how the elites are able with subtlety to institutionalize these enslaving structures by making their decisions, regulations and laws seem innocuous and superficially reasonable. Mitigation of systemic humiliation is particularly challenging, as it operates without easily identifiable agents or humiliators. The authors end with potentially powerful recommendations regarding the adoption of multiple tactics to alleviate suffering.

Lilie Chouliaraki, a well-known critical scholar, traces the shift in the past four decades away from the heart of the moral action of solidarity toward what she calls "ironic solidarity," which is defined by self-centered and consumptive relationships toward vulnerable others. Professor Chouliaraki traces this transformation, by focusing upon three historic trends during this period: the instrumentalization of humanitarianism; the de-politicization of solidarity; and the technologization of communication. The first is driven by a preoccupation with fund raising instead of moral argument; the second trend moves the justification of humanitarian action away from justice and toward minor rewards for the donor; and the third trend re-purposes technology in pursuit of self-expression. To set a new course, the chapter advocates an imperative to care for vulnerable others that listens to the voice of these others and addresses the question of values—of *why* it is important to care. She proposes a new ethics of solidarity that would start by acting upon the shared value of justice as a minimum common pursuit of what it means to be human. Such a course would inevitably improve the frequency and quality of attempts to alleviate human suffering.

Iain Wilkinson, a pioneer in the sociology of social suffering, begins with the premise that using the frame of social suffering has greatly expanded in recent years. Social suffering researchers use a wide variety of evidence to capture the catastrophic burden of those trapped by the human plight of tormenting perplexity. Implicitly if not explicitly, social suffering has come to represent a call to moral responsibility and humanitarian care. After briefly reviewing the history of the acceptance and rejection of humanitarianism as a moral compass for social science research, he argues that this wave will return the social sciences to again recognize the moral power of humanitarianism. Wilkinson concludes that removal of these conceptual and methodological barriers will make possible a wide range of research that will help guide the design of social changes that have the potential to greatly alleviate suffering locally and globally.

Mick Cooper's chapter shows how people (and social systems) suffer excessively because their wants are pulling them in opposite directions. He describes this as dysergetic (conflicting desires) as opposed to synergetic (harmonious desires yielding more than the sum of the individual wants). Two significant conclusions follow from this. One is that dysergetic elements yield suffering, which may be alleviated by transforming some of the wants/desires to more compatible ones. Secondly, this model of synergetic and dysergetic elements applies to interpersonal and societal levels as well as to individuals. The chapter shows how these concepts can be generalized to the interpersonal and societal levels. Cooper argues that suffering can come from a lack of meaningful wants, a belief that one's wants are not attainable, and failure to progress toward one's wants. Among the approaches he suggests for minimizing dysergy, which lead to the alleviation of suffering, are developing a culture of unconditional acceptance of others, helping people to develop communication skills, building a culture of trust, orienting society towards synergetic wants, and maximizing the domains in which people can achieve competence. Overall, the chapter suggests that the concepts of synergies and dysergies are powerful because they can help people and societies find ways to configure elements that ultimately reduce highly afflictive and destructive suffering.

Part II. Quality of Life (QOL), Caring and Suffering-Alleviation

The second section (Part II) moves to two major topics for this volume: the topic of quality of life (QOL) and the topic of care and caregiving. QOL, which is closely allied with human wellbeing, is a research tradition encompassing suffering because suffering is seen by some as the best approach to studying negative qualities of life. Care and caregiving, on the other hand are the principal approaches to personal strategies to try to alleviate individual suffering. Care and caregiving concepts also are used for delivery of aid to large communities or societies. This section begins with an essay by Joseph Sirgy on the usefulness of measuring ill-being concurrently with well-being.

Joseph Sirgy's goal is to make a clear distinction between indicators of well-being and indicators of ill-being at three levels of analyses, namely the individual, the community, and the societal levels. He uses Maslow's hierarchy of needs as a theoretical backdrop to help make these distinctions. Indicators of ill-being reflect satisfaction (or lack of satisfaction) of basic needs (survival-related needs such as biological and safety-related needs), whereas indicators of well-being reflect satisfaction (or lack thereof) of growth needs (social, esteem, self-actualization, intellectual, and aesthetic-related needs). Well-being versus ill-being indicators are identified and clearly distinguished from one another, not only at different levels of analyses (individual, community, and societal) but also between outcome and action indicators. Outcome indicators reflect the desired end state, whereas action indicators reflect indicators of programs and policies designed to influence the outcome. Such distinctions are important for policy-making.

Economist Muhammad Faress Bhuiyan knows Bangladesh first hand and has been studying the forces underlying well-being within their villages. He uses data from three Bangladeshi villages to explore the sources of two types of self-reported mental suffering: feeling worried and feeling depressed. There are three primary findings. First, standard socioeconomic and demographic dimensions do not predict self-reported mental suffering. Second, middle-aged, unhealthy, and never married household heads tend to worry and feel depressed more. Third, individuals who are relatively much better or worse off compared to their neighbors and siblings tend to suffer more. From a policy standpoint, improving health amenities will alleviate mental suffering as well as physical suffering. This study also finds evidence that reducing income inequality alleviates mental suffering.

Caitlin O. Mahoney and Laura M. Harder point out that for alleviating persons, awareness of and attention to suffering combined with a feeling of connection may function as both assets and liabilities. While these capacities enable the galvanization necessary to incite actions aimed at the relief of suffering, they may come at powerful costs, undermining the well-being of advocates and the efficacy of their labors. Personal and social resources have a part to play in how we manage our experience of emotions and our beliefs about social change. Privately, caregivers, advocates, and activists might learn to deliberately recognize and direct their individual capacities for attention, awareness, and connection toward more effective responses. Socially, communities within the advocacy field play an equally imperative role in the emotional experience of its members. Sustainable social change requires an awareness of the ways in which individual beliefs and behaviors, institutional policies, and cultural norms may hamper the alleviation of suffering.

Hye Won Kwon and Rengin Firat demonstrate that altruistic social identities contribute to the development of an altruistic personal identity that results in relieving others' suffering. Previous research has primarily focused on self-values or personal identities in predicting altruistic orientations or behaviors; little empirical research has linked personal values to social identities, and almost no work expands this to explore the implications for altruistic obligations that potentially help alleviate the suffering of others. They address this issue using a new cross-national survey, the Moral Schemas, Cultural Conflict, and Socio-Political Action Survey (2015) that includes data from four countries: United States, France, Turkey and South Korea. Their results mostly support their argument that identifying with groups that value benevolence and caring for others (holding altruistic social identities) contributes to the development of an altruistic personal identity, with some exceptions in Turkey and South Korea. These findings have significant implications for future research on the altruistic self and alleviating suffering in different cultural contexts.

Robert Neimeyer speculates that of all the sources of suffering in human life, the encounter with the tragic deaths of loved ones must be among the most compelling. Adopting the view *that grieving involves the attempt to reaffirm or reconstruct a world of meaning that has been challenged by loss*, he briefly reviews the evidence linking an anguished search for meaning to complicated, prolonged and life-limiting forms of grief. He then presents several concrete implementations of this perspective in case vignettes of work with grieving clients. The chapter closes with a coda on the role and limits of meaning reconstruction as a framework for pluralistic practice in alleviating grief-related suffering.

Paul Rosenblatt begins with the question: Why is it that some people do nothing to help others who are suffering? His chapter offers seven answers to the question, all of which have received considerable attention in the social psychological and sociological research literature. Each answer indicates areas that may be relevant to policy making and possibly productive self-examination that could increase the numbers of people acting to alleviate suffering. The seven categories, ordered on a continuum of resistance easiest to overcome to resistance most difficult to overcome are: (1) not knowing what to do, (2) fear of being inadequate or making mistakes, (3) diffusion of responsibility for helping others in need, (4) obliviousness to the suffering of others, (5) defensive reactions to the suffering of others, (6) reluctance to pay the cost (in money, effort, time, and reputational risk) that could be involved in helping others, and (7) not caring. A major implication of this analysis is that policies and people can change in ways that lead at least some people to take more active and proactive steps to alleviate peoples' suffering.

Part III. Improving Global Development, Healthcare and Poverty Reduction

Part III addresses the topic of global development directly but views it from several different angles. The authors not only deal with the economics of development, but the topics of health and population growth, which take up a lot of the attention of the last two chapters. Of course, the challenge of poverty arises prominently and the Sustainable Development Goals (SDG) are given attention by several authors. Poverty and health get the most attention here, perhaps because these challenging topics arguably have the greatest effect upon increased suffering. It is not surprising that these topics also play the biggest role in strategies for the alleviation of suffering.

Jason Hickel raises the question: Is human suffering increasing or decreasing, in aggregate? One way to answer this question is to look at trends in global poverty and hunger. The World Bank and the United Nations tell us that poverty and hunger have been decreasing over the past few decades. But this narrative relies on misleading statistics. In reality, the problem is much greater than we have been led to believe, with around 4 billion people in poverty today, and around 2 billion people in hunger—and the numbers have been rising over time, not falling. In other words, our current model of international development has failed at its most basic goal. We need to formulate new approaches to alleviating human suffering by addressing the root structural causes of global poverty and hunger, such as the international debt system, structural adjustment, lack of democracy in global governance institutions, unfair trade regimes, poor wages, tax evasion, land grabs, and climate change. This essay makes suggestions toward this end, and concludes that creating a fairer global economy is not sufficient in and of itself. In an era of climate change and resource limits, we also need to rethink the growth imperatives at the core of our system.

Cawo Abdi's chapter considers the suffering of citizens in refugee-hosting nations where extreme inequality and structural violence creates entrenched local misery. Drawing from the experience of refugees and migrants in South Africa, Abdi excavates the denied suffering of poor black South African citizens which inevitably shapes their relationship with refugees who arrive at their shores in search of a safe haven. Her analysis grapples with the contradictions found in South Africa's position as a major refugee-hosting nation and its own reality of having a large segment of its black populations mired in much injustice, violence, exclusion, and apathy. Her aim is ultimately to link the intertwined nature of the suffering for these groups and to argue for interventions that are more holistic to alleviate both groups' suffering.

Mark Lagon and Ryan Kaminski start from the premise that social suffering marks the qualities of suffering that most need alleviation, place their greatest hope in human survival in conceptions of human dignity and the rule of law. *Human dignity*, they argue, consists primarily in (1) promoting human agency to apply their gifts as they so choose, (2) recognizing equal value across all groupings of human beings—despite gender, ethnicity, caste, or race, and (3) supporting institutions that make agency and equality deep and lasting. Their thesis is that the *rule of law* is needed to guarantee human dignity and to empower the world to alleviate social suffering including universal eradication of poverty, violence, injustice, and disrespect. Finally, they conclude that the alleviation of social suffering cannot occur without both human dignity and the rule of law, broadly defined. And they call for mobilizing a pluralistic array of actors in dialogue on dignity and partnering to see it realized.

Joseph Speidel begins with the evidence that nearly all of the world annual population growth of 83 million people is occurring in developing countries where about

40% of pregnancies are unplanned or unwanted. These unintended pregnancies result in either unsafe abortions or births that are high risk and frequently cause the suffering of ill health or premature death. Reproductive health services that provide safe childbirth, modern contraception, and safe abortion care are essential to avoiding and relieving suffering caused by risks to health. Reproductive justice also alleviates the detrimental effects of rapid population growth on the welfare of people and on life-supporting planetary ecosystems. Family planning protects and advances human rights and justice, and enhances personal, family and national economic development. To provide family planning to all women in developing countries who want to end or delay childbearing requires an increase from an estimated $4.1 billion from all sources to $9.4 billion annually. With sufficient political will and devotion of adequate financial and other resources, the high-fertility developing countries (such as those in Sub-Saharan Africa), could make the transition from high to low birth rates, slow their rapid population growth, and achieve social and economic progress.

Andrzej Kulczycki notes that the last few decades have seen substantial progress in reducing preventable maternal mortality and expanding contraceptive use, yet tremendous suffering prevails worldwide due to the continued failure to realize greater reproductive justice, particularly for the world's 1.9 billion women of childbearing age. The vision for reproductive rights has now expanded beyond enabling women and couples to have control over the number and spacing of their children, yet this remains an elusive goal for many. Overall, the burden of poor reproductive health is greatest in Africa where poverty levels are highest, gender equity tends to be relatively low, and effective healthcare is less accessible or affordable. Harmful traditional practices such as child marriage are proving difficult to eradicate, especially where exacerbated by poverty and conflict, but intimate partner violence remains a common behavior in all regions. Everywhere, vulnerable groups include adolescents, poor women, and marginalized ethnic/racial and religious minorities. Kulczycki concludes that achieving universal access to maternal, sexual, and reproductive health services, with a focus on equity and improved quality of care, are critical to fulfill the human rights of women, improve development prospects, and alleviate suffering.

Part IV. Violent Societal Conflict, Human Rights and Justice

This fourth section of the book focus on the role of human rights, in particular freedom from violence. Several chapters tackle genocide, how it can be contained, how reconciliation can follow, the role of the media, and reconciliation processes. Several chapters deal directly with sexual violence, and one of those asks how effective programs have been in aiding recovery of men from sexual violence, particularly during war. The last chapter in this section describes research on attempts to curtail or end sexual exploitation of children.

Samuel Oliner starts with his personal, still-vivid experience of suffering and survival in occupied Poland during the Holocaust years. Then, his narrative shifts to the motivations and characteristics of those who risked their lives and livelihood to help others who were targets of the genocide, whether stranger or friend. Finally, he discusses ways that individuals, groups, and institutions promote altruistic behavior and compassion in the current generation of adults and youth. This is done through the lens of sociology and his lifetime of research into the nature of altruism, apology and forgiveness, caring, and selfless acts of courage. These are some of the ways suffering is reduced if not alleviated.

Adam Muller, Struan Sinclair, and Andrew Woolford provide an overview and comparison of the collective experience of the many different kinds of suffering experienced in both Canadian and American Indigenous Residential Schools (IRS). They are especially concerned with explaining how this suffering diminished important forms of social and cultural capital within Indigenous communities consistent with Raphael Lemkin's conceptualization of genocide. They specify and critically assess the ways in which Canadians have been working to acknowledge IRS harm, especially through a public apology and the Indian Residential School Settlement Agreement (IRSSA), the terms of which specified the creation of a Truth and Reconciliation Commission (TRC). They conclude by reflecting on the possibilities for advancing reconciliation afforded by *Embodying Empathy*, a critical and creative collaboration linking scholars, IRS Survivors, and technologists in an attempt to construct a virtually immersive IRS "storyworld."

Ellen Kennedy argues that women and girls are the heart of a culture and hence are targeted and victimized during genocides and mass atrocities. Such strikes provoke fear and intimidation, prevent the possibility of retaliation, break up families, destroy communities, and change the ethnic identity of subsequent generations. Her chapter explores epidemics of violence against women during some of the major genocides of the twentieth century, including the Armenian genocide during World War I, the Ravensbruck women's concentration camp during the Holocaust, the "rape camps" in Bosnia in the 1990s war, the rape of more than 500,000 Rwandan women during the 1994 genocide, and sexual slavery of Yazidi women and girls in Syria and Iraq by ISIS. She notes that change has occurred from the increased numbers of women prosecutors and judges in national and international tribunals, an increased attention to "gender justice" on a global scale, and clarity of the penalties of such crimes. They all provide deterrence for future sexual violence against women, and promote some measure of justice and the alleviation of suffering.

Élise Féron found that the extent of suffering generated by sexual violence against men in conflict zones is increasingly recognized by the international community and especially by the United Nations High Commissioner for Refugees (UNHCR), which issued guidelines in July 2012 on how to identify and support male victims of rape and other sexual violence in conflict and displacement situations. Specific support mechanisms for male survivors are almost nonexistent in conflict zones; most humanitarian organizations focus on female survivors of sexual violence. Only a few survivors' groups have spearheaded programs directly and specifically addressing the suffering induced by sexual violence against men. Relief is often privileged over long-term prevention, which would require working on how masculinities are built in times of war, and addressing conflict dynamics themselves. The risk that many of these programs are running is to over-focus on sexual violence and hence neglect other forms of violence that are perpetrated during times of conflict, and to which sexual violence is tightly linked. It seems equally important to understand and tackle sexual violence inflicted upon both men and women as interconnected phenomena, while acknowledging male and female survivors' specific suffering and needs.

Elizabeth Heger Boyle and Joseph Svec in their research discovered that female genital cutting (FGC) practices, which affect nearly 100 million girls and women worldwide (Yoder et al. 2013), cause immediate and long-term suffering. Fortunately, there has been a dramatic reduction in FGC in recent decades, and the downward trend is continuing, alleviating pain and negative health consequences for future generations of girls. The lessons learned from the successful case of FGC reduction have implications for reducing other types of suffering. They elaborate how reductions in FGC became possible, first, in terms of social policies adopted at the international level and, second, in terms of health, development, and education programs at the community level. Finally, they outline the ways in which the characteristics of FGC overlap with the characteristics of many forms of suffering, making FGC change a promising model for successful reforms in other areas.

Joachim Savelsberg notes that in the late nineteenth and twentieth centuries some actions that caused mass violence have been redefined from heroic deeds to criminal acts, including war crimes and genocide. His chapter outlines dimensions of mass violence in recent history and describes how new institutions such as the International Criminal Court (ICC) and Amnesty International have sought to define actions producing mass violence as criminal acts. Special attention and research detail are given to recent events in Darfur, derived in large part from the author's research on inter-nation media content over the course of the Darfur conflict. If the described, relevant institutional changes persist, we can be optimistic about being on a path that relieves some kinds of world suffering.

Richard Estes, after reviewing the evidence, finds that the sexual exploitation of children is not new, but in the last quarter of the twentieth century to the present day, this set of horrific practices has continued to grow. The phenomenon is worldwide and exists as a continuum of sex crimes committed against children. This phenomenon annually brings suffering to the lives of tens of thousands of children between the ages of 7 and 19 in the North American region, i.e., Canada, Mexico, and the United States. This chapter explores the nature, extent, and severity of sexual exploitation (in all of its forms) for the youth in these three countries. His chapter also presents a series of recommendations designed to reduce the suffering associated with both commercial and non-commercial child sexual exploitation.

Part V. Preventing Future Suffering

The theme of the final section (Part V) centers on the future, applying several different themes. One is the most obvious question of how to prevent future suffering. Another is how to balance a combination of immediate needs with needs of future generations. These challenging questions emerge within discussions of education, economics, preventative medicine and climate change. We should not forget that the alleviation of suffering does not have to be limited to the present tense. Alleviation is just as useful as a guiding principal for the future as it is for the present. That is true not only for issues like climate change that very clearly extend into the future, but it is also true for suffering-producing problems that might appear in the future. Thus part of alleviation encompasses prevention of suffering. We can prepare for the future by helping to shape the future so that suffering is minimized for all sectors and levels of society.

Meg Wilkes Karraker argues that homelessness is a critical issue facing societies around the world. The scale of human suffering around homelessness stretches beyond shelter insecurity to include hunger and malnutrition, lack of healthcare, greatly increased crime victimization, deprivation from job markets, and embarrassingly visible marginality within society. Using data from a small, longitudinal study of undergraduate students at a medium-sized Catholic university in the upper Midwestern United States, her chapter considers the potential role of higher education in socializing undergraduate college students to engage in community-based learning around social justice for people who are homeless. Student attitudes tended to persist between the pre- and post-tests, with small to moderate changes in the direction of less negative stereotypes regarding the homeless and more accurate knowledge following the sociology course. While the findings are not as dramatic as community-based learning advocates might like to see, this research suggests how higher education has the potential to promote attitudes conducive to relieving suffering.

Lea Hagoel believes that scientific developments have expanded the struggle against cancer beyond diagnosed patients too large, targeted populations of asymptomatic individuals invited for cancer screening. Medicine offers these individuals procedures aimed at the detection of cancer in its early stages to improve recovery and survival. She views this process within the frame of risk assessment, the risk assigned to 'healthy' individuals, which carries significant implications. On the Healthy-Sick axis, their "healthy" status is questioned without defining them as "sick," but it may lead to questions, doubts, and even suffering. The resulting uncertainly has new meanings assigned to health, personal futures, hopes, and life itself. The person defined at risk is in "limbo" and may cause a sense of helplessness, hopelessness, and hence, existential suffering. Recognition of this complex situation may alleviate individual existential suffering. Individuals may be able to benefit from the experience through meaning-centered reflection about their lives, as suggested by Viktor Frankl's logotherapy, and through adjustment to the reality of a risk-society.

Mehmet Kocaoğlu and Rhonda Phillips begin from the assumption that a caring economy is one that supports policies and rules based on the value of caring for ourselves, others, and nature. The ideas around caring for ourselves and our environment, and caregiving to others, are instrumental to the underlying ethos of caring economics. Market-based economics tend not to explicitly address issues around compassion, caring, empathy, or well-being. Instead, its focus is on self-interest, which presumably is necessary for rational decision-making by maximizing an individual's utility. Or is it? Some challenge this assumption and describe ways that compassion and empathy can be taught, can be integrated into structures of business, organizations, and communities, and essentially push toward more caring economies. Suffering is often directly tied to economic well-being so the implications are significant for many. This chapter explores ideas about caring economies and approaches that may help alleviate suffering.

Ronald Anderson found that many institutions, including the World Bank, have recognized that climate change produces not only climate-based disasters but it gets in the way of reducing world poverty, promoting education, and other crucial social objectives. While the solution would seem to be that international development should be advocated, this essay compares international development to "local partnership," which is an approach that utilizes community organization to guide its growth. The Ecovillage movement exemplifies how community can succeed where international development has failed. Recent climate disasters around the world reveal that disadvantaged social groups, such as the poor and the elderly, stand to lose far more than those in mainstream demographic categories. In fact, those disadvantaged groups can be said to personally suffer from climate disasters far more than mainstream groups. This helps resolve the dilemma of whether to focus efforts to alleviate suffering in the present or to attend to future sufferers. By working toward alleviating the suffering of currently victimized groups, we not only relieve their hurt, but point toward the injustice of failure to mitigate climate change.

Conclusion

In the chapters that follow, the reader will discover surprisingly wide diversity in approaches to discussing suffering-alleviation. Broad coverage and great depth are needed in conceptualizing suffering-alleviation so that it can more effectively guide our thought and behavior, improving our quality of life. At the beginning of this chapter, I made the claim that "Alleviation of suffering lies at the core of caring for others, humanitarian relief, civil society, social solidarity, and social welfare policy. For many people and some societies, suffering is the essence of human purpose, and for some it is the source of greatest meaning in their lives."

If indeed alleviation of suffering lies at the hub of human purpose, it surely will remain as such into the short-term future. The last chapter of this book takes an inter-generational perspective and argues for acting to alleviate suffering of the future and future generations. Such a view implies that the future should be taken more seriously in the present and as we move forward. Then, not only will we hold greater concern for the well-being of future generations, but we will take more seriously the challenge to improve the quality of our lives around the world, not only now but into the future.

References

Amnesty International. (2015). *Human rights facts and figures for 2014*. https://www.amnesty.org/en/latest/news/2015/02/annual-report-201415-facts-and-figures/. Accessed 11 Aug 2016.

Anderson, R. E. (2015). Introduction to thought and research on world suffering. In R. E. Anderson (Ed.), *World suffering and the quality of life* (pp. 3–29). NY: Springer.

Arneson, R. (2000). Luck, egalitarianism and prioritarianism. *Ethics, 110*(2), 339–349. doi:10.1086/233272.

Armstrong, K. (2011). *Twelve steps to a compassionate life*. New York: Anchor.

Aswegan, A. L. (2007). Our ethical duty is to relieve pain and suffering. *ACEP News* (September). https://www.acep.org/Clinical---Practice-Management/Our-Ethical-Duty-Is-to-Relieve-Pain-and-Suffering/. Accessed 10 Oct 2016.

Baumeister, R. F., Bratslavsky, E., Fiknkenauer, C., & Vohs, K. D. (2011). Bad is stronger than good. *Review of General Psychology, 5*(4), 323–370.

Bowker, J. (1970). *Problems of suffering in religions of the world*. Cambridge: Cambridge University Press.

CDC. (2016). *Family caregiving: The facts*. Atlanta: Center for Disease Control and Prevention (CDC). http://www.cdc.gov/aging/caregiving/facts.htm Accessed 6 Oct 2016.

Chouliaraki, L. (2013). *The ironic spectator: Solidarity in the age of post-humanitarianism*. Cambridge: Polity Press.

Darley, J. M., & Latane, B. (1970). *The unresponsive bystander: Why doesn't he help?* New York: Appleton Century Crofts.

Etzioni, A. (2009, Winter/Spring). The common good and rights: A neo-communitarian approach. *Georgetown Journal of International Affairs, 10*, 113–119.

Farmer, P. (1996). On suffering and structural violence: A view from below. *Daedalus, 125*(1), 261–283.

Farmer, P., et al. (2013). *Reimagining global health: An introduction*. Berkeley: University of California Press.

Gallup, Inc. (2015a) *Gallup.com home page*. http://www.gallup.com/Home.aspx. Accessed 18 Aug 2015.

Gallup, Inc. (2015b) *Gallup world poll*. http://www.gallup.com/poll/105226/world-poll-methodology.aspx?version=print. Accessed 18 Aug 2015.

Glenn, E. N. (2010). *Forced to care – Coercion and caregiving in America*. Cambridge: Harvard University Press.

Hickel, J. (2017). Addressing the structural causes of world suffering. In: R. E. Anderson (Ed.), *Alleviating world suffering* (pp. 2–10). Cham: Springer.

Ivtzan, I., Lomas, T., Hefferon, K., & Worth, P. (2015). *Second wave positive psychology: Embracing the dark side of life*. NY: Routledge.

Jimeniz, J. A., et al. (2014). *Social policy and social change: Toward the creation of social and economic justice*. Newberry Park: Sage Publications.

Johnston, N., & Schollar-Jaquish, A. (Eds.). (2007). *Meaning in suffering—Caring practices in the health professions*. Madison: University of Wisconsin Press.

Jordan, T. E. (2012). *Quality of life and mortality among children*. New York: Springer Briefs.

Kleinman, A. (2010a). Caregiving: Its role in medicine and society in America and China. *Aging International, 35*(2), 96–108.
Kleinman, A. (2010b). Four social theories for global health. *The Lancet, 375*(9725), 1518–1519.
Kleinman, A., & van der Geest, S. (2009). 'Care' in health care: Remaking the moral world of medicine. *Medische Antropologie, 21*(1), 159–168.
Korten, D. (2016). *Global civil society*. http://livingeconomiesforum.org/global-civil-society. Accessed 10 Sept 2016.
Land, K. C., Michalos, A. C., & Sirgy, M. J. (2012). The development and evolution of research on social indicators and quality of life. In K. C. Land et al. (Eds.), *Handbook of social indicators and quality of life research* (pp. 1–2). New York: Springer.
Larson, K. (2012). *Where the heart beats: John Cage, Zen Buddhism, and the inner life of artists*. New York: Penguin Books.
MacAskill, W. (2016). *Doing good better: How effective altruism can help you help others, do work that matters, and make smarter choices about giving back*. New York: Avery.
Mayerfeld, J. (2005). *Suffering and moral responsibility*. NY: Oxford University Press.
McGonigal, K. (2015). *The upside of stress: Why stress is good for you, and how to get good at it*. New York: Penguin Publishing Group.
Mukherjee, R. (1989). *The quality of life—Valuation in social research*. Newbury Park: Sage.
Ohlen, J. (2002). Practical wisdom: Competencies required in alleviating suffering in palliative care. *Journal of Palliative Care, 18*(4), 293–299.
OnGood. (2016). Facts and stats about NGOs worldwide. *OnGood*. https://www.ongood.ngo/portal/facts-and-stats-about-ngos-worldwide. Accessed 10 Sept 2016.
Peerman, G. (2008). *Blessed relief: What Christians can learn from buddhists about suffering*. Woodstock: Skylight Paths Publishing.
Popper, K. (1952). *The open society and its enemies*. Princeton: Princeton University Press.
Pruett, G. E. (1987). *The meaning and end of suffering for Freud and the Buddhist tradition*. Lanham: University Press of America.
Seligman, M. E. P. (2011). *Flourish: A visionary new understanding of happiness and well-being*. New York: The Free Press.
Singer, P. (2009). *The life you can save – Acting now to end world poverty*. New York: Random House.
Singer, P. (2015). *The most good you can do: How effective altruism is changing ideas about living ethically*. New Haven: Yale University Press.
Tronto, J. C. (1993). *Moral boundaries: A political argument for an ethic of care*. New York: Routledge.
Tugend, A. (2012). Praise is fleeting, but brickbats we recall. *New York Times* (March 23), p. B5.
UN. (2016a). *Outcome of the world humanitarian summit – Report of the secretary-general*. New York City: United Nations. https://www.worldhumanitariansummit.org/key-documents#chairsummary-linking. Accessed 10 Oct 2016.
UN. (2016b). *Ending conflict, alleviating suffering will require new levels of solidarity, compassion for one another, secretary-general tells awards reception*. Press Release, New York City: United Nations. http://www.un.org/press/en/2016/sgsm18132.doc.htm. Accessed 10 Oct 2016.
UNODC. (2013). *Global study on homicide*. New York: United Nations Office on Drugs and Crime (UNODC).
U.S. Census. (2013). *America's families and living arrangements: 2012*. https://www.census.gov/prod/2013pubs/p20-570.pdf Accessed 6 Oct 2016.
U.S. Congress. (1921). *Proceedings of a hearing on "Relief of suffering populations of the world, stricken by war, famine, and pestilence." Committee on Foreign Affairs*. Washington, DC: Government Printing Office. Reprinted in 2012 by Forgotten Books. www.forgottenbooks.org. Accessed 22 May 2013.
WHO. (1995). The World Health Report 1995- Bridging the Gaps. World Health Organization (WHO). http://www.who.int/whr/1995/media_centre/executive_summary1/en/. Accessed 10 Jan 2017.

Wilkinson, I., & Kleinman, K. (2016). *A passion for society: How we think about human suffering*. Berkeley: University of California Press.

Williams, C. R. (2008). Compassion, suffering and the self: A moral psychology of social justice. *Current Sociology, 56*(5), 5–24.

World Bank. (2005). *Empowering people by transforming institutions: Social development in World Bank operations*. Washington, DC: World Bank. http://documents.worldbank.org/curated/en/563751468780547056/Empowering-people-by-transforming-institutions-social-development-in-World-Bank-operations. Accessed 10 Oct 2016.

World Bank. (2016). *Defining civil society*. Washington, DC: World Bank. http://web.worldbank.org/WBSITE/EXTERNAL/TOPICS/CSO/0,,contentMDK:20101499~menuPK:244752~pagePK:220503~piPK:220476~theSitePK:228717,00.html. Accessed 10 Sept 2016.

Chapter 2
Systemic Humiliation as Daily Social Suffering

Daniel Rothbart and Poul Poder

Introduction

Almost everyone has felt humiliated at some time in life. Humiliation is closely associated with a wide range of social emotions: disgrace, affront, condescension, degradation, dishonor and indignity, loss of face, mortification, self-abasement, shame, and submission (Taylor 1989, p. 59). The pain from humiliation can be as innocuous as a pin prick or as serious as a rupture to one's core sense of self. The innocuous sort is commonplace. It might occur when someone is insulted for some social indiscretion, such as dressing improperly at a funeral, interrupting a speaker at a public event, or driving too slowly on the highway. Of course, the insulted person may take the high road by shaking off the insult as silly and completely unwarranted. This person may even reverse the direction of accusation by castigating in public the agent of the insult for having committed an act of verbal violence. These hypothetical examples illustrate a critical difference between humiliation and shame. A humiliated person refuses to accept the legitimacy of the attempted debasement by others (Fernández et al. 2015); a person experiencing shame takes their own debasement as well-deserved, acknowledging their indiscretion or offense and so conceding the validity to their degradation in the eyes of others (Miller 1993, p. 43).

In the context of intergroup relations, humiliation experienced by low-power groups can be quite severe, causing long-term suffering and animosity. We are

D. Rothbart (✉)
School for Conflict Analysis and Resolution (S-CAR), George Mason University,
3351 North Fairfax Dr, Arlington, VA 22201, USA
e-mail: drothbar@gmu.edu

P. Poder
Centre for Resolution of International Conflict, Department of Political Science, University of Copenhagen, Copenhagen, Denmark
e-mail: pp@cric.ku.dk

R.E. Anderson (ed.), *Alleviating World Suffering*, Social Indicators Research
Series 67, DOI 10.1007/978-3-319-51391-1_2

referring to social systems, defined by a set of norms, rules, and behavior patterns that in effect undermine the group members' dignity, diminish their accomplishments, degrade the symbols of their identity, and impose excessive burdens that are not shared by high-power groups. Such suffering comes from mechanisms that are embedded within the power dynamics between social groups—mechanisms that are strategically designed to impact how low-power groups think, feel and behave. Some of these mechanisms are active, whereby an agent engages in denigrating behavior towards another person or group; other mechanisms are passive, whereby the agent of humiliation withholds the respect that is due to another person or group as human beings who deserve the esteem of others.

In this chapter, we show how severe forms of humiliation go beyond visible interaction between an individual perpetrator and an individual target. We introduce the notion of systemic humiliation, which can be understood as a set of norms, rules, and patterns of behavior that have the effect of warping the thoughts and emotions of a targeted population by directly or indirectly injuring their sense of self, affecting their thoughts about society's elites, and determining their behavior. Systemic humiliation involves structural, subjective, and normative processes that are deployed by elites in societies of extreme social inequality, deploying mechanisms to control marginalized groups by instilling in them a sense of inferiority, insinuating that they are unworthy of the esteem of high-power groups. In such societies, the systemic accumulation of experiences of humiliation tends to weaken the subjugated people's resolve to demand civil, political, or human rights, since they lack resources and social support in order to act on their feelings of humiliation. The mechanisms of systemic humiliation are embedded in the social fabric, evade the subjective consciousness of targeted group members, and are strategically designed to control and manipulate.

In this chapter, we explain in the section "Introduction" how humiliation leads to physical, social, and moral suffering. In the section "Humiliation as physical, social, and moral suffering" we give depth to the notion of systemic humiliation by identifying five instruments that are deployed in many societies of stark power imbalance. We conclude in the section "Systemic humiliation" with recommendations for a multi-perspective orientation to alleviate suffering from such humiliation.

Humiliation as Physical, Social, and Moral Suffering

Rather than causing momentary discomfort from an embarrassing indiscretion, humiliation can lead to suffering that is situated in one's core sense of self, affecting an individual's relatively stable identity (Hartling and Luchetta 1999, p. 263). Humiliation tends to be experienced as painful social suffering (Barash and Lipton 2011; Hartling 2007; MacDonald and Leary 2005; Wilkinson 2005). Given the depth of its impact, the suffering is often long lasting (Hartling 2007). Under certain conditions, humiliation can prompt retaliation, which can lead to a downward cycle of denigration; one humiliated party inflicts humiliation on another, and so the suffering can circulate endlessly (Barash and Lipton 2011; Fuller 2004; Hartling 2007; Lindner 2006).

Experimental psychologists have recently found some striking similarities between the neurochemistry of physical pain and that of social pain, including humiliation (Eisenberger 2012) They examined the neurochemical processes of subjects who were undergoing feelings of social rejection, forced exclusion, and diminished value in the eyes of others and discovered that the regions of the brain that are activated by a painful physical injury, which are called the anterior cingulate cortex [dACC] and the anterior insula [AI], are also activated by such painful social experiences (Eisenberger 2012; Eisenberger and Lieberman 2005; Eisenberger et al. 2003). Underpinning both kinds of pain is a similar, although not identical, process of neural circuitry. Moreover, researchers discovered a causal link between social pain and aggression, indicating that the kind of violence associated with physical pain is replicated in the violent reaction to social pain (Gaertner et al. 2008; Leary et al. 2006; Twenge et al. 2001).

Humiliation is an emotion of contested judgment about one's value, worth, status, or power. It is experienced as an attack on one's character, identity, and worth—an attack that can have an enduring impact on one's consciousness and relations with others. Such attacks represent injury to the moral plane of life, that is, an existential malaise that comes with a sickening feeling of having diminished worth in the eyes of others. The moral plane of life is the dimension of life in which one's sense of self is interlinked with moral bonds with members of one's identity group: family, nation, social class, or religious order. With such bonds come normative discriminations between what is morally good or bad, right and wrong, and valuable or trivial. Such discriminations are thoroughly embedded in the sense of self—of one's bonds with, and breaks from, others (Taylor 1989, p 28).

Insight into the moral plane of life, and to moral injury, comes from an unexpected source: the recent findings of clinical psychologists exploring the trauma experienced by war veterans (Litz et al. 2009). Psychologists discovered that the diagnosis of post-traumatic stress disorder [PTSD] does not fully capture the veterans' feelings of humiliation as a result of their participation in wartime violence. While the diagnosis of PTSD centers on the subject's psyche as the primary locus of the trauma, many veterans experience a different kind of trauma regarding their relational identity as members of the military. The PTSD diagnosis fails to capture the intense feelings of worthlessness, despair, guilt, humiliation, or shame. Their responses to wartime experiences include the painful sense that they are disvalued, denigrated, or diminished in status by the public (Kilner 2010, p. 60). Some soldiers become deeply distressed as a result of witnessing, committing, or failing to stop acts that they perceive as inhumane, cruel, depraved, or unjustified (Drescher et al. 2011, p. 9), and such disturbances represents an ailment that invades the ways in which they see, think, and feel about themselves in relation to others. For some veterans, such experiences shake their core beliefs about humanity (Litz et al. 2009, p. 700). This distress comes with a strong sense of shame and humiliation that fosters a sense of uncertainty about their place, value, and relative worth as a soldier. With this reflection, they ask, "Was my action morally just? Am I diminished as a person because of such an action? Should I adjust my sense of who I am in relation to others?" This is a rupture of the moral plane of one's life—a moral injury. In sum, humiliation is painful in personal, social, and moral ways.

Systemic Humiliation

Humiliation can also be found in mechanisms of collective domination, where one population group lives under control of another group, determining the allocation of rights, resources, and responsibilities. These mechanisms are woven seamlessly into a system's operations and embedded usually in routine functions of institutions. This is a well-worn topic of social scientists, such as followers of Marx, Foucault, and Goffman, who probed the pernicious mechanisms of control of marginalized segments of the population. With the operation of such mechanisms, the preconditions for structural violence are set in place. Structural violence refers to a system's faceless forms of inequality, where one category of people benefits while the other category of people suffers. The result is some form of direct violence, such as extreme poverty, high mortality rate, suppression of freedoms, physical brutality, psychological trauma, or other human rights abuses (Galtung 1969). Some of the mechanisms of control are virtually depersonalized, lacking a fixed point—or person—of origin. Such mechanisms are deployed when, for example, corporate leaders render "reasonable" decisions, government administrators establish "essential" directives, and office bureaucrats follow "common sense" policies. The source of systemic humiliation is not caused by any particular agent, but comes from structurally violent systems that limit opportunities and impose excessive hardships with a force of insidious control over certain population groups.

Such instruments reflect a capacity to distort the victims' thoughts, feelings, and desires in order to serve the interests of the elite group (Lukes 2005). This is the power to invade the psyche of group members, warping their desires and influencing their behavior. As Steven Lukes argues, this technique of mind control disguises, suppresses, distorts, buries, or fabricates aspects of "reality" in ways that prefigure acceptance of systems of domination (Lukes 2005, pp. 27–28). When deployed effectively, such power has the impact of a poisonous self-denigration that diminishes the soul, making one feel debased and relegated as a lesser being. This power allows colonial rulers, for example, to get under the skin of marginalized people and to rule, control, and dominate them (Galtung 1975, p. 268), making them feel grateful to be lorded over and satisfied with their positions of servitude to the elites. In such contexts, systemic humiliation is deployed for the strategic purpose of weakening their resolve to rebel by reducing them to isolated beings who fear the next abuse, attack, or assault. The strategy is for the colonized people to embrace their status, to acquiesce to controls placed upon them, and to tacitly act as compliant and complicit subjects of their own domination. Such rulers would bristle at the effrontery of their "ungrateful subjects" to think that they have the right to protest their status. The strategy of deploying such power is not merely to deny these people a particular civil right, for example, to vote, to move freely in society, or to engage in political contestation without threats of reprisal. The true strategy of such deployment for colonized people is for the people themselves to self-define as unworthy of even making a claim for basic rights so that they undermine their right to demand redress of suffering at the hands of society's elites.

We identify five instruments of systemic humiliation: directives, ideology, language, image, and cultural symbols.

Discriminatory State Directives

One form of systemic humiliation is realized through directives: laws by legislative bodies, decisions by governmental leaders, or operational norms by state agencies and bureaucracy. For example, in the United States, the laws of the Jim Crow South established racial segregation of public spaces, such as hotels, restrooms, restaurants, theaters, prisons, hospitals, schools, and housing. Conjoined with these laws were social norms for the "proper behavior" of Blacks. They must never assert that a White person is dishonest, ignorant, or cruel (Kennedy 1990, Chapter 1). Humiliation accumulates from repetition of insults: bureaucrats who implement special rules for "coloreds," welfare officers asking intrusive questions about a recipient's personal life, a police officer who inspects an African American by asking to remove his or her clothes, or an employer who mistreats non-White employees while offering special benefits to Whites. Whites rarely used courteous titles of respect, such as Mr., Mrs., Miss, Sir, or Ma'am, when referring to Blacks. And a Black person was never to remark on the appearance of a White female. Civil rights leaders recognized the prolonged psychic injury that results from generations of indignities, that is, from the scars, lynching, and brutal treatment at the hands of Whites. In their campaign to expose racial injustice, Black nationalists argued that racism is not limited to the Jim Crow South but is embedded structurally in layers of "non-racialized" directives—social norms, bureaucratic procedures, and government policies. Railing against such insidious forms of bigotry, Malcolm X, for example, implored Blacks to rebel against the stigma of being lesser than Whites, insisting that Blacks should demand from White society a recognition of their dignity, moral character, past glories, and future potential.[1]

Today, many activists for racial justice see racist practices in the 'non-racialized' criminal justice system, where, for example, police officers are given wide discretion

[1] The accounts of routine humiliations experienced by Blacks are conveyed with exquisite clarity through the recent publication of Ta-Nehisi Coates' in *Between the World and Me*. Like all the writers cited above, Coates seeks to resist the forces of abuse, violence, and humiliation. Uplifting his son's self-image, Coates declares that "You have value. You have every right to wear your hoodie, to play your music as loud as you want. You have every right to be you."

to interpret behaviors, gestures, clothing, and odd gestures with suspicion. Within the system's logic, ghetto residents are cast as pre-criminals and so become suitable targets for disciplinary controls. They are, in effect, target worthy. We will not find the term *target-worthy subjects* in any legal statute, nor does the term appear in any governmental directive or mission statement. However, as the state does not actively counteract the police force's operation in terms of "target-worthy subjects," it can be considered an informal directive. Being target worthy means that the body is subject to micro-inspections of various kinds and cast as objects of the system's disciplinary technologies. Target-worthy subjects receive the scrutiny of police officers, who are trained to be vigilant for the indicators of criminality: loose or baggy clothing, angry facial expressions, or hand-held objects that look like weapons. Such indicators create, in the officer's mind, the "reasonable presumption" of danger, which authorizes the deployment of forceful restraints.

The consequences of being targeted are quite severe. According to a study conducted by the *Washington Post*, police officers shot and killed 965 civilians in 2015 (Kindy and Fisher 2015). While Black men comprise only 6% of the total population of the U.S., they comprised 40% of the unarmed civilians shot and killed by police officers in 2015. Based on this disproportionality of fatalities, the rate of killings of Black men represents more than six times their proportional size in the US. For those civilians who exhibited non-threatening behavior in the presence of a police officer, three out of every five of them were Black or Hispanic (Kindy and Fisher 2015, pp. 12–13). Non-Whites are cast as objects of suspicion, which in turn represents a denigration that goes to the core of their dignity and self-esteem.

Ideologies of Rank-Ordering

A second instrument of systemic humiliation centers on ideologies of rank around the categories of race, religion, gender, ethnicity, or national origin. The advocates of such ideologies accept the 'social reality' of the pure, advanced race, exceptional nation, chosen people, more intelligent gender or culturally superior ethnic group. Those ranked lower in society tend to be stigmatized, as if tainted as impure, unexceptional, unchosen, ignorant, or uncivilized. This is the taint of debasement, inferiority, and indignity of those who are, presumably, unworthy of the equal rewards of society and more vulnerable to its dangers in relation to the high-ranking group. Of course, the activists for the rights movements throughout the world seek to expose such ideologies for the wide-ranging crimes that are committed in their name, as illustrated above in the movement of Black nationalists in the United States.

Consider the ideology of the central leadership of Sudan, which holds the reins of power in and around Khartoum and over a majority of the Sudanese that are living at the periphery. Dominating the central government in Khartoum, the National Congress Party (NCP) advances an ideology of Arabism that divides the nation into two categories: pure citizens and dangerous subjects. For advocates of this ideology, the genuine Sudanese citizen is Arab and not African, speaks in a single language (Arabic), embraces an extreme form of Islam that includes Sharia Law, and lives according to the Arab-Muslim culture (Sharkey 2008, p. 28). Sudanese Arabs are presumably naturally destined to rule over "primitive" Africans, who are cast as alien, dangerous, and unworthy of protection (Idris 2010, p. 205). Government officials have embarked on a campaign to impose such a rank ordering in every village, school, and clinic (de Waal and Flint 2008, p. 28).

Essentializing Language

A particularly insidious form of humiliation centers on the deceptive power of words to solidify notions of a group's inferiority. Such power is more duplicitous than the well-documented technique of war propagandists to demonize the enemy, casting them as, for example, vicious, uncivilized, wicked, depraved or satanic. We are referring to the discursive power that comes from innuendo, double meanings and disguised imagery. Such a power can be likened to a magician's trick of drawing one's gaze away from processes that are hidden from the viewers' line of sight. Consider for example the meanings of terms that are used to categorize a particular population group. In some societies such terms reflect an ideologically-driven strategy to divide and control a people by imposing rigid notions about the prevailing social order. We know, for example, how the nineteenth century European rulers of the colonies in Africa would cast the indigenous people as 'primitives,' 'savages,' and 'tribes,' all of which were used to advance agendas of domination.

In like measure certain governments in Africa today craft categorical terms for purposes of population control. Consider again the case of Sudan. In the earlier years of his presidency, Omar Bashir launched in 1990 a campaign to impose an Arab-African rank ordering throughout the nation, targeting every village, school, and clinic according to Arab-Islamic practices. Such a campaign included policies about language; the central government adopted Arabic as the primary language for all of the nation's institutions, such as those of education, governance and the economy. Those Darfurians who speak only an indigenous language are excluded from participation in such institutions. Even specific categorical terms were changed. For example, the duality of "Arab-African" represents a change in the categorical terms for certain non-Arab tribes. By the time non-Arab groups led by the Fur, Zaghawa, and Massalit engaged in military conflict with the central government in 2003, the term "Arab-African" became widely circulated throughout the nation, replacing the traditional term for non-Arabs. This change reflects the government's divisive tactics (Flint 2009, p. 17). Yet, there are no purely objective indicators to distinguish between all so-called Sudanese Arabs and Sudanese Africans. While this change seems trivial to many Sudanese, it comes with sub-conscious associations to narratives of "the Africans'" disgraced history of enslavement, these narratives that foster stereotypes about their behavior, character traits and capacities or incapacities. Through this tacit linkage between the categorical term "African" and dominant narratives about who 'they' are, and are not, the categorical terms foster the impression of capturing the essence of these non-Arabs groups, as if to objectify them as permanently tainted by impact of their disgraced past.

Stereotypical Images

Another mechanism of humiliation centers on the use of images. In general, an image is a cognitive perception of something in which complexity is reduced, variability is suppressed, and perceptions of others are distorted. When used to characterize a group of people, images can be psychologically appealing because of the simplification yet reflect a myopic understanding of group members. An image offers a stereotypical picture of their character traits, behaviors, and capabilities, or lack thereof. Some degrading images center on the notion of dirt, as with images that a population group is contaminated, decayed, filthy, grimy, and unclear. Other degrading images rely on the idea of disease—that 'those people' are sickly, tainted, contaminated, poisonous, decrepit, or decayed. For example, in the lead-up to the Rwandan genocide in 1994, propagandists of Hutu extremism portrayed Tutsis through images of insects, snakes, and cockroaches, which were invoked by propagandists to create a revulsion of Tutsis among Hutus. Such imagery conveys the message that all Tutsis are inherently secretive, malicious, and treacherous. Such imagery had clear normative meaning. Hutus were implored to "get to work," "clear the bush," and "clean around their houses," all of which were euphemisms for killing Tutsis.

Of course, war propaganda is replete with stunning imagery of the enemy.[2] The images associated with the so-called war on terror depict terrorists as vicious, sinister, and evil. Such stereotypes have been deployed with demands for vigilance, sacrifice, and obedience in the face of such threats, representing categorical humiliation that dehumanizes enemy militants.

A more indirect stereotyping image is illustrated in what urbanist and sociologist Elijah Anderson calls the iconic ghetto, which refers to our cultural imaginary of the ghetto as inhabited by Black people, characterized by poverty, aggression, and criminality. Rather than a concert image of an acre of land, the iconic ghetto conveys negative images of social groups to many Americans, including Blacks who have elevated their social and economic standing well above ghetto residents (Anderson 2016). The iconic ghetto is revealed differently depending on race. Anderson contends that the urban space in American cities is divided into White spaces and Black spaces that are conjoined to some cosmopolitan spaces where both Blacks and Whites locate themselves quite comfortably. In contrast to the Black spaces, which Whites rarely pass through, urban Blacks have to navigate Whites' spaces as they attend university campuses, formal buildings of city authorities,

[2] Images have been recognized by international relations scholars as a psychologically powerful way in which one nation stereotypes another nation (Alexander et al. 2005).

city squares, and similar places. Blacks are often under surveillance in such spaces, presumably for the security needs of the city residents. Black people are well aware of being racially profiled, which often invokes a sense of degradation and at times fear. Yet many White residents are unaware of such racially-charged surveillance methods, believing that the campus and the city square are equally accessible to all people. Such methods illustrate modes of disgrace, that is, a form of humiliation that is embedded in the systems of urban security. Such surveillance may not occur in conjunction with the brute force of a security guard's club it but operates with the known gaze of authorities, representing an indirect form of humiliation.

Destructive Cultural Symbols

A fifth instrument of humiliation occurs when the defining symbols of a particular identity group are destroyed. For example, pictures of the target group's iconic figures are torn down, sacred texts are burned, and places of worth are vandalized. In addition to these forms of cultural violence, we identify the violence of suppressing from the collective consciousness any memory of past injustices against a targeted group. In such cases, the episodes of mass brutality, suffering, or injustice experienced by the subordinate groups are wiped clean from society's defining narrative, as if such episodes never occurred. The effect of this collective amnesia is for the dominant group to enjoy the symbols of their glory, pride, and purity (Galtung 1975, p. 292). Such practices include the following:

- Proclamation by the nation's political leaders that the nation is comprised of "one people," with the same place of national origin or race, as South American countries that diminish the status of indigenous people;
- Distortion of the nation's education curricula, including history textbooks, as illustrated in the case of the school boards in Texas that minimize the suffering of slaves before the Civil War;
- Imposition of a single religion as mandatory for society members, as in the case of the campaign among the national leadership of Sudan to impose Sharia Law;
- Imposition of a single set of cultural practices—rituals, clothing, celebrations of holidays—that have the effect of nullifying the distinctive customs of a targeted group, as in the laws prohibiting Muslim women from wearing headdresses;
- Showcasing the achievements of the nation's sacred figures while disguising the suffering of the low-rank group members at the hands of these figures, such as praise by many Americans to Andrew Jackson's conquest of Spanish Florida while ignoring the brutality that he brought to the Seminoles for harboring fugitive slaves.

In sum we have identified five mechanisms of systemic humiliation: (1) state directives such as laws, decisions, regulations, and commands; (2) supremacist ideology that is used to rationalize such directives; (3) language that underpins this ideology; (4) images that give visual form to the language of elite supremacy over the targeted group; and (5) symbols of degeneracy. The deployment of such instruments often sparks counter-reaction, leading to cycles of suffering (Barash and Lipton 2011). Again, we can recognize the deeply pernicious nature of systematic humiliation to weaken the will of a targeted group to resist, rebel, and retaliate against their dominant elites.

Alleviating the Impact of Systemic Humiliation

Recognizing the depth and breadth of systemic humiliation in layers of social interactions, we believe that the alleviation of suffering should not be limited to one sector of society but calls for initiatives on multiple spheres of social life. In our concluding observations, we argue that such alleviation demands serious attention to three distinct perspectives—political, social, and human rights. These perspectives can be operative in unison within multiple sectors of society.

Political Perspective

Within the political domain, alleviation implies government programs, policies, and initiatives that are designed to reverse the impact of the mechanisms of humiliation presented above while seeking to promote the dignity of all citizens. We offer three such examples of these mechanisms.

First, in the area of education, the government can set policies to develop history textbooks that avoid the trappings of supremacist ideologies, such as the omission of accounts of the painful past, regarding stories of suffering, destruction of cultural symbols and experiences of inequity. A second example is the removal of humiliating language. The government can legislate the elimination of terms in all government agencies that are perceived to be offensive to certain minority groups. Consider the recent bill issued by the Obama Administration to replace the terms "Negro" and "Oriental" with "African American" and "Asian American." This bill passed both the U.S. House of Representatives and Senate without serious objection. Third, regarding certain symbols of humiliation, the federal government can identify and remove those federal holidays that are perceived to be offensive to certain minority groups. The removal of the U.S. holiday of Columbus Day, which is humiliating to Native Americans, would represent an example of indirect apology for past indignities experienced by this group (Mayer 2012, p. 132).

Social Perspective

Alleviation calls for a reconciliation of broken relationships by changing the ways in which such groups interact, promoting trust and mutual understanding. This is not reconciliation in the sense of a return to some past mode of interaction; such a return is unattainable given the trauma experienced by those affected by the systematic humiliation.

Certain measures in civil society can be deployed to recognize and undermine the impact of such humiliation and promote constructs of dignity for all group members. Civil society organizations can establish a commitment to improve broken relations by recognizing and avoiding offensive language. For a nation that promotes freedom of speech, such as the United States, the central government cannot legislate change in language use without serious political resistance. Yet a recognition in civil society of humiliating language can foster positive change. For example, certain museums in Europe have removed descriptions of pictures that were interpreted as offensive to certain minority groups. Also, filmmakers can become more sensitized to the pernicious impact of movies and avoid negative stereotyping of members of minority groups. Television producers can stop exploiting humiliation as it is done in many entertainment programs today (Fuller 2006, pp. 177–178). Outside of the realm of mass media, symbolic gestures of recognition can be quite influential, such as creating memorials to past suffering, honoring those figure who resisted systems of injustice, and publicly expressing regret and possibly apology by political leaders for past injustices.

Human Rights Perspective

As we argue above, the suffering from systemic humiliation constitutes a moral injury to the targeted group members, degrading them as beings who are worthy of esteem. A human rights perspective to alleviation rests on the moral principle of the inherent worth of all people; as described in the Universal Declaration of Human Rights, "all members of the human family are born with dignity, equality and inalienable rights" (United Nations 2009). While this principle is subject to a wide range of objections from many quarters, the framing of alleviation as redress to human rights violations draws attention to a wide range of possible correctives. Consider, for example, the new Sustainable Development Goals [SDGs] of the 2030 Agenda for Sustainable Development, which was approved by the United Nations Assembly, September, 2015. (For a comprehensive analysis of SDGs, see Lagon and Kaminski 2017). The SDGs are developed to alleviate human suffering by promoting, what can be called, a dignitarian perspective to human rights.

For example, institutional support and enforcement of international human rights codes should be advanced by the European Union (Smith 2006). Certain measures can be put in place to promote a racial break with norms of systemic humiliation

(Fuller 2004, 2006; Barash and Lipton 2011). Particular attention could be given to programs for revealing the truth about the painful past, exposing a history of suffering of groups targeted for humiliation, and identifying the individuals and institutions responsible for such suffering. The truth about the past demands attention to a critical approach to history, which necessitates a commitment to expose human rights violations, identifying its perpetrators and giving voice to its victims. (For example, see Muller et al. 2017 who offers a compelling argument for the ways in which empathy with victims can be engendered through virtual engagement with their past experiences.) Interlinked to dilemmas of redefining national identity are those associated with transitional justice. Yet, within this domain, it is critical to adopt norms of dignity for all others associated with the systemic humiliation. In other words, dignity should be shown even to those who contribute to, or were complicit in, practices of denigration. The downward spiral of humiliation, going back and forth between groups, must stop.[3]

To be sure, such commissions are presented by their architects as above the fray of partisan politics but have been accused of promoting a subterranean strategy of inter-group partisanship. The truths and reconciliation commissions (TRCs), for example, are accused of exposing only those truths that legitimize the political leadership, contributing to their orthodoxy, which systematically silences members of the groups that are marginalized in post-violent society.

Conclusion

In this chapter we identify the locus of humiliation in systems of inequality, each of which has its rules, norms, and patterns of acceptable behavior. Suffering from systemic humiliation goes to the core of intergroup relations, promoting constructs of collective difference that are charged with normative meaning about supremacy and inferiority. The three perspectives of alleviation of suffering—political, social, and human rights—address domains that are critical for transforming society into one that promotes the dignity of all.

References

Alexander, M. G., Levin, S., & Henry, P. J. (2005). Individual motives underlying international images. *Political Psychology, 26*(1), 27–45.

Anderson, E. (2016). *Police violence and the iconic ghetto*. Social interaction and theory: A conference in honor of Prof. Randall Collins, 7–8 April 2016, University of Pennsylvania.

Barash, D. P., & Lipton, J. E. (2011). *Payback – Why we retaliate, redirect aggression and take revenge*. Oxford: Oxford University Press.

[3] Evelyn Lindner writes: "When humiliating people is no longer legitimate, humiliating humiliators is no longer legitimate either" (Lindner 2007, p. 30).

de Waal, A., & Flint, J. (2008). *Darfur-a new history of a long war*. London/New York: International African Institute, the Royal African Society and Social Science Research Council.
Drescher, K., Foy, D., Kelly, C., Leshner, A., Schutz, A., & Litz, B. T. (2011). An exploration of the viability and usefulness of the construct of moral injury in war veterans. *Traumatology, 17*(1), 8–13.
Eisenberger, N. I. (2012). The pain of social disconnection: Examining the shared neural underpinnings of physical and social pain. *Nature Reviews Neuroscience, 13*, 421–434.
Eisenberger, N. I., & Lieberman, M. D. (2005). Why it hurts to be left out: The neurocognitive overlap between physical and social pain. In K. D. Williams, J. P. Forgas, & W. von Hippel (Eds.), *The social outcast: Ostracism, social exclusion, rejection, and bullying* (pp. 109–127). New York: Psychology Press.
Eisenberger, N. I., Lieberman, M. D., & Williams, K. D. (2003). Does rejection hurt? An fMRI study of social exclusion. *Science, 302*(5643), 290–292.
Fernández, S., Saguy, T., & Halperin, E. (2015). The paradox of humiliation: The acceptance of an unjust devaluation of the self. *Personality and Social Psychology Bulletin, 41*(7), 976–988.
Flint, J. (2009). *Beyond 'Janjaweed': Understanding the militias of Darfur*. Geneva: Small Arms Survey, Graduate Institute of International and Development Studies. http://www.smallarmssurveysudan.org/pdfs/HSBA-SWP-17-Beyond-Janjaweed.pdf. Accessed 25 July 2016.
Fuller, R. W. (2004). *Somebodies and nobodies – Overcoming the abuse of rank*. Vancouver: New Society Publishers.
Fuller, R. W. (2006). *All rise – Somebodies, nobodies and the politics of dignity*. San Francisco: Berrett-Koehler Publishers.
Gaertner, L., Iuzzini, J., & O'Mara, E. M. (2008). When rejection by one fosters aggression against many: Multiple-victim aggression as a consequence of social rejection and perceived groupness. *Journal of Experimental Social Psychology, 44*(4), 958–970.
Galtung, J. (1969). Violence, peace and peace research. *Journal of Peace Research, 6*(3), 167–191.
Galtung, J. (1975). Is peaceful research possible: On the methodology of peace research. In J. Galtung (Ed.), *Peace: Research, education, action: Essays in peace research, Volume I* (pp. 263–279). Ejlers: Copenhagen.
Hartling, L. M. (2007). Humiliation: Real pain, a pathway to violence. *Brazilian Journal of Sociology of Emotion, 6*(17), 466–479.
Hartling, L. M., & Luchetta, T. (1999). Humiliation: Assessing the impact of derision, degradation and debasement. *Journal of Primary Prevention, 19*(4), 259–278. doi:10.1023/a:1022622422521.
Idris, A. (2010). Beyond "African" and "Arab". In F. Deng (Ed.), *New Sudan in the making?* (pp. 195–214). Trenton: Red Sea Press, Inc..
Kennedy, S. (1990). *Jim crow guide: The way it was*. Gainesville: University Press of Florida.
Kilner, P. (2010). A moral justification for killing in war. *Army Magazine*, February, 55–60.
Kindy K. & Fisher, M. (2015, December 27). Officers fatally shoot 965: Tally more than twice FBI's usual count. *The Washington Post*.
Lagon, M. P., & Kaminski, R. T. (2017). Dignity and rule of Law: Governance and the alleviation of social suffering. In R. E. Anderson (Ed.), *Alleviation of world suffering: The challenge of negative quality of life*. New York: Springer.
Leary, M. R., Twenge, J. M., & Quinlivan, E. (2006). Interpersonal rejection as a determinant of anger & aggression. *Personality and Social Psychology Review, 10*(2), 111–132.
Lindner, E. G. (2006). *Making enemies – Humiliation & international conflict*. London: Preager Security International.
Lindner, E. G. (2007). Dynamics of humiliation in a globalized world. *International Journal on World Peace, 24*(3), 15–52.
Litz, B. T., Stein, N., Delaney, E., Lebowitz, L., Nash, W. P., Silva, C., et al. (2009). Moral injury & moral repair in war veterans: A preliminary model & intervention strategy. *Clinical Psychology Review, 29*(8), 695–706.
Lukes, S. (2005). *Power: A radical view* (2nd ed.). New York: Palgrave MacMillan.

MacDonald, G., & Leary, M. R. (2005). Why does social exclusion hurt? The relationship between social & physical pain. *Psychological Bulletin, 131*(2), 202–223.

Mayer, B. (2012). *The dynamics of conflict – A guide to engagement & intervention*. San Francisco: Jossey-Bass.

Miller, W. I. (1993). *Humiliation & other essays on honor, social discomfort, & violence*. Ithaca: Cornell University Press.

Muller, A., Sinclair, S., & Woolford, A. (2017). Digitized suffering, actual healing: Empathy, reconciliation, and redress through a virtual Indian residential school. In R. E. Anderson (Ed.), *Alleviation of world suffering: The challenge of negative quality of life*. New York: Springer.

Sharkey, H. (2008). Arab identity & ideology in Sudan: The politics of language, ethnicity & race. *African Affairs, 107*, 21–43.

Smith, D. (2006). *Globalization – The hidden agenda*. Oxford: Polity Press.

Taylor, C. (1989). *Sources of the self*. Cambridge, MA: Harvard University Press.

Twenge, J. M., Baumeister, R. F., Tice, D. M., & Stucke, T. S. (2001). If you can't join them, beat them: Effects of social exclusion on aggressive behavior. *Journal of Personality and Social Psychology, 81*(6), 1058–1069.

United Nations (2009). *Universal declaration of human rights*. http://www.un.org/en/documents/udhr/index.shtml. Accessed 20 June 2016.

Wilkinson, I. M. (2005). *Suffering: A sociological introduction*. Oxford: Polity Press.

Chapter 3
Suffering and the Ethics of Solidarity

Lilie Chouliaraki

> *'If you are also feeling the pain for all those who have no access to cure, buy the Pastilles, join your voice with MSF's kai scream. Scream now! Some will hear you. Many will be able to get cure* (MSF 2011).

Introduction

'Javier Bardem Screams with Medecins Sans Frontiers' (MSF 2011) was a 30-s video that invited us to mimic the Hollywood actor's reaction towards the devastating pain and suffering of millions of vulnerable people around the world. Capitalizing on the actor's capacity to express intense emotion and his potential for affective identification with his audiences, the video urged us to scream with him as, for instance, we are driving our car, in our own city streets. It also invited us to buy a commercial product and connect with MSF. In this way, the 'Scream' campaign sought to both maximize our solidarity towards the misfortunes of faraway others and guarantee our attachment to a powerful NGO brand.

It is the relationship between 'how I feel' and 'what I can do' about distant others, so clearly thrown into relief in the MSF appeal, that concerns me in this chapter[1]. There is no doubt that emotion has always played a central role in the communication of solidarity, yet, I argue, there is something distinct about the ways in which the self figures in contemporary humanitarianism. This is obvious when we consider Red Cross appeals, for instance, where the question of 'what I can do' is raised through shocking images of emaciated children or Amnesty International

[1] http://sofii.org/case-study/medicos-sin-fronteras-medicine-for-someone-elses-pain.

L. Chouliaraki (✉)
Faculty of Media and Communications, London School of Economics and Political Science, Houghton Street, London WC2A 2AE, UK
e-mail: L.Chouliaraki@lse.ac.uk

R.E. Anderson (ed.), *Alleviating World Suffering*, Social Indicators Research Series 67, DOI 10.1007/978-3-319-51391-1_3

ones, where the question is answered through a call to personalized letter-writing for the liberation of prisoners of conscience. Neither of these two examples returns the imperative to act on vulnerable strangers to ourselves, asking us to get in touch with our feelings in order to express our solidarity with them.

Taking my point of departure in this new emotionality, here I explore the factors through which the communication of solidarity has changed in the course of the past four decades. A crucial period for humanitarianism, the 1970–2010 timespan is characterized by three major, seemingly unconnected but ultimately intersecting, transformations: the instrumentalization of the aid and development field; the retreat of the 'grand narratives' of solidarity; and the increasing technologization of communication. Whilst each transformation has been extensively explored in its own right, the co-articulation of the three and, importantly, the implications of this co-articulation for the changing meaning of solidarity have remained relatively untouched.

In drawing attention to the new emotionality of the '*Scream*' appeal, what I propose is that the meaning of solidarity today should be approached as simultaneously defined, or over-determined, by the branding strategies of MSF, by a generalized reluctance to accept 'common humanity' as the motivation for our actions and by the interactive possibilities of online media. It is, I argue, only when we examine solidarity as a problem of communication, that is as a moral claim seeking to reconcile the competing demands of market, politics and the media, that we can better understand how the spectacle of suffering is subtly but surely turning the West into a specific kind of public actor – the ironic spectator of vulnerable others.

Irony refers to a disposition of detached knowingness, a self-conscious suspicion vis a vis all claims to truth, which comes from acknowledging that there is always a disjunction between what is said and what exists – that there are no longer 'grand narratives' to hold the two together (Rorty 1989).

The ironic spectator is, in this sense, an impure or ambivalent figure that stands, at once, skeptical towards any moral appeal to solidary action and, yet, open to doing something about those who suffer.

In following the mutations of these communicative practices across time, the story of this article is essentially a story of how changes in the aesthetics of humanitarian communication are also changes in the ethics of solidarity. It is a story about how the move from an objective representation of suffering, as something separate from us that invites us to contemplate the condition of distant others, towards a subjective representation of suffering, as something inseparable from our own 'truths' that invites contemplation on our own condition; it is also a move from an ethics of *pity* to an ethics of *irony*. This is an epistemic shift in the communication of solidarity, I contend, in that it signals the retreat of an other-oriented morality, where doing good to others is about our common humanity and asks nothing back, and the emergence of a self-oriented morality, where doing good to others is about 'how I feel' and must, therefore, be rewarded by minor gratifications to the self – the new emotionality of the quiz, the confessions of our favorite celebrity, the thrill of the rock concert and twitter journalism being only some of its manifestations.

Whilst all ethics of solidarity involves an element of 'egoistic altruism', ironic solidarity differs from other versions in that it explicitly situates the pleasures of the self at the heart of moral action, thereby rendering solidarity a contingent ethics that no longer aspires to a reflexive engagement with the political conditions of human vulnerability. The decline of grand narratives has undoubtedly contributed to the rise of the ironic disposition, but, as I show below, this contingent ethics of solidarity has a more complex history that forces us to examine all three dimensions of its emergence – not only the political, but also the professional and the technological. At the heart of these aesthetic and ethical transformations, I conclude, lies a fundamental mutation in the communicative structure of humanitarianism. This is the retreat of the theatrical structure of solidarity, where the encounter between Western spectator and vulnerable other takes place as an ethical and political event, in favor of a mirror structure, where this encounter is reduced to an often narcissistic self-reflection that involves people like 'us'.

But first things first. Let me now sketch out this change in the communicative structure of solidarity by introducing each of the three key dimensions of this its communication: the *institutional*, where I discuss the implications of the radical expansion and concomitant instrumentalization of the aid and development field; the *political*, where I address the end of grand narratives and the ensuing rise of individualist morality as a motivation for action; and the *technological*, where I show how the new media have facilitated an unprecedented explosion of public self-expression, thereby also changing the premises upon which solidarity is communicated. It is, as I have said, only in the light of these three dimensions that we can begin to make sense of the shift from the objectivity of the theatre to the new emotionality of the mirror as a paradigmatic shift in the very meaning of solidarity.

The Instrumentalization of Humanitarianism

The '*Scream*' appeal is informed by an emphasis on *'inspiration'* that, as Richard Turner, Action Aid's ex-Head of Fundraising, put it, focuses on making people *'feel great if they give, but don't make them feel rotten if they* don't' (www.professionalfundraising.co.uk October 2009). Leaving the needs-based iconography of poverty behind for inducing negative feelings of guilt, the inspiration-based approach is about inducing positive, warm feelings and, in so doing, aims at motivating longer-term support for the organization's cause: *'we'd like to think'*, as Turner continues, *'that the kind of supporters we attract are likely to give to us for longer and give more than if we'd increased our response rate with hard-hitting, more needs-based advertising'*.

Reflecting a general tendency in the aid and development field, this is the language of corporate communication that, instead of traditional strategies of dissemination, prioritizes the strategy of branding: the cultivation of a deep emotional attachment to a particular commodity, the NGO brand, with a view to guaranteeing customer loyalty to this brand.

Humanitarianism has, of course, never been antithetical to the market and has, in fact, been theorized as a quintessentially liberal idea born out of capitalism, for instance as the benign face of the expansion of labor markets beyond the West (Friedman 2003). Yet, the contemporary articulation of humanitarianism with the market is a rather recent development that reflects a shift within capitalism from, what Boltanski and Chiapello call, a classical liberal to a neo-liberal conception of public morality (2005). In the light of this shift, we may argue that whereas modern humanitarianism was grounded on the crucial separation between a public logic of economic utilitarianism, applicable in the sphere of commodity exchange, and a private logic of sentimental obligation towards vulnerable others, applicable in the sphere of individual altruism and increasingly in institutionalized philanthropy, late modern humanitarianism, what I here theorize as *post-humanitarianism*, increasingly blurs the boundary between the two. In so doing, it manages both to turn the ever-expanding realm of economic exchange into a realm of private emotion and self-expression and, in a dialectical move, to simultaneously commodify private emotion and philanthropic obligation.

Starting in the 1980s and gaining full momentum in the early 1990s, two developments have brought about this shift towards, what Cheah (2006) calls, the *instrumentalization* of the aid and development field – that is, the subordination of the other-oriented aims to save lives and change societies to the self-oriented imperative of profitable performance in the humanitarian sector itself. These are the *marketization* of humanitarian practice and the *production of administrative knowledge* in the discipline of Development Studies.

The *marketization of humanitarian practice* is a consequence of the explosion of International Organizations (IOs) and International NGOs (INGOs), in the aid and development sector. Aid agencies, for instance, expanded their operations by 150% in the 1985–1995 decade whereas, in the USA alone, their numbers rose by a hundred in the 1980–1990 decade (from 167 to 267) and almost doubled in the subsequent one, 1990–2000 (from 267 to 436).[2] Marketization has, in this sense, emerged from these organizations' strong competition for survival, in a sector that has not only become more densely populated[3] but has also come to depend primarily on project-based funding by transnational intermediaries and state donors. In the 1990–2000 decade, to give an example, funding levels rose nearly threefold, from $2,1 million to $5,9 million, reaching more than $10 million by 2005–2006, whilst the distribution of these funds has increasingly shifted to depend on bilateral aid and state budgets' earmarking, thereby rendering strong state interests a key criterion for INGO fund-raising (Smillie & Minear 2004: 8–10, 195; Barnett 2005: 723–40; Barnett and Weiss 2009: 33–35).

Even though the proliferation of humanitarian agencies has been hailed as contributing to the cosmopolitan ethos of global civil society, in that INGOs '*breed new*

[2] See McCleary and Barro (2007) and Barnett and Weiss (2008) for these numbers and for discussions on the significance of this increase in the humanitarian sector.

[3] See Natsios (1995); Simmons (1998) and Cooley and Ron (2002) for the density argument in the sector.

ideas, advocate, protest, and mobilize public support, as Mathews's argues, and, in the process, further *'shape, implement, monitor, and enforce national and international commitments'* (1997: 52–3), we can clearly see that such proliferation entails a major risk. Insofar as it takes place within an economy of scarcity, where many agencies bid for limited funding, the competition for resources inevitably tends to foster compliance with the rules of the Western donor market rather than with real priorities in the global South. Indeed, despite the expansion of the field and the provision of '*... more aid than ever before*', as Barnett and Weiss claim, *'the bulk of resources (are) controlled by a few donor countries that (are) more inclined to impose conditions and direct aid towards their priorities'* so that, they conclude, *'the least fortunate are getting the least of attention'* (2008: 34).

Despite, therefore, its benign objectives of maximising efficiency and increasing accountability to donors, the financial regime of the aid and development field ultimately legitimizes a neo-liberal logic of governance that turns the cosmopolitan aspirations of humanitarianism into the corporate aspirations of the West and, in so doing, not only fails to serve the ideal of global civil society but bears harmful effects on vulnerable others.

If the instrumentalization of humanitarianism is enacted through institutional practices on the ground, it is primarily legitimized through the *scientific knowledge produced in the field of Development Studies*. Born in the 1960s, as a response to the need to study the processes of de-colonization and the evolution of the new states, Development Studies has always been marked by a key tension between normative theory, showing how ideal societies or states would look like, and best practice, making concrete policy recommendations that are applicable in the here-and-now (Schuurman 2009). Even though this has historically been a productive tension that propelled critical research in the field, there has recently been, according to theorists, a definitive tip in the balance towards policy rather than normative theory (Biel 2000; Kothari 2005).

This means that Development Studies is today largely abandoning the critical perspectives of political economy, which thematized inequality as a systemic cause of under-development and linked inequality to non-economic issues – thus further connecting Development Studies to the disciplines of Politics, Sociology or History and Anthropology. Instead, what today dominates the field is, what Fine (2009) calls, *'new development economics'*: the neo-liberal economics of the (post) Washington Consensus, which favors micro-economic, rather than macro- or structural economic, approaches to development, and methodological positivist, rather than critical reflexive, research designs.

What this discussion suggests is that, whilst substantial critical work on the instrumentalization of both the practice and knowledge production of humanitarianism already exists, little that has been said on the impact of instrumentalization on the communication of solidarity itself. And yet, as we saw, the shift from advocacy-based communication strategies to outsourced campaigns designed by advertising agencies, and the concomitant turn towards 'consumer loyalty', 'product branding' or 'client-driven inspirational campaigns' are a major part of this instrumentalization that demands urgent critical scrutiny. Let me now turn from the institutional to the political dimension of humanitarianism in order to discuss how the meaning of solidarity itself has been changing, as a result of the post-Cold War collapse of ideologies.

Solidarity Without Grand Narratives

The new emotionality of humanitarian appeals is not simply due to the new instrumentalism of advocacy communication. Rather, it also has its roots in a fundamental change in the political culture of solidarity, after the end of the Cold War. Indeed, the idea of solidarity has a long and complex history (Rorty 1989; Boltanski 1999; Eagleton 2009) and it is worth looking back to work out how it has been mutating in time. In its contemporary secular form solidarity dates as far back as the eighteenth century and the rise of the 'culture of sympathy'. This was the time when the rise of modern capitalism generated a new moral discourse on the inherent goodness of human nature and on the importance of treating distant others not as enemies but as 'cordial strangers' (Hyde 1999; Hutchinson 1996).

The founding father of the economic liberalism of modernity, Adam Smith, is an instrumental figure in this discourse in that he both celebrated benevolence towards vulnerable others as a fundamental moral property of the human psyche, in his *Theory of Moral Sentiments* (1759), and advocated the regulation of society by the amoral 'invisible hand' of commercial activity, in his *Wealth of Nations* (1778; and see Shapiro 2002 for the 'Smith effect' upon Western modernity).

It is, I argue, this instability between humanity and inhumanity, between benevolence and violence, that has propelled the historical variations of the meaning of solidarity in the course of modernity. Two of these variations are relevant to my discussion on humanitarianism: *solidarity as salvation*, or the humanitarian solidarity of the Dunantean project, and *solidarity as revolution*, or the political solidarity of Marxian militantism. Whereas the former is associated with humanitarianism 'proper', in that it was born as a moral response to the atrocities of war and aspired to save lives and comfort suffering humanity, the latter is associated with a social critique of the conditions of suffering and aspired to change the social relations of economic exploitation that made suffering possible, in the first place.

Despite their profound differences, these two forms of solidarity, salvation and revolution, are nonetheless informed by similarly universal norms of morality. Humanitarian solidarity is informed by a morality of altruistic benevolence, which had both Christian and secular roots (Boltanski 1999), whilst political solidarity is informed by a morality of social justice, which relied on Marxian and anti-colonial theory (Calhoun 2009; Moyn 2010). Like all forms of universalism, however, neither of the two solidarities was ultimately able to avoid the accusation that its moral certainties were doing more harm than good to the societies they were applied to: '*solidarity*', in Gilroy's words, has become '*suspect*' (2006: 70).

Ultimately, what these critiques of universalism towards both forms of solidarity, salvation and revolution, problematize is the traditional relationship between politics and solidarity. The former, the critique of salvation, points to the fact that there can be no pure humanitarianism, in that all choices to save lives are ultimately political choices about which suffering is worth alleviating and who is to blame for it. It is, at least partly, in response to the re-definition of the morality of salvation as ultimately a political morality, that the field has sought to instrumentalize its institutional practices through scientific methodologies and, in so doing, to sustain the claim that its practices remain neutral, beyond political interest. Rather than succeeding, however, humanitarianism is today accused of a double compromise –not only of being *'undertaken in a variety of circumstances that challenge its moral clarity'* but, as Calhoun observes, also of being undertaken *'in complex organizations that demand instrumental orientations to action'* (2008: 96).

In parallel to this attempt to defend the de-politicization of the solidarity of salvation, there is a simultaneous marginalization of the politics of justice in the solidarity of revolution. Symptomatic of the post-Cold War decline of narratives of social change, the retreat from justice has its roots in the New Left, which, already in the late 1960s, challenged its *'Marxist predecessors'* precisely for being *'guilty... of inhumane behaviour in the name of the revolution and the better society that awaits humanity in the far-off, distant future'* (Rifkin 2009: 416). The significance of this position, to be radicalized in the post-Cold War era, is not only historical, in that it produced a scathing attack of the inhumanity of the Soviet model of social justice, but, importantly, intellectual, in that it replaced the Marxian critique of class injustice with a new focus on the human condition – what Boltanski and Chiapello call, a *'critique of authenticity'* (2005).

Fully resonating with, albeit not restricted to, the post-modernist celebration of the death of meta-narratives, this intellectual shift towards 'authenticity' rather than social justice further signals a new political focus not on the suffering society as a pathology of the capitalist system but on the individual suffering self as a generalized pathology of all systems of power: *'Loneliness, estrangement, isolation describe the vast distance between man and man today... We oppose the depersonalization that reduces human beings to the status of things. If anything, the brutalities of the 20th century teach us that means and ends are intimately related, that vague appeals to "posterity" cannot justify the mutilations of the present...'* (Roszak 1995: 58 cited in Rifkin 2009: 416).

Similarly to Moyn's (2010) subjects of solidarity who are treated as individual holders of rights disembedded from structures of injustice, I argue that the publics of solidarity, too, are today called to enact solidarity as an individualist project of contingent values and consumerist activisms – ironic solidarity being precisely a solidarity that, in recognising the limits of its own legitimacy and efficacy, avoids politics and rewards the self. Even though the philosophical contours of this emerging practice of solidarity has been imaginatively conceptualized in Rorty's seminal treatise on irony as a condition of solidarity, as early as in 1989, the precise content of this practice, its articulation with the market and technology as well as its implications for public morality have not as yet become the focus of critical inquiry.

The Technologization of Communication

The question of solidarity and its historical mutations, it follows, cannot be examined separately from the communicative structure that has made this moral discourse available to us, in the first place. The '*Scream*' appeal, to return to our example, is interesting precisely because its structure does not resemble earlier proposals to solidarity, in at least two ways. First, it uses the interactive affordances of the internet so as to talk about distant others, yet it ultimately communicates something about 'us', and second, it invites us to connect with the MSF website as a response to the question of 'what to do', yet it avoids the question of 'why we should act'. It is these two features, the invitation to self-expression and the absence of normative morality, which, I suggest, define the technologization of humanitarianism today. Let me address each of them in turn, before I reformulate anew the main concerns of my research.

The first, the *invitation to self-expression*, is a key feature of new media, in that digital technologies have provided the necessary infrastructure to turn media users into producers, rather than only consumers, of public communication. Whereas the MSF appeal capitalized on the interactive potential of online sites to generate personalized profiles of its users, other practices of humanitarian communication rely on mobile phones, blogs and convergent journalism platforms, to involve increasingly more people into the production of their messages. The technologization of solidarity refers, in this sense, to the capacity of digital media to incorporate the moral imperative to act on vulnerable others within technological platforms that render solidarity a matter of twittering personal emotion, downloading the message of our favorite celebrity, web-streaming our preferred Live 8 bands, clicking on the donation link of MSF or clicking 'like' on a Facebook wall (Fenton 2007, 2008).

It is this capacity of the new media to engage people in unprecedented forms of public self-presentation that, according to Rifkin, has defined our 'empathic civilization' as simultaneously the age of a '*new dramaturgical consciousness*' – the consciousness of our capacity to act ourselves out in front of unknown others (2010: 555–560; see also Thumim 2009). Dramaturgical consciousness, becomes, in this account, paramount in the formation of cosmopolitan dispositions, precisely because the planetary connectivity of the new media have now turned the world into a new 'theatrum mundi' – a theatre, whose moralising force lies in the fact that we do not only passively watch distant others but we can also enter their own reality as actors: '*the whole world might be a stage*', Rifkin says echoing the Shakespearean metaphor, '*but during the twentieth century most of the people were in the audience, whereas in the twenty-first century everyone is onstage and in front of the spotlights, thanks to YouTube, MySpace, Facebook, the blogosphere etc.*' (2009: 555).

Whilst the quality of cosmopolitan dispositions that the digital media are able to mobilize is fiercely debated, what interests me here is the fact that the cosmopolitanizing potential of these media relies on their capacity to act both as sites of self-expression: '*Young people today*', Rifkin continues his description of the West as an empathic civilization, '*are in front of the screen or on the screen, spending much of their waking day in virtual worlds ... choreographing virtually every aspect of their lives – hoping that millions of others will log on and follow along.*' (2009: 558). What this account leaves out is the potential of these media to not only turn outwards to the world but also inwards to the self, encouraging a narcissistic preoccupation with 'me' and others like 'me' (Fuchs 2014).

At the same time, this humanitarian turn to self-expression is also a practical response to compassion fatigue, the publics' apathy to traditional iconographies of suffering. Demonstrating a high degree of institutional reflexivity, as Vestergaard (2010) argues, major INGOs are today experimenting with a new aesthetics of solidarity that, in line with market research, is driven by the preferences of public polling – as, for instance, in Action Aid: '*The charity's direction*', as Turner says, speaking of the new emotionality of appeals, '*is the result of extensive consultation with donors and focus groups*' (2009).

Motivated by the diagnosis of compassion fatigue, this focus on the brand capitalizes on the mature market of humanitarianism, so as to take our familiarity with major INGOs for granted and avoid explicit messages of solidarity that may fuel fatigue towards grand narratives – for instance, towards the solidarity of salvation through iconographies of starving babies (McLagan 2003; Vestergaard 2010). Yet, even though branding builds upon a rather confident view of Western publics as already familiar with the morality of solidarity, the engagement of these publics with specific humanitarian brands can by no means be taken for granted. This is because, as recent UK-based research shows, Western publics may accept that helping the poor is our 'human obligation' but, at the same time, appear reluctant to prioritize poverty in the South over poverty at home and, in fact, provide support, albeit limited, to cuts in humanitarian aid; such results, as Henson and Lindstrom put it, '*are, on the one hand, quite heartening. Even in times of austerity*' they argue, '*there are quite strong views that we have a moral obligation to help the poor in the world. On the other,*' they continue, '*when it comes to support for spending on aid, such values appear to be undermined by domestic priorities ... the view seems to be that when times are tough, we cannot afford to waste money and must focus on problems closer to home*' (2010: 3).

Conclusion

Historical change in the ethics of solidarity, I have argued in this chapter, is a complex matter that should be approached in its institutional, political and technological dimensions. Whilst it is impossible to produce a perfect narrative that encompasses all three in equal measure, my ambition was rather to approach the communicative practices of humanitarianism as sites of articulation, where all three dimensions intersect with and overdetermine one another, in ways that variously come to define solidarity, at different points in time.

This focus on communication is of course not new. The humanitarian field has always focused on the impact of its messages on public attitudes to solidarity – for instance, in the reflexive aesthetics of inspiration-oriented rather than needs-based discourse. More often than not, however, such concerns have failed to go beyond the instrumental question of how to maximize donor funding and to address the real question of how the communication of solidarity may shape longer-term perceptions of the West as a moral actor. This neglect of the performative force of humanitarian communication, not only in the direct sense of acting out dispositions of solidarity but, in so doing, also in the sense of producing the publics it addresses rather than simply referring to them, has given rise to a *'persistent problem'* in the field: the problem of engagement. Whilst, according to research, INGO donations have today reached an all-time high, the quality of public engagement appears to have fallen at its lowest point ever: *'the disjuncture between the two sets of data* (donations/engagement, LC)*'*, Darnton comments, *'sparks some serious questions about how long the prevailing business model for development NGOs can continue, and what the implications are for the quality of public engagement'* (2011: 13).

At the heart of these questions lies the problem of the ethics of solidarity, insofar as the decline in public engagement reflects, more substantially, a weakening in the public appeal of the imperative to care for vulnerable others. The humanitarian field rightly approaches this problem of engagement as a communication problem, seeking to replace the 'transaction' model of communication with a 'values' model and so to introduce new interpretative 'frames' for its messages of solidarity (Darnton with Martin 2011). My view is, however, that the paradox of engagement cannot be addressed simply by shifting around the wording of messages or moving across a continuum of given values. Far from underestimating the power of words, what I suggest here is that, instead of manipulating messages, we need to establish the deeper causes that have led to the deterioration of a collective sense of altruistic commitment. This, in turn, requires a more holistic understanding of humanitarian communication not simply as linguistic practice but also as historical practice – as the gradual convergence of three longer-term social processes, the instrumentalization, de-politicization and mediatization of care. Such an understanding, as I showed, enables us to see the decline of engagement as a complex synergy between these three processes and thus to explain the decline in the context of a new ethics of solidarity. This is an ethics that informs acts of good-doing not because of an unwavering belief in 'our' common humanity but because of a belief in the effortless, albeit minor, self-gratifications of Western, consumerist lifestyles – what I referred to as a shift from a solidarity of pity to a solidarity of irony.

Understanding the deeper causes of the decline of public engagement in the West could further enable us to complement such diagnostic claims with normative ones, with alternative imaginations of solidarity that challenge both the sentimentalism of pity and the instrumentalism of irony. Rather than an over-reliance on either emotion, as in the pity-driven campaigns of emaciated children, or on reflexive self-expression, as in the celebrity-driven performances of people like 'us', alternative imaginations of solidarity can and should aim at fulfilling two communicative requirements. First, they should include the figure of the distant other so that they can be seen, heard and recognized; and second, they should address the question of why it is important that we act on their vulnerability – a question that makes the critique of power and the pursuit of justice a part of our public practice of solidarity.

Far from pure idealism, this new ethics of solidarity is feasible and realistic, I believe, insofar as it is grounded on the same historical legacy as the two current paradigms of solidarity are: the 'culture of sympathy'. This alternative ethics would, however, avoid both the certainties of this legacy, that is pity's 'salvation' or 'revolution', *and* the suspicion against all of its values, as in the self-centredness of irony. Solidarity would, instead, start from justice as a minimum 'common pursuit' that recognizes certain shared presumptions about what it means to be a human being and conceives of solidarity as a fundamentally political project: *'We could have been creatures incapable of sympathy, unmoved by the pain and humiliation of others, uncaring of freedom and – no less significant- unable to reason, argue, disagree and concur'*, Sen powerfully argues; yet, he continues, *'the strong presence of these features in human lives ... does indicate that the general pursuit of justice might be hard to eradicate in human society, even through we can go about that pursuit in different ways'* (2009: 415). Anchored, I suggest, upon our fundamental human abilities both to empathize and to judge, this ethics of solidarity should be less about branding and more about our engagement with the voices of vulnerability and with the values that may inform our action upon it. Indeed, in a world divided by systemic divisions between West and the global South, any attempt to imagine bonds of solidarity with vulnerable others can be grounded on nothing less but a persistent pursuit of the meaning of justice.

References

Barnett, M. (2005). Humanitarianism transformed. *Perspectives on Politics, 3*(4), 723–740.

Barnett, M., & Weiss, T. G. (Eds.). (2008). *Humanitarianism in question: Politics, power, ethics*. Ithaca: Cornell University Press.

Barnett, M., & Weiss, T. (Eds.). (2009). *Humanitarianism in question: Politics, power, ethics*. Ithaca: Cornell University Press.

Biel, R. (2000). *The new imperialism: Crisis and contradictions in North-South relations*. London: Zed Books.

Boltanski, L. (1999). *Distant suffering: Politics, morality and the media*. Cambridge: Cambridge University Press.

Boltanski, L., & Chiapello, E. (2005). *The new spirit of capitalism* (G. Elliott, Trans.). London: Verso.

Calhoun, C. (2008). Cosmopolitanism in the modern social imaginary. *Daedalus, 137*(3), 105–114.

Calhoun, C. (2009). The imperative to reduce suffering: Charity, progress and emrgencies in the field of humanitarian action. In M. Barnett & T. Weiss (Eds.), *Humanitarianism in question: Politics, power, ethics*. Ithaca: Cornell University Press.

Cheah, P. (2006). *Inhuman conditions: On cosmopolitanism and human rights*. Cambridge, MA: Harvard University Press.

Cooley, A., & Ron, J. (2002). The NGO scramble: Organizational insecurity and the political economy of transnational action. *International Security, 27*(1), 5–39.

Darnton, A. with Martin, K. (2011). *Finding frames: New ways to engage the UK public in global poverty*. London: Bond.

Eagleton, T. (2009). *Trouble with strangers: A study of ethics*. Chichester/Malden: Wiley-Blackwell Publishing.
Fenton, N. (2007). Contesting global capital, new media, solidarity, and the role of a social imaginary. In N. Carpentier & B. Cammaerts (Eds.), *Reclaiming the media: Communication rights and democratic media roles* (pp. 225–242). London: Intellect Books.
Fenton, N. (2008). Mediating solidarity. *Global Media and Communication, 4*(1), 37–57.
Fine, B. (2009). Development as zombieeconomics in the age of neo-liberalism. *Third World Quarterly, 30*(5), 885–904.
Friedman, L. J. (2003). Philanthropy in America: Historicism and its discontents. In L. J. Friedman & M. D. McGarvie (Eds.), *Charity, philanthropy and civility in American History* (pp. 1–21). Cambridge: Cambridge University Press.
Fuchs, C. (2014). *Social media. A critical introduction*. London: Sage.
Gilroy, P. (2006). *Postcolonial melancholia*. New York: Columbia University Press.
Henson, S., & Lindstrom, J. (2010). *Aid to developing countries: Where does the UK public stand? Results and analysis from the UK public opinion monitor [online]*. Institute of Development Studies: Brighton.
Hutchinson, J. F. (1996). *Champions of charity: War and the rise of the red cross*. Boulder/Oxford: Westview Press.
Hyde, L. (1999). *The gift: Imagination and the erotic life of property*. London: Vintage.
Kothari, U. (Ed.). (2005). *A radical history of development studies: Individuals, institutions and ideologies*. London: Zed Books.
Mathews, J. T. (1997). Power shift. *Foreign Affairs, 76*(1), 50–66.
McCleary, R. M., & Barro, R. J. (2007). *U.S.-based private voluntary organizations: Religious and secular PVOs engaged in international relief and development, 1939–2004*. American Political Science Association Annual Conference, 30 August–2 September 2007, Chicago.
McLagan, M. (2003). Human rights, testimony and transnational publicity. *S & F Online, 2*(1). Available at: http://barnard.edu/sfonline/ps/mclagan.htm#section1. Accessed 8 Aug 2011.
Moyn, S. (2010). *The last utopia: Human rights in history*. Cambridge, MA: Harvard University Press.
MSF. (2011). *Javier Bardem Screams with Medecins Sans Frontiers (video)*. Medecins Sans Frontieres (MSF) (AKA Doctors without Borders.) Available at: http://sofii.org/case-study/medicos-sin-fronteras-medicine-for-someone-elses-pain
Natsios, A. S. (1995). NGOs and the UN system in complex humanitarian emergencies: Conflict or cooperation? *Third World Quarterly, 16*(3), 405–420.
Rifkin, J. (2009). *The empathic civilization: The race to global consciousness in a world in crisis*. New York: Jeremy P. Tarcher/Penguin.
Rifkin, J. (2010). *The empathic civilization: The race to global consciousness in a world in crisis*. New York: Penguin.
Rorty, R. (1989). *Contingency, irony and solidarity*. Cambridge: Cambridge University Press.
Schuurman, F. (2009). Critical development theory: Moving out of the twilight zone. *Third World Quarterly, 30*(5), 831–848.
Shapiro, M. J. (2002). *Reading Adam Smith: Desire, history and value*. Oxford: Rowman & Littlefield Publishers.
Simmons, P. J. (1998). Learning to live with NGOs. *Foreign Policy, 112*(Autumn), 82–96.
Smillie, I., & Minear, L. (2004). *The charity of nations: Humanitarian action in a calculating world*. Bloomfield: Kumarian Press.
Smith, A. (1759). *The Theory of Moral Sentiments*. New York: Prometheus Books.
Smith, A. (1778). *Wealth of nations*. London: W. Strahan and T. Cadell.
Thumim, N. (2009). 'Everyone has a story to tell'. Mediation and self-representation in two UK institutions. *International Journal of Cultural Studies, 12*(6), 617–638.
Vestergaard, A. (2010). Identity and appeal in the humanitarian brand. In L. Chouliaraki & M. Morsing (Eds.), *Media, organizations and identity* (pp. 168–184). London: Palgrave MacMillan.

Chapter 4
Social Suffering and the Enigma of Humanitarianism

Iain Wilkinson

Introduction

In the social sciences, a major wave of published research has been using the frame of social suffering, which is the broadest and deepest form of human suffering. Social suffering promotes capturing the essence of how peoples' suffering is produced and conditioned by society. Social suffering researchers use a wide variety of evidence to capture the catastrophic burden of those trapped by the human plight of horrendous suffering. Implicitly if not explicitly, social suffering has come to represent a call to moral responsibility and humanitarian care. After briefly reviewing the history of the acceptance and rejection of humanitarianism as a moral compass for social science research, in this chapter I argue that this wave will return the social sciences to again recognize the moral power of humanitarianism. This discussion ends with recent developments that tend to reverse researchers' rejection of humanitarianism in academic life. Removal of these conceptual and methodological barriers will make possible a wide range of research that will help guide the design of social changes that have the potential to greatly alleviate suffering.

Problems of social suffering are attracting increasing amounts of scholarly interest and critical debate. Arguably this represents a significant new development in contemporary social research. Much of this work is committed to understand the social and cultural conditions that cause human suffering. In many instances researchers are also interested to explore the possible contribution that social science might make to people's healing and recovery and repair. There is concern to move beyond the work of understanding so as to be engaged with practices of humanitarian care. This courts great controversy, for there have been many occasions in the history of Western social science where humanitarian culture and politics have been portrayed as misguided fanaticisms or as wedded to moral crusades

I. Wilkinson (✉)
School of Social Policy, Sociology, University of Kent, North East Canterbury CT2 7NF, UK
e-mail: I.M.Wilkinson@kent.ac.uk

R.E. Anderson (ed.), *Alleviating World Suffering*, Social Indicators Research Series 67, DOI 10.1007/978-3-319-51391-1_4

that are set to cause yet further harm. I argue, however, that such outright hostility towards modern humanitarianism should be questioned on the grounds that it leaves social science with little else offer but critique. In contrast to a complete critical dismissal of humanitarianism I contend that a more productive line of inquiry lies in exploring the genealogy of the conventions of critique by which humanitarian thought and action is set in question and held up for judgement. I further explore some of the way in which those involved in research and writing on social suffering are seeking to critically recondition a humanitarian response to social suffering that allies social science with practices of caregiving.

The New Wave of Research on Social Suffering

The social sciences of the twenty first century have a new found concern with problems of social suffering. Over the last twenty years or so an unprecedented number of published studies have featured social suffering as a headline concern (cf. Bourgois 2003; Bourdieu et al. 1999; Das et al. 2001; Frost and Hoggett 2008; Kleinman et al. 1997; Renault 2008, 2010; Wilkinson and Kleinman 2016). The labeling of social problems and forms of social experience as 'social suffering' signals a commitment to understand how human suffering is caused and conditioned by society. In this regard, it calls select forms of social organization and uneven distributions of socio-economic resources into critical debate on account of the harms and social suffering produced. At the same time, those concerned with documenting people's social suffering tend to operate with the understanding that much that matters within 'the social' components of people's life experience is not readily grasped or easily understood. By carefully attending to the ways individuals voice their distress, and to how they embody their pains, researchers understand themselves to be gathering important data on how social life takes place as a distinctly moral experience (Kleinman 1998). We are invited to dwell on how adverse social events and conditions are borne by people and to attend to the damage done to their human dignity and personhood. This documentation of experiences of social suffering offers a porthole onto the lived experience of social life and as an opportunity to question its moral character and human meaning.

This marks a return to traditions of social inquiry that guide social understanding through 'fellow feeling' (Frazer 2010; Mullan 1988). Accordingly, the documentation of social suffering tends to incorporate styles of writing, forms of text and imagery designed to convey subjective standpoints, corporeal situations and the flow of sentiment. Documents of social life make us feel for people's predicaments and to care for what happens to individuals in situations of adversity. We are asked to pay heed to how individuals articulate their suffering on the understanding that the many frustrations borne through failing to find an adequate means to describe 'how it feels' or to explain 'what it all means' expose some part of the social contradictions they inhabit and the cultural deficits they bear. Visual materials are frequently deployed as a means to provide us with insights into the social environments in which people respond to what is happening to them and carry this suffering both within and upon their bodies.

This approach to social research operates in sharp contrast to traditions that seek to expunge moral feelings from the conduct of social science. A 'scientizing' approach in sociology and anthropology has often operated from the premise that moral feelings occlude rationality and deny sound judgement (Bannister 1991; Haskell 2000; Mazlish 1989; Poovey 1995, 1998). By contrast in research and writing on social suffering, moral feelings are understood to be a necessary part of the effort to make adequate sense of how people experience society. Social life takes place in enactments of substantive moral values that greatly matter for people. Here we are encouraged to empathize with the moral conflicts that individuals inhabit and with the moral frustrations they bear giving us an understanding that these are forms of experience in which the moral character of social life is revealed.

In many instances, documents from social suffering also commit to humanitarian projects of social reform. Furthermore, humanitarian cultures and politics are understood to be aligned with movements of social inquiry and the endeavor of social understanding. Humanitarian care for people is identified with care for human society as such; and further, by our participation in acts of caregiving. We come to understand how human social life is made possible, and in particular the forms of social life which make possible pro-social human relationships (Wilkinson and Kleinman 2016: 161–87). This is the approach that sustained what Jane Addams referred to as 'doing sociology' in the context of the activities of the progressive era Chicago settlement community of Hull-House (Addams 1965 [1892]; Addams 1998 [1910], 2002a [1902]). More recently it has been rekindled in the humanitarian medical anthropology of Philip Bourgois, Paul Farmer, Arthur Kleinman and Nancy Scheper-Hughes (Bourgois 2002; Bourgois and Schonberg 2009; Farmer 1992, 1999, 2006, 2013; Kleinman 1980, 2006; Scheper-Hughes 1992, 1998, 2005, 2011).

In what follows I outline some of the possible explanations for this revitalization of research and writing on social suffering in our times. I argue that this is operating to return social scientists to an arena of debate where the character, substance and practice of humanitarianism regains a center of attention. Along with others I contend that this calls for a more theoretically and historically refined account of the social forces that inspire and sustain humanitarian culture and its politics. I further argue that it requires us to explore the genealogy of the conventions of critique by which humanitarianism is questioned and held in judgement within social science. I suggest that the overall effect is not only to set social science up for debate as a moral practice, but also to underline the urgency of the requirement to better understand the connections between modern humanitarianism and the development of human sociality and sociological learning. There is no space here do to these arguments justice. This essay is only designed to initiate dialogue and debate. I conclude by outlining some of the challenges that are hereby set for social theory and the practice of social research.

Emerging Segregation Between the Social Sciences and Humanitarianism

This brief historical overview of sociology and social science research reveals some of the academic conflicts and intellectual tensions that in the early part of the twentieth century led large numbers of social scientists to distance themselves from the culture and politics of humanitarianism. In a largely forgotten article published in 1884 Lester Frank Ward, the first president of the American Sociological Association, cautioned his readers against adopting a wholly hostile relationship towards humanitarianism. He advised that American sociologists should be wary of adopting a British tendency that readily dismisses 'the sentiment of humanity' as a matter not worthy of serious sociological investigation. Ward urged them to critically question the narrowly conceived intellectualism that treats humanitarianism as no more than a 'fanaticism' for social reform. He argued that sociologists should approach humanitarian sentiment as 'the object of deep study' so as to better understand how society might prove itself 'capable of caring for the most unfortunate of its members in a manner that shall not work demoralization' (Ward 1884: 571).

Under the influence of Ward, Albion Small further promoted the view that sociology should be working to compliment and promote humanitarian agendas. While many of the social scientists of his day stood opposed to 'do-gooder confusion' and openly disparaged its 'sentimentalism', Small held out the hope that sociology might still operate as the handmaid to humanitarian social reform (Becker 1971). However, as he witnessed the advance of academic sociology and the extent to which its practitioners hankered for scientific accreditation, he came to view this as a lost cause. Increasingly it appeared that the culture of social science within the American academy was set antagonistically opposed to humanitarianism.

No doubt for Small this was a message brought home through his ill-fated attempts to establish a collaborative partnership between the newly formed Department of Sociology at the University of Chicago and Jane Addams' social reform work at Hull-House. Mary Jo Deegan records that it was not only the case that as academic sociology became the preserve of 'disinterested' scientific experts that Jane Addams sought to combat the public portrayal of her work as a sociological laboratory experiment, but also, that powerful interest groups in the University of Chicago were concerned to disassociate themselves from Addams' campaign work and politics. Deegan notes that insofar as Hull-House became known for its support for sweatshop workers' rights, women's suffrage, campaigns against corrupt landlords and movements to promote world peace through the First World War, then it came to be increasingly identified with value commitments that operated against the political and economic interests of those funding the university (Deegan 1988). By the 1920s it seemed all too clear that professional social science could not be allied with humanitarian movements for social reform; and indeed, that in their cultural values and social practices social scientists and humanitarians operated to undermine one another's favored standpoints on how to relate to the social world and our human predicament.

Historians of social science are now inclined to portray individuals such as Lester Frank Ward, Albion Small and Jane Addams as operating against the tide of their times. Whilst these three were torchbearers for an older tradition of social inquiry that held that moral sentiment was a guide to social understanding and that our critical reasoning about human states and social conditions should pay heed to humanitarian feeling, most of their contemporaries took opposing views. By the turn of the twentieth century there appeared to be little doubt in the minds of most social scientists, and especially those working in the United States and Britain, that humanitarianism should have no part in processes of rational deliberation, and further that it was a fanaticism that gave ground to 'indiscriminate charity' and a socially volatile politics of feeling.

In her famous essay on *The Social Question,* Hannah Arendt documents some of the worries that underpinned these views where she holds 'the passion of compassion' responsible for Robespierre's reign of terror (Arendt 1963). Here humanitarian feeling is portrayed as an anathema to reasoned debate and as a force that can be used to persuade people to take violent actions to achieve their aims. Aside from the fear that humanitarianism serves as an encouragement to mob rule, its sentimentality was also understood to obstruct the planning and implementation of social policy by utilitarian principle. It is now observed that many of the pioneers of modern social policy operated with the understanding that they should remove expressions of personal feeling from their documentation of social problems, for moral sentiment was readily associated with political naivety (Englander and O'Day 1995; Harrison 1982; Yeo 1996).

New Roles for Humanitarianism in Social Research

In the twenty-first century there are movements in social science that are set on renegotiating and reevaluating its relationship with humanitarianism. Certainly in the context of research and writing on social suffering, practitioners openly express humanitarian commitments and seek to associate their work with humanitarian agendas. These trends can be seen most blatantly in the number of book titles recently published with claims to 'Public Sociology' and 'Engaged social research.' When compared to the tenor of sociological and anthropological debates at the turn of the previous century, it seems that there has been something of a radical volte-face. How can we begin to explain this?

A range of factors appear to be involved. Firstly, and perhaps most obviously one might point to the extraordinary growth and spread of humanitarian organizations through the twentieth century; and especially over the last fifty years or so (Barnett 2011; Barnett and Weiss 2008). Never before in human history has there been such a large scale institutional and professionalized humanitarian response to people's social needs; and especially those of individuals trapped in situations of extreme adversity. Indeed, it is now impossible to understand the modern nation state and is concerns with human welfare without taking into consideration how its culture and operations have come under the direction of humanitarian imperatives. On this score, there can be no doubt that the humanitarianism of the twenty-first century is far better resourced, more politically influential and institutionally well-established than it was a century ago. No longer can it be dismissed as a mere fanaticism for social reform; rather it has become an increasingly important and powerful component of modern statecraft and politics.

Secondly, on many accounts a renewed engagement with humanitarian agendas and commitments appear to be connected to some of the radical and far-reaching transformations that have taken place in modern processes of cultural reproduction and exchange; and especially in connection with communication media. Through television and the internet, we are now routinely set to gaze from a 'mediatized' distance upon scenes of violence, war, famine and mass destruction (Boltanski 1999). In this regard, the cultural experience of people living through the last fifty years of human history is quite different to that of any other time or place (Thompson 1995). Arguably, one of the overall effects is an amplification of the presence of human suffering as a planetary condition so that a negotiation with its meaning and consequences is made a pressing collective concern. Indeed, it can be argued that such experience is now significantly altering the ways we relate to others and ourselves and that the cultural and political dimensions of human subjectivity are undergoing changes that we scarcely recognize or understand (Biehl et al. 2007).

Thirdly, in some quarters it is argued that an increased concern to reform and revise the ways social science responds to humanitarianism is a result of its feminization. Feminist critiques of academic culture and its cultural history have drawn attention to the extent to which its portrayals of humanitarian culture and politics reflect gender biases and promote patriarchal ideology. Accordingly, critics such as Laurent Berlant contend that the earlier academic hostility towards humanitarianism at the turn of the twentieth century was connected to a wider derogation of women's culture (Berlant 2004, 2008). Certainly, this was already recognized by Jane Addams in her day (Addams 2002b, 2007; Koven ans Michel 2013). It is now the case, however, that on many accounts this understanding is operating to draw cultures of modern rationality and processes of rationalization into critical debate out of a concern to expose the ideological effects of the values that thereby set into practice. In this context, the critique of humanitarianism is held under suspicion on account of the ways that it can be shown to have operated through early modern history as an adjunct to processes of gender discrimination.

Fourthly, the worry that rational cultures, while presenting themselves as standing above the fray of morality and politics, are actually operating to promote values and interests that do harm to people can also be identified as giving ground to a humanitarian critique of modern medicine. There is no doubt, moreover, that in the minds of medical anthropologists engaged in documenting problems of social suffering, that this is a guiding motivation and a matter of professional concern (Kleinman 1988, 2006). Indeed, as far as social science is concerned it may well be in relation to the sheer volume of research that is now committed to expose the suffering done to people through processes of 'medicalization' that there is a newfound concern to question the values governing the conduct of modern rationality; and here, moreover, a focus is brought to how these are set opposed to humanitarian principle and sentiment (Abramowitz et al. 2015).

This is a complex matter and there are many other factors beyond the four mentioned above that are contributing to the reconfiguration of social science so that it is made to question the terms under which it relates and responds to humanitarian concerns. Here I am not so much concerned with providing readers with a fully detailed and well analyzed account of this point in our cultural history. My interests lie, rather, in establishing that there is a distinctly new context in which we need to work, understanding the social forces and moral values that are incorporated within our modes of thought and practice; and further, that these are operating to set the character, conditions and consequences of contemporary humanitarianism as a pressing matter for further sociological and anthropological debate.

Going Forward: Humanitarian Research Responds to Human Suffering

Contemporary debates on modern humanitarianism tend to reflect the disciplinary concerns and critical agendas of the academic field of International Relations. Here a 'conventional narrative' features as a means to set limits on what is understood by humanitarianism and its practice. Humanitarianism is understood to be the inspiration of Henri Dunant and the work of the Red Cross. It is narrowly conceived as a specific form of civil action; one guided by principles of impartiality (the quality and quantity of aid is set to correspond with human needs), neutrality (humanitarian action is motivated by a direct response to human suffering and nothing else besides), and independence (humanitarian action operates above the fray of politics). In this context, commentators are largely concerned with detailing how, whilst incorporated within UN systems of global governance and following its connections to military interventions and counterterrorism, Dunant's founding vision has been betrayed. Humanitarianism is cast under suspicion as a political ideology that operates to establish and sustain relations of domination; and here moreover, it is frequently portrayed as caught up within a spiraling crisis of legitimacy (Barnett and Weiss 2008; Rieff 2002).

Some have further sought to associate research and writing on social suffering with an uncritical adoption of humanitarian agendas that serve to promote unequal power relations and discriminatory ideas and practices (Chouliaraki 2006, 2013; Fassin 2012). In this regard, social science is left mimicking, whilst also redeveloping, many age-old critiques of humanitarianism where it is identified with a lust for sensationalism, forms of promiscuous voyeurism and the moral crusades of sectional groups intent on imposing disciplinary regimes of moral order upon society (Fiering 1976; Halttunen 1995; Mintz 1995). In addition to this, insofar as it is held to be motivated by compassionate feelings that obstruct the work of critical reason, then it is cast in an all too familiar role as standing opposed to processes of utilitarian deliberation and rational debate (Calhoun 2004; Käpylä and Kennedy 2014; Ticktin 2011).

Those committed to research and writing on social suffering tend to openly acknowledge the risks inherent in documents of social life that court moral feeling. Here there is renewed commitment to the understanding that an 'eruption of moral sympathetic feeling' is a necessary part of the process whereby people are animated with concern for human rights (Wilkinson and Kleinman 2016: 148); and while there is always a danger that such feelings can be enjoyed as an end in themselves or serve as an encouragement to extreme behavior, nevertheless, they are taken as required for bringing focus to questions of humanity. As Pierre Bourdieu explains, the greater worry here is that through our dispassion and rationality we engage in acts of 'symbolic violence' that 'gloss' over the human experience of suffering so as to leave it unacknowledged and beyond concern (Bourdieu 1999). It is also the case that here practitioners tend to be wary of critique when this is presented as the main goal or end purpose of social analysis. People's social suffering is understood to require far more than a response of critique; rather it is understood to issue a demand for human care. It is in terms of its capacity to meet this need and its contribution to the alleviation of people's suffering that social science is held out for debate.

There are no positions to occupy here that are exempt from political controversy and moral strife. The brute fact of suffering itself declares that there is too much that matters for people's lives. It may well be the case, moreover, that as far as our collective involvement with humanitarianism is concerned we are, as Charles Taylor puts it, dealing with 'a big and deep story' that 'no one can claim to understand ... fully' (Taylor 1984: 155). Research and writing on social suffering calls us to reexamine and reevaluate the conduct of social science in face of many humanitarian dilemmas. It also draws the disciplinary conventions of social science into debate as distinct forms of moral practice. Here, perhaps more than ever before, the values we enact though our writing and research activities are set to court conflict; yet this may well be a necessary part of the process whereby these are made better oriented to human needs and the value of humanity itself (Wilkinson 2016).

Our end goal is not merely to spread a critically reconditioned humanitarianism across the horizons of researchers and policy makers, but it concerns the alleviation of suffering itself, especially social suffering. Removal of conceptual and methodological barriers will make possible a wide range of research that will help guide changes that have the potential to substantially alleviate suffering globally. A more complete understanding of pathways out of intractable social suffering will undoubtedly include a fuller understanding of social practices of care and the many ways this functions to alleviate social suffering.

References

Abramowitz, S., Marten, M., & Panter-Brick, C. (2015). Medical humanitarianism: Anthropologists speak out on policy and practice. *Medical Anthropology Quarterly, 29*(1), 1–23.

Addams, J. (1965). The subjective necessity for the social settlements. In C. Lasch (Ed.), *The social thought of Jane Addams*. Indianapolis: The Bobbs-Merrill Company.

Addams, J. (1998). *Twenty years at hull house*. New York: Penguin.

Addams, J. (2002a). 1902 *Democracy and social ethics*. Urbana/Chicago: University of Illinois.

Addams, J. (2002b). *The long road of woman's memory*. Urbana/Chicago: University of Illinois.

Addams, J. (2007). *Newer ideals of peace*. Urbana/Chicago: University of Illinois.

Arendt, H. (1963). The social question. In*On revolution*. Harmondsworth: Penguin.

Bannister, R. C. (1991). *Sociology and scientism: The American quest for objectivity, 1880–1940*. Chapel Hill: University of North Carolina Press.

Barnett, M. (2011). *Empire of humanity: A history of humanitarianism*. Ithaca: Cornell University Press.

Barnett, M., & Weiss, T. G. (Eds.). (2008). *Humanitarianism in question*. Ithaca: Cornell University Press.

Becker, E. (1971). *The lost science of man*. New York: George Braille.

Berlant, L. (Ed.). (2004). *Compassion: The culture and politics of an emotion*. New York: Routledge.

Berlant, L. (2008). *The female complaint: The unfinished business of sentimentality in American culture*. Durham: Duke University Press.

Biehl, J., Good, B., & Kleinman, A. (Eds.). (2007). *Subjectivity: Ethnographic investigations*. Berkeley: University of California Press.

Boltanski, L. (1999). *Distant suffering: Morality media and politics*. Cambridge: Cambridge University Press.

Bourdieu, P. (1999). Understanding. In P. Bourdieu et al. (Eds.), *The weight of the world: Social suffering contemporary society*. Cambridge: Polity Press.

Bourdieu, P., et al. (1999). *The weight of the world: Social suffering contemporary society*. Cambridge: Polity Press.

Bourgois, P. I. (2002). *In search of respect: Selling crack in El Barrio*. Cambridge: Cambridge University Press.

Bourgois, P. (2003). Crack and the political economy of social suffering. *Addiction Research & Theory, 11*(1), 31–37.

Bourgois, P. I., & Schonberg, J. (2009). *Righteous dopefiend*. Berkeley: University of California Press.

Calhoun, C. (2004). A world of emergencies: Fear, intervention, and the limits of cosmopolitan order. *Canadian Review of Sociology, 41*(4), 373–395.

Chouliaraki, L. (2006). *The spectatorship of suffering*. London: Sage Publications.

Chouliaraki, L. (2013). *The ironic spectator: Solidarity in the age of post-humanitarianism*. Cambridge: Polity Press.

Das, V., Kleinman, A., Lock, M. M., Ramphele, M., & Reynolds, P. (Eds.). (2001). *Remaking a world: Violence, social suffering, and recovery*. Berkeley: University of California Press.

Deegan, M. J. (1988). *Jane Addams and the men of the Chicago School, 1892–1918*. New Brunswick: Transaction Books.

Englander, D., & O'Day, R. (Eds.). (1995). *Retrieved riches: Social investigation in Britain, 1840–1914*. Aldershot: Scolar Press.

Farmer, P. (1992). *Aids and accusation: Haiti and the geography of blame*. Berkeley: University of California Press.

Farmer, P. (1999). *Infections and inequalities: The modern plagues*. Berkeley: University of California Press.

Farmer, P. (2003). *Pathologies of power: Health, human rights and the new war on the poor*. Berkeley: University of California Press.

Farmer, P. (2006). Never again? Reflections on human values and human rights. In G. B. Peterson (Ed.), *Tanner lectures on human values* (Vol. 26). Salt Lake City: University of Utah Press.

Farmer, P. (2013). Conversation in the time of cholera: A reflection on structural violence and social change. In M. Griffin & J. W. Block (Eds.), *In the company of the poor: Conversations with Dr Paul farmer and Fr Gustavo Gutierrez*. New York: Orbis Books.

Fassin, D. (2012). *Humanitarian reason: A moral history of the present*. Berkeley: University of California Press.

Fiering, N. S. (1976). Irresistible compassion: An aspect of eighteenth-century sympathy and humanitarianism. *Journal of the History of Ideas, 37*(2), 195–218.

Frazer, M. L. (2010). *The enlightenment of sympathy: Justice and the moral sentiments in the eighteenth century and today*. Oxford: Oxford University Press.

Frost, L., & Hoggett, P. (2008). Human agency and social suffering. *Critical Social Policy, 28*(4), 438–460.

Halttunen, K. (1995). Humanitarianism and the pornography of pain in anglo-American culture. *The American Historical Review, 100*(2), 303–334.

Harrison, B. (1982). *Peaceable kingdom: stability and change in modern Britain*. Oxford: Clarendon Press.

Haskell, T. L. (2000). *The emergence of professional social science: The American Social Science Association and the crisis of authority*. Baltimore: John Hopkins University Press.

Käpylä, J., & Kennedy, D. (2014). Cruel to care? Investigating the governance of compassion in the humanitarian imaginary. *International Theory, 6*(2), 255–292.

Kleinman, A. (1980). *Patients and healers in the context of culture: An exploration of the borderland between anthropology, medicine, and psychiatry*. Berkeley: University of California Press.

Kleinman, A. (1988). *The illness narratives: Suffering, healing and the human condition*. New York: Basic Books.

Kleinman, A., Das, V., & Lock, M. (Eds.). (1997). *Social suffering*. Berkeley: University of California Press.

Kleinman, A. (2006). *What really matters: Living a moral life amidst uncertainty and danger*. New York: Oxford University Press.

Koven, S., & Michel, S. (2013). *Mothers of a new world: Maternalist politics and the origins of welfare states*. London: Routledge.

Mintz, S. (1995). *Moralists and modernizers: America's pre-civil war reformers*. Baltimore: The John Hopkins Press.

Mullan, J. (1988). *Sentiment and sociability: The language of feeling in the eighteenth century*. London: Clarendon Press.

Mazlish, B. (1989). *A new science: The breakdown of connections and the birth of sociology*. New York: Oxford University Press.

Poovey, M. (1995). *Making a social body: British cultural formation 1830–1864*. Chicago: University of Chicago Press.

Poovey, M. (1998). *A history of the modern fact: Problems of knowledge in the sciences of wealth and society*. Chicago: Chicago University Press.

Renault, E. (2008). *Souffrances dociales*. Paris: La Découverte.

Renault, E. (2010). A critical theory of social suffering. *Critical Horizons, 11*(2), 221–241.

Rieff, D. (2002). *A bed for the night: Humanitarianism in crisis*. London: Vintage.

Scheper-Hughes, N. (1992). *Death without weeping: The violence of everyday life in Brazil*. Berkeley: University of California Press.

Scheper-Hughes, N. (1998). Undoing: Social suffering and the politics of remorse in the New South Africa. *Social Justice, 24*(4), 114–142.

Scheper-Hughes, N. (2005). *The last commodity: Post-human ethics and the global traffic in "Fresh" organs*. New York: Blackwell Publishing.

Scheper-Hughes, N. (2011). Mr Tati's Holiday and João's Safari-seeing the world through transplant tourism. *Body & Society, 17*(2–3), 55–92.

Scheper-Hughes, N., & Wacquant, L. (Eds.). (2002). *Commodifying bodies*. London: Sage.
Taylor, C. (1984). Foucault on freedom and truth. *Political Theory, 12*(2), 152–183.
Thompson, J. B. (1995). *The media and modernity: A social theory of the media*. Cambridge: Polity.
Ticktin, M. I. (2011). *Casualties of care: immigration and the politics of humanitarianism in France*. Berkeley: University of California Press.
Ward, L. F. (1884). Mind as a social factor. *Mind, 9*(36), 563–573.
Wilkinson, I. (2016). The problem of understanding modern humanitarianism and its sociological value. *International Social Science Journal, 65*(215–216), 65–78.
Wilkinson, I., & Kleinman, K. (2016). *A passion for society: How we think about human suffering*. Berkeley: University of California Press.
Yeo, E. (1996). *The contest for social science: Relations and representations of gender and class*. London: Rivers Oram Press.

Chapter 5
Synergy, Dysergy and the Alleviation of Preventable Suffering

Mick Cooper

Introduction

Some forms of suffering are unpreventable (Anderson 2015). Indeed, as existential philosophers and psychotherapists have argued (e.g., Camus 1955; Frankl 1986), the inevitability of suffering is woven in to the very fabric of human existence. And yet, at each level of suffering-physical, mental, interpersonal and social (Anderson 2015)-there are forms of threat, loss and damage that seem eminently avoidable. Two teenage girls are stoned to death in Syria for committing "adultery", a morbidly obese man cannot stand for more than 30 min and is confined to his bed-these are forms of extreme suffering that seem like they could be otherwise. Preventable suffering, in some respects, is the worst form of suffering, because it is so unnecessary. And yet, paradoxically, it also offers the greatest hope, because it is the pathway through which suffering can genuinely be alleviated.

Anderson (2015, p. 7) writes that suffering comes from three places-"individuals, social institutions, and forces of nature", and that preventable suffering comes from "human choices". This chapter focuses on one particular form of choosing-and failure to choose-that can be seen at the root of many forms of preventable suffering. This is *dysergies*, defined as relationships between two forces in which the wholes are less than the sums of the parts (Cooper 2012). In dysergetic relationships, two forces engage in "interfering", "conflicting", "competing" or "lose-lose" ways (Austin and Vancouver 1996; Axelrod 1984; Cooper 2012; Michalak and Grosse Holtfort 2006; Wiese and Salmela-Aro 2008), such that there is a net loss of total effect. In this chapter, I will show how the concept of dysergies can help to account for, and draw into a unified framework, different forms of mental, interpersonal, and social suffering. On this basis, I will argue that the development of *synergies*-"win-win"

M. Cooper (✉)
Department of Psychology, University of Roehampton,
Holybourne Avenue, London SW15 1JD, UK
e-mail: mick.cooper@roehampton.ac.uk

R.E. Anderson (ed.), *Alleviating World Suffering*, Social Indicators Research Series 67, DOI 10.1007/978-3-319-51391-1_5

relationships between different forces-may be an effective means towards the alleviation of preventable suffering, and suggest concrete ways in which this can be achieved.

Teleological and Telic Foundations

As suggested above, the concepts of dysergy and synergy necessitate an understanding of people as force-like, dynamic entities. More specifically, as with contemporary motivational theorists, the model developed in this chapter understands people as purposive, intentional and future-oriented, organizing their activities towards the actualization of "goals" (e.g., Moskowitz and Grant 2009), "personal projects" (e.g., Little et al. 2007), "personal strivings" (e.g., Emmons 1986), or "wants" (Cooper 2012). These wants can be conceptualized as existing in a hierarchical framework (Powers 1973), with lower order wants (e.g., "to eat a pizza") understood as means of attaining higher order wants (e.g., "to satiate hunger", "to enjoy time with friends"). Ultimately, all wants are understood as leading up to the highest order, most foundational wants, such as "to survive"; or self-determination theory's autonomy, competence and relatedness (Ryan and Deci 2000).

This *teleological* understanding of human being forms the basis for *telic* theories of human wellbeing, suffering and affect. These propose that people's feelings are closely connected to the extent with which people *actualize* their wants (Emmons 1986). Empirical evidence suggests that this is in four main respects (Wiese 2007). First, people tend to feel better when they have a greater awareness of their higher order wants, and a belief that these are meaningful and important (Emmons 1986; Little et al. 2007; Steger 2013). For instance, Frankl (1986) and other meaning-centered therapists (e.g., Breitbart et al. 2010) have argued that people can experience profound psychological suffering when they do not have a sense of meaning and purpose in life. Second, higher levels of wellbeing are associated with a belief that one's wants are attainable (Emmons 1986). That is, people who feel that there is no way of achieving their goals may feel profound hopelessness, futility and frustration. Third, positive affect is associated with progress towards personally meaningful goals (Koestner et al. 2002); with negative affect linked to feeling "stuck", or that one's goals are rapidly receding. Finally, people feel good when they achieve the things that they want (Emmons and Diener 1986). Hence, they can suffer if they consistently fail to achieve the goals that they have set for themselves. From a telic standpoint, then, a principal component of wellbeing is *want-actualization*: awareness of, confidence in achieving, progress towards, and attainment of, personally meaningful goals.

Dysergy and Synergy at the Individual Level

If people are understood, however, as purposeful, goal-directed beings, how is it that they can fail to do exactly that: to actualize their wants? In many cases, this may be because an individual's environment does not have the resources to meet their wants. A person, for instance, wants physical safety, but they live in war-torn Sudan; or they want motherly love and comfort, but their mother has died.

In such cases, the failure to actualize wants, and the subsequent suffering, may be unpreventable at the individual level. However, another possible reason why people may fail to actualize particular wants, and consequently experience suffering and distress, is because other wants are pulling them in an opposite direction. An example of this might be the person suffering from morbid obesity. Although, in part, this may be due to genetic factors; it is also possible that their difficulties emerge because they are acting towards wants that are pulling them away from their desire for health and weight loss. For instance, the person may be over-eating as a way of trying to suppress emotional pain, or as a form of self-punishment. Another example might be a young woman who feels desperately lonely in her life, but who is also scared of losing control. Here, as a purpose-oriented being, she strives to ensure that she does not become too dependent on another person but, in doing so, she pulls against the very intimacy that she craves. This hypothesized relationship between goal conflict and distress is strongly supported by the empirical research, which shows that greater levels of conflict are associated with lower levels of psychological functioning, affect, mobilization, and life satisfaction (Austin and Vancouver 1996; Cox and Klinger 2002; Emmons 1986; Emmons and King 1988; Karoly 1999; Kelly et al. 2015; Riediger 2007; Riediger and Freund 2004).

The other side of this coin is the hypothesis that "harmony and integrated functioning among one's goals are essential for subjective well-being" (Emmons 1986, p. 1065). That is, it has been widely argued-in both the psychological (e.g., Cooper 2012) and psychotherapeutic literature (e.g., Ferrucci 1982)-that wellbeing is associated with the existence of synergetic (Corning 1998), or "facilitative" (Riediger and Freund 2004), intergoal relationships. Indeed, I have argued previously that all psychotherapies, in essence, strive to help clients overcome intrapersonal dysergies, and move towards more synergetic intrapersonal relationships (Cooper 2012). So, for instance, the morbidly obese man learns that he can deal with his emotions by talking about them, rather than over-eating-a strategy which is much more compatible with his desire to lose weight. Or the young woman learns, through a deep therapeutic encounter, that relating closely to others can actually bring about greater feelings of control.

Dysergy and Synergy at the Interpersonal and Social Level

Within the psychological literature, there has been a tendency to conceptualize goal conflict at the intrapersonal level only. However, to a certain extent, dysergies are always dependent on an external context. For instance, the morbidly obese man's conflict between being healthy and over-eating exists because food contains calories. Were it calorie-free, there would be no conflict here. Another example: a woman wants to actualize her sexual desires towards other women, but she also desperately craves the approval of those around her. Here, again, whether these goals are synergetic or dysergetic is strongly related to her external, social environment. If others are accepting or prizing of her sexuality then she can fully actualize her lesbian wishes and still be valued by others. However, if others are judgmental or condemning of it, then she may be forced to choose between one want or the other. Now, the choice is between sexual satisfaction accompanied by intense feelings of isolation, shame or self-loathing; or social "acceptance" accompanied by a deep sexual frustration. In this respect, we can say that an individual's environment sets the context for whether their goals are likely to be brought into conflict with each other, or have the potential to be synergetically actualized (or are simply independent). Another way of conceptualizing this is to say that, as the *resources* in a person's environment-whether economic, material or interpersonal-become more limited, so their goals are more likely to come into conflict. That is, if a person has everything available to them-for instance, love, time, and financial resources- they have the possibility of actualizing multiple goals concurrently. But as resources get more restricted, so their wants are more likely to be brought into conflict with each other. Now the actualization of one want is more likely to necessitate the sacrifice of others. Crucially, however, whatever the limits to a person's resources, it is always likely that they can find some more synergetic ways of configuring their wants. For instance, the woman might come to see the homophobia in others as a sign of *their* vulnerability, rather than as a judgment on her. Now, she may find it easier to feel accepted, in her essence, by others; while developing her sexuality in the way that she wants to.

The interpersonal and social planes, however, not only set the context for intrapersonal synergies and dysergies; they can also be understood as levels of analysis in which synergies and dysergies, themselves, operate. That is, we can also consider the extent to which dyads, groups, or societies as a whole, have wants that are synergetic with, dysergetic with, or independent of, each other. Such dynamics have been explored in detail within "game theory", where people are conceptualized as relating to others in "win-win" ("non-zero-sum"), "win-lose" ("zero-sum") or "lose-lose" ways (Axelrod 1984; Wright 2000). An example of a dysergetic interpersonal relationship: An Iranian refugee flees to the UK because she wants to feel "safe", but her presence evokes feelings of threat in a UK national. The latter strives to reduce these feelings through acting towards the refugee in aggressive and racist ways. This, then, creates greater feelings of fear in the refugee, who then acts in more defensive ways towards the UK national, creating a vicious cycle of mutual distrust, fear and mental suffering. Compare this with a more synergetic configuration in which the UK national, feeling threatened by the alienness of the refugeee, decides to address this by learning more about the refugeee's culture and political context. Now, she responds to the refugee in a more compassionate and understanding way, evoking a more open and warmer response to the UK national. Here, a virtuous cycle may be evoked, with both parties learning and benefitting from the other, and an overall increase in wellbeing.

As at the individual level, we can understand the roots of interpersonal and social dysergies in terms of limited resources. The greater the available resources (for instance, if there was a plethora of well-paid jobs in the UK), the lower the likelihood that different people's wants would come into conflict (cf., "realistic conflict theory", Sherif and Sherif 1953). However, as at the individual plane, there is always likely to be some possibility for reconfiguration: for greater or lesser degrees of synergy, even with the same set of resources. As in the example of the refugee and the UK national above, for instance, within the same circumstances, two people can suffer in fear and hatred; or they can thrive, learn and grow.

Towards Mental, Interpersonal and Social Synergies

This final section of the chapter looks at a range of strategies that may help to enhance synergetic relationships, at both the mental and interpersonal or social level. The list is not exhaustive, but an attempt to consider some of the implications for the analysis developed in this chapter.

Developing a Culture of Unconditional Acceptance

Research suggests that one of the highest order human wants is for relatedness to others (e.g., Ryan and Deci 2000). If this is the case, then the conditions under which that is realized is likely to be a powerful determinant of synergies-and consequently of wellbeing and suffering-at both the mental, interpersonal and social level. If an individual can feel loved and accepted for whoever and however they are, then there is the potential for maximizing the extent to which they can actualize *all* their desires, without compromising their need to be loved. By contrast, a limited pool of acceptance within a society-as with the lesbian woman discussed earlier-means that the striving for approval necessitates the sacrificing of other wants. Needless suffering is evoked. Of course, what is being suggested here is not the unconditional acceptance of another's acts, however destructive or harmful they might be. Clearly, that could lead to an overall reduction in interpersonal or social wellbeing. But an unconditional acceptance of the other's "internal world" essentially "costs" nothing. That is, to accept and value the others' experiences, feelings and desires takes nothing away from the self, but means that that other can more fully actualize their wants. This is the basis of a Rogerian approach to therapy (Rogers 1957, 1961), which strives to provide clients with an unconditionally accepting therapeutic relationship such that they can come to acknowledge and integrate their many different experiences. It is also closely linked to an attitude of celebrating diversity, in which heterogeneity and difference are engaged as positive qualities to be prized. Valuing diversity in others maximizes those others' opportunities to thrive; it is a pool of interpersonal resources which allows that other to flourish along multiple trajectories.

Helping People to Develop Communication Skills

In game theory (e.g., Wright 2000) as well as in couple and family therapies (e.g., Evans 2012), communication across positions is the key to "negotiating coordinated strategies" (Fisher 2008, p. 75), and developing improved relationships. The same could be said of individual psychotherapy, where people learn about, and begin to talk and negotiate across, multiple wants. Through open and authentic communication, people may be more able to see the higher order desires that are driving lower order wants, and this may lead to greater empathy, as the person sees the essentially human desires underpinning the other's actions. In communicating across higher order wants, people are also more able to work out synergistic solutions: ways of engaging that can help each person actualize their higher order wants. Through open and honest communication, for instance, the British nationalist may come to see that what drives the Iranian refugee is not a desire to overrun the UK, but for safety and security. This, then, evokes less of a defensive-dysergetic-response. And in understanding this, as well as the needs of the UK national, there is the possibility of seeking solutions that are genuinely fulfilling for both parties. How can two people from different cultures, for instance, feel safe and unthreatened in the same locality? Such questions may not be easy to answer, but the act of communication and dialogue gives the best possibility of finding mutually satisfactory, and beneficial, solutions.

Developing Trust

Closely related to communication skills is the development of trust. One of the key findings that comes out of research on the "prisoner's dilemma" game (in which two players have to decide whether to cooperate with, or defect on, each other) is the centrality of trust to win-win, synergetic relationship (Axelrod 1984; Wright 2000). Fisher (2008, p. 129) writes, 'If we could find ways to trust each other, we could then find win-win solutions to many of our most serious problems.' Synergies can be likened to an arch bridge, which cannot be built up one side at a time (Cooper 2016). Rather, synergies require both sides to be prepared, and to trust and have faith that the other side will be ready to meet them. Once the synergy is established, like the setting of a key stone in the arch bridge, they can be extremely strong; but until that time they are highly vulnerable to collapse. It may feel much "safer", for instance, for the British national to deal with her fear of the refugee through racism and aggression. It requires nothing of the other: here, the British national is entirely self-sufficient. The development of synergetic possibilities, by contrast, requires the British national to open herself out: to take the risk of needing and being reliant on the other. The rewards from such actions can be immense but, like the activation energy required for a chemical reaction, the person may first need to invest energy and resources in overcoming distrust.

Orientating Society to Synergetic Wants

In establishing synergetic relationships between people, it is also important to note that some wants may have more synergetic potential than others (Cooper 2016). The desire for deep connections with others, for instance, may have high synergetic potential, because, by definition, it is a mutual act: we can only experience it when we feel the other experiences it towards us too (Mearns and Cooper 2005). "Love begets love, friendship fosters friendship, community draws out communal feelings in others" (Cooper 2016, p. 6). In other words, the desire for relatedness has the potential to support the actualization of this same desire in others. This also extends to many other relational desires. For instance, the desire to care for others, or be compassionate and altruistic towards them, all have high synergetic potential; as does the desire for sexual intimacy. Indeed, perhaps sex has the potential to be the most synergetic of all acts: where our deep, intense pleasure has the capacity to evoke the same intense feelings in another.

Achieving Competence Without Leaving Others Feeling Incompetent

Other desires, however, may have less synergetic potential, or actively lean towards dysergy. The desire for competence may be a particularly important instance here: another of self-determination theory's three highest order needs (Ryan and Deci 2000). In comparison to relatedness, which requires the relatedness of another, competence tends to be defined *relative to* the competence of others (Morse and Gergen 1970). Hence, for instance, if people around me are highly successful, it can leave me feeling more insecure about my own achievements. In many instances, such as college grades or sports, my achievement is also directly opposed to the achievement of others: if I win, they lose, and vice versa.

Yet from a self-determination theory perspective, we cannot simply eradicate the desire to feel good about ourselves. So how might a society allow more people to achieve more feelings of competence more of the time? Here, one of the problems with contemporary western society may be that success tends to be judged according to only a very few criteria. Hence, we are constantly thrown up against each other to determine who, for instance, is the richest, thinnest, or most cited. Compare this with a culture in which there are multiple ways in which people can achieve:

> So, for instance, people are not just venerated for being rich or beautiful; but also for being loyal friends, or skilled baristas, or talented bus drivers. Every walk of life has the potential to have areas in which people can excel, and can be recognized for excelling. And such a society also needs to support a growing specialization of activities. So it is not just, for instance, that people are beer makers; but makers of porter, or lambic beers, or cream ales. And within each one of these specialties grows sub-specialties that people can excel in. (Cooper 2016, p. 8)

Central to the functioning of such a specialized society would be a prioritizing of creativity. Creativity generates new possibilities, new domains, and new areas for growth: "not only porters and cream ales, for instance, but coconut lagers, midnight blue beers, and Sumerian-inspired Stone Age ales" (Cooper 2016, p. 8). And, with each of these developments, comes the potential for new specializations, new creative evolutions. Through fostering creativity, a society has greater potential to branch out and grow. And, in doing so, it can create more pathways in which more people can succeed more of the time. In other words, just as the valuing of diversity has the potential to reduce intrapersonal dysergies, so it has the potential to reduce dysergies at the interpersonal and social level: fostering a culture in which the attainment of one adds to-rather than subtracts from-the attainment of others.

Discussion

Synergies, I have suggested, can be fostered by developing a culture that prizes others and otherness, and in which people learn communication skills and the capacity to trust. Schools seem an ideal place to begin nurturing such competences, and there are many programs that can support this process, such as empathy training and emotional literacy work. For such programs to be widely disseminated, however, there is a need for a society to believe in the value of trust over fear, and cooperation over ruthless competition. The framework developed in this chapter can, perhaps, help make such an argument, by setting out a common metric by which all policies and practices can be judged, and by showing how synergies are one means of getting there. Here, a "good" society is one in which as many people get as much of what they want as much of the time, and a "good" social policy or practice is one that can contribute to-rather than take away from-this overall actualization of wants. By this definition, actions like communication, tolerance and compassion are all "good" things because, through their synergetic potential, they can increase this net wants-actualization (i.e., the extent to which people in a society, as a whole, actualize their wants). Acting compassionately, for instance, helps some people feel good because they experience the pleasure of reaching out, and it helps other people feel good because they experience the pleasure of being helped and supported in their lives. By contrast, actions like intolerance, racism and homophobia are "bad" because they reduce the net actualization of wants. Homophobia, for instance, reduces the capacity of its many victims to feel good about themselves; without actualizing anything of enduring worth for anyone else. Understanding society in these terms, we can begin to develop a robust argument for why such values and actions as compassion, altruism and trust are the basis for a thriving society. Not because they are simply "nice" or "kind", but because they are the best way of all us getting what we want.

As a theory of human suffering, two further aspects of this model can be highlighted. First, its understanding of people as agentic, purposive and intelligible is well-suited to the humanitarian agenda it is trying to develop. Too often, attempts to address the causes and consequences of human suffering are based on psychologies that derogate the very human beings that they are trying to help. The lay assumption, for instance, that human beings cause suffering to others out of some inherent "badness" invokes a Hobbesian model of human being as selfish, brutal and nasty. Similarly, positivist psychological and social theories-in their striving for universalized laws and understandings-strip human beings of their individuality and "radical otherness" (Levinas 1969); reducing them down to mechanistic, passively-determined "its" (Buber 1958). Second, the framework developed in this chapter bridges a mental, interpersonal and social divide, and outlines concepts and process that can be seen as operating at all three levels. This may be helpful because it means we can talk about common processes of positive, and negative, change; and learn from different domains. For instance, dialogue has been promoted as a powerful, synergistic force at the interpersonal level, but what would this look like intrapersonally? Psychological theorists, drawing on the interpersonal dialogic writings of Bakhtin (1973) and Buber (1947), are beginning to ask such questions, and help develop more effective strategies for addressing dysergies at the intrapersonal plane (Cooper et al. 2012; Rowan 2010).

Conclusion

To summarize, in this chapter, I have argued that the notions of dysergy and synergy can be powerful tools in helping us conceptualize, and develop means of addressing, preventable human suffering. Here, intelligible, purpose-oriented beings are seen as coming into conflict with themselves, and each other, as they strive towards the things that they want. Social improvement, in this framework, can come from helping people to reconfigure their wants in more synergistic ways: through communication and trust, through prioritizing goals that have high synergetic potential, and through a deep appreciation of the diversity across-and within-people. This approach does not neglect the importance of external resources, per se: it is clear that people need such things as food, housing and respect to actualize their wants. But within any one set of resources, there is always the possibility of more or less want-actualization, depending on how synergetically or dysergetically activities are configured. Synergies allow people to come together-both in the intra and interpersonal sense-and make the most of what they do have. They cannot eradicate suffering, but they can be considered an underlying principle of what helps to make a less suffering world.

References

Anderson, R. E. (2015). Implications of world suffering for human progress. In R. E. Anderson (Ed.), *World suffering and quality of life* (pp. 3–29). Dordrecht: Springer.

Austin, J. T., & Vancouver, J. B. (1996). Goal constructs in psychology: Structure, process, and content. *Psychological Bulletin, 120*(3), 338–375. doi:10.1037/0033-2909.120.3.338.

Axelrod, R. (1984). *The evolution of cooperation*. New York: Basic.

Bakhtin, M. (1973). *Problems of Doestoevsky's poetics* (R. W. Rostel, Trans., 2nd ed.). Ann Arbor: Ardis.

Breitbart, W., Rosenfeld, B., Gibson, C., Pessin, H., Poppito, S., Nelson, C., et al. (2010). Meaning-centered group psychotherapy for patients with advanced cancer: A pilot randomized controlled trial. *Psycho-Oncology, 19*(1), 21–28.

Buber, M. (1947). Dialogue (R. G. Smith, Trans.) *Between man and man* (pp. 17–59). London: Fontana.

Buber, M. (1958). *I and thou* (R. G. Smith, Trans., 2nd ed.). Edinburgh: T & T Clark Ltd.

Camus, A. (1955). *The myth of sisyphus* (J. O'Brien, Trans.). London: Penguin.

Cooper, M. (2012). *A hierarchy of wants: Towards an integrative framework for counselling, psychotherapy and social change*. Glasgow: University of Strathclyde. Retrieved from download from pure.strath.ac.uk/portal

Cooper, M. (2016). The fully functioning society: A humanistic-existential vision of an actualizing, socially-just future. *Journal of Humanistic Psychology*. doi:10.1177/0022167816659755.

Cooper, M., Chak, A., Cornish, F., & Gillespie, A. (2012). Dialogue: Bridging personal, community and social transformation. *Journal of Humanistic Psychology, 53*(1), 70–93. doi:10.1177/0022167812447298.

Corning, P. A. (1998). "The synergism hypothesis": On the concept of synergy and its role in the evolution of complex systems. *Journal of Social and Evolutionary Systems, 21*(2), 133–172. doi:10.1016/S1061-7361(00)80003-X.

Cox, W. M., & Klinger, E. (2002). Motivational structure: Relationships with substance use and processes of change. *Addictive Behaviors, 27*(6), 925–940. doi:10.1016/S0306-4603(02)00290-3.

Emmons, R. A. (1986). Personal strivings: An approach to personality and subjective well-being. *Journal of Personality and Social Psychology, 51*(5), 1058–1068. doi:10.1037/0022-3514.51.5.1058.

Emmons, R. A., & Diener, E. (1986). A goal-affect analysis of everyday situational choices. *Journal of Research in Personality, 20*(3), 309–326.

Emmons, R. A., & King, L. A. (1988). Conflict among personal strivings: Immediate and long-term implications for psychological and physical well-being. *Journal of Personality and Social Psychology, 54*(6), 1040–1048. doi:10.1037/0022-3514.54.6.1040.

Evans, G. (2012). Couple counselling. In C. Feltham & I. Horton (Eds.), *The Sage handbook of counselling and psychotherapy* (pp. 581–589). London: Sage.

Ferrucci, P. (1982). *What we may be*. London: Aquarian.

Fisher, L. (2008). *Rock, paper, scissors: Game theory in everyday life*. London: Basic Books.

Frankl, V. E. (1986). *The Doctor and the soul: From psychotherapy to logotherapy* (R. Winston & C. Winston, Trans., 3rd ed.). New York: Vintage Books.

Karoly, P. (1999). A goal systems–self-regulatory perspective on personality, psychopathology, and change. *Review of General Psychology, 3*(4), 264–291. doi:10.1037/1089-2680.3.4.264.
Kelly, R. E., Mansell, W., & Wood, A. M. (2015). Goal conflict and well-being: A review and hierarchical model of goal conflict, ambivalence, self-discrepancy and self-concordance. *Personality and Individual Differences, 85*, 212–229.
Koestner, R., Lekes, N., Powers, T. A., & Chicoine, E. (2002). Attaining personal goals: Self-concordance plus implementation intentions equals success. *Journal of Personality and Social Psychology, 83*(1), 231–244. doi:10.1037/0022-3514.83.1.231.
Levinas, E. (1969). *Totality and infinity: An essay on exteriority* (A. Lingis, Trans.). Pittsburgh: Duquesne University Press.
Little, B. R., Salmela-Aro, K., & Phillips, S. D. (Eds.). (2007). *Personal project pursuit: Goals, action, and human flourishing*. Mahwah: Lawrence Erlbaum Associates Publishers.
Mearns, D., & Cooper, M. (2005). *Working at relational depth in counselling and psychotherapy*. London: Sage.
Michalak, J., & Grosse Holtfort, M. (2006). Where do we go from here? The goal perspective in psychotherapy. *Clinical Psychology: Science and Practice, 13*(4), 346–365.
Morse, S., & Gergen, K. (1970). Social comparison, self-consistency, and the concept of the self. *Journal of Personality and Social Psychology, 16*(1), 148–156.
Moskowitz, G. B., & Grant, H. (Eds.). (2009). *The psychology of goals*. New York: Guilford Press.
Powers, W. T. (1973). *Behaviour: The control of perception*. Chicago: Aldine.
Riediger, M. (2007). Interference and facilitation among personal goals: Age differences and associations with well-being and behavior. In B. R. Little, K. Salmela-Aro, & S. D. Phillips (Eds.), *Personal project pursuit: Goals, action, and human flourishing* (pp. 119–143). Mahwah: Lawrence Erlbaum Associates Publishers.
Riediger, M., & Freund, A. M. (2004). Interference and facilitation among personal goals: Differential associations with subjective well-being and persistent goal pursuit. *Personality and Social Psychology Bulletin, 30*(12), 1511–1523. doi:10.1177/0146167204271184.
Rogers, C. R. (1957). The necessary and sufficient conditions of therapeutic personality change. *Journal of Consulting Psychology, 21*(2), 95–103.
Rogers, C. R. (1961). *On becoming a person: A therapist's view of therapy*. London: Constable and Co..
Rowan, J. (2010). *Personification: Using the dialogical self in psychotherapy and counselling*. New York: Routledge/Taylor & Francis Group.
Ryan, R. M., & Deci, E. L. (2000). Self-determination theory and the facilitation of intrinsic motivation, social development, and well-being. *American Psychologist, 55*(1), 68–78.
Sherif, M., & Sherif, C. W. (1953). *Groups in harmony and tension; an integration of studies of intergroup relations*. Oxford: Harper.
Steger, M. F. (2013). Experiencing meaning in life. In P. T. P. Wong (Ed.), *The human quest for meaning: Theories, research, and applications* (2nd ed., pp. 165–184). New York: Routledge.
Wiese, B. S. (2007). Successful pursuit of personal goals and subjective well-being. In B. R. Little, K. Salmela-Aro, & S. D. Phillips (Eds.), *Personal project pursuit: Goals, action, and human flourishing* (pp. 301–328). Mahwah: Lawrence Erlbaum Associates Publishers.
Wiese, B. S., & Salmela-Aro, K. (2008). Goal conflict and facilitation as predictors of work-family satisfaction and engagement. *Journal of Vocational Behavior, 73*(3), 490–497. doi:10.1016/j.jvb.2008.09.007.
Wright, R. (2000). *Nonzero: The logic of human destiny*. New York: Vintage Books.

Part II
Quality of Life (QOL), Caring and Suffering Alleviation

Chapter 6
Distinguishing Indicators of Well-Being from Indicators of Ill-Being

M. Joseph Sirgy

Introduction

The study of well-being comprises substantial bodies of empirical work done by scientists working across many disciplines. The international and interdisciplinary natures of this field of social science theory and research (from the natural and social sciences to the arts, humanities, the nature and social sciences, as well as the performing arts) are captured by Alex Michalos in his 12-volume *Encyclopedia of Quality of Life and Well-Being Research* (Michalos 2014). The field of study documents progress in enhancing human well-being and the reduction of well-being through indicators. Hence, much of the focus of quality-of-life and well-being research is on the use of *indicators* to chronicle progress and development. These indicators tend to promote a fuller understanding of the social, political, and economic dynamics that contribute to human well-being and ill-being. In addition, there are significant public policy implications of research on indicators to advance well-being (and reduce ill-being) in individuals, families, communities, entire countries, geopolitical regions, and the world as a whole (Hagerty et al. 2002).

In the field of quality-of-life studies, Headey et al. (1984) made the distinction between well-being and ill-being in their seminal article titled *Well-Being and Ill-Being: Different Dimensions*. The authors presented evidence that the construct of well-being is distinct from that of ill-being (i.e., the two constructs are not unidimensional). The authors were able to confirm this distinction using survey data that involved four measures of well-being: Life-as-a-Whole Index, the Self-Fulfillment Index, the 3-point Happy Scale, Bradburn's (1969) Positive Affect Scale; and three measures of ill-being: Bradburn's (1969) Negative Affect Scale, the Worries Index, and the Somatic Complaints Index. More recently, Lee and Oguzoglu

M.J. Sirgy (✉)
Virginia Tech Real Estate Professor of Marketing, Virginia Polytechnic Institute & State University, Blacksburg, VA 24061, USA
e-mail: sirgy@vt.edu

R.E. Anderson (ed.), *Alleviating World Suffering*, Social Indicators Research Series 67, DOI 10.1007/978-3-319-51391-1_6

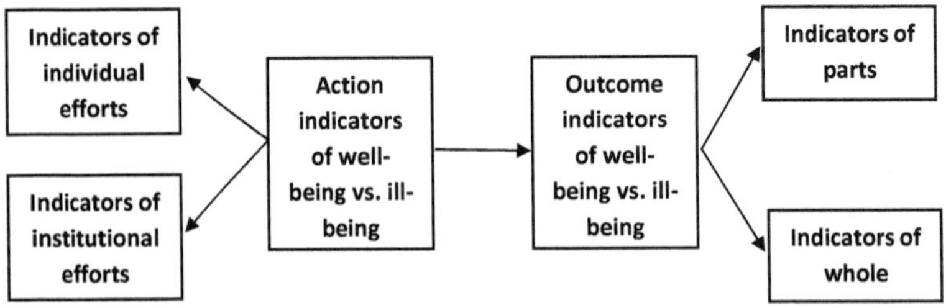

Fig. 6.1 Indicators of well-being versus ill-being embedded in outcome versus action indicators, which are further embedded…

(2004) used longitudinal survey data from the Household, Income, and Labour Dynamics in Australia Survey to demonstrate the same point—that well-being and ill-being are not opposite ends of the same continuum. Their study found that while past ill-being had a significant impact on current well-being the reverse relationship is not true, i.e., past well-being did not have a significant effect on current ill-being.

In *Human Suffering and Quality of Life*, Anderson (2014, p. 10) defined suffering as "perceived threat or damage to a sense of self," and "distress resulting from threat or damage to one's body or self-identity." This may include distress from threat or damage to the physical self as in physical suffering, and distress as in the psychological self as in mental suffering, as well as distress to social identity or social suffering. In Anderson's (2015, p. 4) edited book on *World Suffering and Quality of Life*, he made an all-encompassing distinction among all forms of human suffering: physical, mental, interpersonal, and social. My definition of *ill-being* is consistent with Anderson's definition of human suffering but it is broader in scope in the sense that it includes Anderson's four types of human suffering and beyond to encompass *meta-level concepts* of ill-being at the community and societal[1] levels. Anderson addresses human suffering at the community and societal levels in terms of *social suffering*. However, his definition of social suffering of communities and societies is based on individuals' experiences. I go beyond his definition of social suffering as reflected by the individual. Meta-constructs of ill-being apply equally to communities and societies at large in which the unit of analysis is not necessarily the individual. As such, the goal of this chapter is to make a clear distinction of indicators of well-being from indicators of ill-being at several levels of analyses, namely the individual level, the community level, and the societal level. Further, a distinction between outcome and action indicators is made. Outcome indicators reflect the desired end state, whereas action indicators reflect indicators of programs and policies designed to influence the outcome states. Such distinctions are important for policy-making (see Fig. 6.1).

[1] I make multiple references to "societal-level analysis" throughout the chapter. Societal in this context means country or state. To be distinguished from individual and community-level analyses.

Indicators of Well-Being and Ill-Being

Quality-of-life data tend to be *complementary in that some capture dimensions of quality of life that we would like to increase (enhancement of positive states—well-being), whereas others capture dimensions that we would like to decrease (reduction of negative states—ill-being).* That is, an effective quality-of-life narrative about individual, community, or country uses indicators and data that capture both positive and negative states of quality of life. For example, domains concerning functional status or human suffering reflect negative states that naturally should be reduced. When these indicators are used in a quality-of-life index, they tend to be counterbalanced with indicators that capture positive states. This issue is important because quality-of-life measures are designed to capture the comprehensive totality of life experiences, both positive and negative.

For example, Argyle (1996) argued that subjective well-being is determined by three factors: (1) happiness, (2) life satisfaction, and (3) absence of ill-being. He argued that subjective well-being cannot be experienced when people experience ill-being in the form of depression or anxiety. I (Sirgy 2011) also elaborated on the distinction between positive and negative states by equating this distinction with basic versus growth needs. That is, indicators reflecting positive states tend to focus on growth needs, whereas indicators focusing on negative states tend to reflect basic needs (Maslow 1954). Human development needs comprise a hierarchy of basic and growth needs. Health, safety, and economic needs are essentially basic needs (i.e., needs related to human survival). Social, esteem, actualization, knowledge, and aesthetics needs are growth needs (i.e., needs related to human flourishing). Basic needs are more pre-potent and salient than growth needs.

Hence, quality-of-life indicators should capture the full spectrum of human development, both well-being and ill-being as a snapshot and as a process. For the less-developed countries, capturing well-being in terms of basic needs (i.e., ill-being indicators capturing the negative states) is more important than focusing on growth needs (i.e., well-being indicators capturing the positive states). It is difficult to achieve growth needs without first attending to basic needs. Many quality-of-life scholars have argued this point. For example, Veenhoven (1988, 1991) made the distinction between basic need satisfaction and subjective well-being. People with higher income levels can easily satisfy their basic needs (food, housing, health) and therefore are more likely to focus on experiences that lead to higher levels of subjective well-being. Customarily, much of the research on poverty equates poverty with disease; high rate of infant mortality; low average life expectancy; malnutrition; hunger; and lack of access to water, education, knowledge, public and private resources, housing, clothes, and security. Similarly, the Human Development Index (HDI) is the average of three human development dimensions: living standard (measured through GDP per capita), health (measured in terms of life expectancy at birth), and education (calculated through adult literacy for one-third and the average years of school enrollment of adults above 25 years for the remaining two-thirds). These indicators reflect negative states in the sense that they focus on basic needs (i.e., ill-being), not well-being *per se*. Most indicators of children well-being reflect ill-being, not well-being. Examples include infant mortality rate (deaths between birth and age 1 per 1000 live births), under age 5 mortality (per 1000 live births), and children under age 5 who are underweight for their age (Land et al. 2015).

To achieve a high level of quality of life, people have to satisfy the full spectrum of their developmental needs—both basic needs (reducing ill-being) and growth needs (increasing well-being). Indicators capturing the full spectrum of needs satisfaction would allow for the assessment and monitoring of progress toward that end. Thus, quality-of-life indicators should capture both basic and growth needs satisfaction. Indicators related to basic needs (negative states or ill-being) may include environmental pollution, disease incidence, crime, housing, unemployment, poverty and homelessness, cost of living, community infrastructure, and illiteracy and lack of job skills. In contrast, indicators related to growth needs (positive states or well-being) include work productivity and income, consumption of no basic goods and services, leisure and recreational activities, professional development, community landscape, arts and cultural activities, intellectual activities, and spiritual activities.

Many indicators projects are developed with a special focus on growth needs (or well-being). For example, Lloyd and Auld (2002) and Michalos and Zumbo (2003) conducted an indicators project focused on leisure and its relationship to quality of life.

To appreciate the distinction between well-being and ill-being indicators, the reader has to become familiar with other distinctions among indicators given the fact in the context of how quality-of-life researchers use indicators to capture quality of life of individuals, communities, and countries. These distinctions include outcome versus action indicators. Within outcome indicators, quality-of-life researchers make distinctions between indicators capturing the state of well-being/ill-being as a whole versus its constituent parts. Conversely, within action indicators researchers have traditionally made distinctions between indicators reflecting individual efforts and indicators reflecting institutional efforts. These distinctions will be discussed further in the sections below.

Outcome Versus Action Indicators

When studying the well-being/ill-being of individuals, communities, and countries, quality-of-life scholars capture well-being and ill-being using a variety of indicators that are complementary to one another. These indicators can best be viewed in terms of *action (efforts)* and *outcomes (results)* indicators. Outcome indicators of well-being versus ill-being are traditionally expressed in terms of parts versus whole. Specifically, these outcome indicators can also be expressed in terms of parts versus whole. An outcome well-being indicator focusing on the "whole" means that the indicator is designed to capture quality of life in a holistic manner (e.g., personal happiness). The focus is on the totality of quality-of-life of an individual, community, or society at large. In contrast, "parts" indicators reflect specific elements that comprise the "whole." Customarily, quality-of-life researchers develop quality-of-life indices involving various dimensions of well-being and/or ill-being (e.g., education, health, income). Furthermore, outcome indicators of well-being and ill-being are usually expressed through subjective versus objective constructs. Subjective outcome indicators reflect the personal voice of those in the direct line of experience, with all the inherent personal biases and associated methodological inconsistencies in generalizing such perspectives to the target population. In contrast, objective outcome indicators are more impartial, such as changes in average years of life expectancy, in infant and child death rates, and in rates of criminal activities. Many of these data are collected and disseminated by official government agencies and bodies.

Action indicators describe broad-based forces operating in the microenvironments that influence the well-being and ill-being of people individually and collectively. For example, if a country that was funding prenatal care for pregnant women wanted to measure the overall effectiveness of its efforts on the well-being/ill-being of women, it could compare the dollar amount of the financial investment (action indicator) to both a subjective indicator (how well pregnant women felt they were treated by the prenatal care team) and an objective indicator (the number of live births). Such indicators include public and private investments in achieving particular outcomes; the creation of policies that encourage people and organizations to act in a particular way; and the varieties of physical, social, and technological infrastructures that promote societal investments in particular areas or processes.

Outcome Indicators

Outcome indicators are designed to *capture the state of well-being and ill-being of individuals, communities, and countries at large.* An example of an overall health outcome indicator is life expectancy, which many argue is a good indicator of overall health status. There are many other examples of outcome indicators from well-established indicator systems. The HDI is an example of an outcome indicator at the country level that has three dimensions (income, education, and health); hence, it captures each part of the whole, as well as the whole (the composite index captures the whole). These quality-of-life indicators at the societal level are objective indicators.

One can find many other large-scale national and international surveys directly related to subjective well-being or life satisfaction (Sirgy 2012). Common throughout these large-scale surveys and indices are indicators that seek to capture the subjective experience of the totality of life at the individual level (i.e., satisfaction with life overall) and satisfaction with life domains (satisfaction with material life, family life, social life, community life, cultural life, work life). Hundreds of studies have been conducted using these primary indicators of the human quality of life. Again, these indicators can be considered outcome indicators of well-being capturing the whole (at the individual level).

Quality-of-life researchers refer to the theoretical underpinning of this research as "bottom-up theory" (e.g., Diener 1984; Sirgy 2012), in that satisfaction from various life domains (namely, domain satisfaction) spills over to influence overall life satisfaction. Specifically, the theory argues that, in the minds of people, satisfaction experiences are organized in memory in a hierarchy varying from the abstract to the concrete. At the most abstract level, there is overall life satisfaction—a judgment that a person makes about his or her life overall varying from "very unhappy with my life" to "very happy with my life." Below the most abstract level is the domain satisfaction, which captures one's feelings about well-being in specific domains such as work life, social life, family life, spiritual life, financial life, community life, marital life, or love life. Bottom-up theory asserts that domain satisfaction influences life satisfaction moderated by domain salience. That is, if a person feels that work life is most important relative to other domains (e.g., social life, leisure life, and community life), then increases (or decreases) in work life satisfaction are likely to induce increases (or decreases) in overall life satisfaction. Those life domains that are less important are not likely to have much influence on overall life satisfaction. At the most concrete level of the satisfaction hierarchy are satisfaction memories involving concrete events (i.e., specific objects, people, and issues). Satisfaction at the most concrete level influences domain satisfaction. For example, a reprimand from the boss at work is likely to generate negative affect that can adversely influence one's overall sense of work well-being. The influential well-being research conducted using bottom-up theory includes the large-scale surveys of quality of life in the United States by Andrews and Withey (1976) and Campbell et al. (1975).

As such, domain satisfaction indicators are considered outcome indicators at the individual level that are subjective and focusing on the parts, not the whole. Hence, I make a distinction between indicators capturing parts (i.e., ill-being and well-being in specific life domains) versus whole (i.e., ill-being and well-being reflective of the whole individual). Furthermore, the vast majority of ill-being/well-being indicators systems that are well-established in the literature reflect individuals' experiences (see Chaaban et al. 2016 for a more recent review of these indicators systems) are based on individual scores of well-being and ill-being. Even at the community and societal levels, quality-of-life indices are developed by aggregating individual-level scores of ill-being and well-being (by life domain such as "health" or the individual as a whole such as "life overall"). This does not preclude the fact that other indicator systems are not based on individual experiences but community or society's experiences at an emergent level. For example, the economic well-being dimension of the UN Human Development Index is based on GDP per capita. This measure of economic well-being (or ill-being) captures the level of economic development of countries at an emergent level (i.e., the country as a whole, not based on the country's citizens' level of personal or household income). Hence, the reader should recognize that indicators of well-being and ill-being are based on indices involving experiences that can be captured at three levels of analysis: individual, community, and societal level. See Tables 6.1 and 6.2 for a complete list of outcome indicators broken down by well-being versus ill-being and parts versus whole at three levels of analyses, namely the individual level, community level, and societal level.

Table 6.1 Outcome indicators of ill-being at various levels of analysis

Indicators of ill-being	Domain	Individual level	Community level	Societal level
Parts (capturing specific dimensions of ill-being)	**Social ill-being**	Formative indicators of social ill-being of individuals (e.g., social isolation, social disengagement, social avoidance, social shyness, personal victimization)	Aggregation of individual level social ill-being scores of community members	Aggregation of individual or community level social ill-being scores for a given country
		Indicators of social ill-being of individuals (e.g., loneliness)	Indicators of social ill-being of communities (e.g., community strife, crime)	Indicators of social ill-being of countries (e.g., national strife, corruption)
	Leisure ill-being	Formative indicators of leisure ill-being of individuals (e.g., level of personal disengagement in leisure, sports, and recreational activities)	Aggregation of individual level leisure ill-being scores of community members	Aggregation of individual or community level leisure ill-being scores for a given country
		Indicators of leisure ill-being of individuals (e.g., personal boredom)	Indicators of leisure ill-being of communities (e.g., community's leisure deficit)	Indicators of leisure ill-being of countries (e.g., the country's leisure deficit)
	Work ill-being	Formative indicators of work-ill-being of individuals (e.g., job hopping, career deficit, lack of job-related skills, unemployment, work-related apathy, job burnout)	Aggregation of work ill-being scores of community members	Aggregation of individual or community level scores of work ill-being for a given country
		Indicators of work ill-being of individuals (e.g., work alienation)	Indicators of work ill-being of communities (e.g., level of unemployment in a given community, lack of job skills)	Indicators of work ill-being of countries (e.g., national unemployment rate)

(continued)

Table 6.1 (continued)

Indicators of ill-being	Domain	Individual level	Community level	Societal level
	Culture ill-being	Formative indicators of culture ill-being of individuals (e.g., lack of knowledge of culture-related topics such as history, music, and arts)	Aggregation of cultural ill-being scores of community members	Aggregation of individual or community level scores of culture ill-being for a given country
		Indicators of culture ill-being of individuals (e.g., cultural illiteracy)	Indicators of culture ill-being of communities (e.g., community cultural deficit, illiteracy)	Indicators of culture ill-being of countries (e.g., national ignorance)
	Spiritual ill-being	Formative indicators of spiritual ill-being of individuals (e.g., narcissistic behaviors, self-centeredness, antisocial behavior)	Aggregation of spiritual ill-being scores of community members	Aggregation of individual or community level scores of spiritual ill-being for a given country
		Indicators of spiritual ill-being of individuals (e.g., moral apathy)	Indicators of spiritual ill-being of communities (e.g., community decadence and lack of moral values)	Indicators of spiritual ill-being of countries (e.g., national decadence and lack of moral values)
	Financial well-being	Formative indicators of financial ill-being of individuals (e.g., income sufficiency, financial debt, poor credit rating, lack of personal savings for retirement, financial bankruptcy, lack of insurance protection—home, life, auto, basic material possessions, etc.)	Aggregation of financial ill-being scores of community members	Aggregation of individual or community level scores of financial ill-being for a given country
		Indicators of financial well-ill-being of individuals (e.g., poverty)	Indicators of financial ill-being of communities (e.g., level of poverty in a community)	Indicators of financial ill-being of countries (e.g., country level of poverty)

(continued)

Table 6.1 (continued)

Indicators of ill-being	Domain	Individual level	Community level	Societal level
	Shopping ill-being	Formative indicators of shopping ill-being of individuals (e.g., lack of personal access to shopping and acquisition of basic goods and services, amount of time and effort spent on shopping for basic goods and services daily)	Aggregation of shopping ill-being scores of community members	Aggregation of individual or community level scores of shopping ill-being for a given country
		Indicators of shopping ill-being of individuals (e.g., shopping exhaustion)	Indicators of shopping ill-being of communities (e.g., shopping deserts, "outshopping" for necessity goods)	Indicators of shopping ill-being of countries (e.g., country imports of necessity goods; humanitarian aid coming in to a country)
	Health ill-being	Formative indicators of health ill-being of individuals (e.g., disease incidence, physical frailty, disability, pain sensation, physical injury, psychopathology)	Aggregation of health ill-being scores of community members	Aggregation of individual or community level scores of health ill-being of a given country
		Indicators of health ill-being of individuals (e.g., self-ratings of personal health)	Indicators of health ill-being of communities (e.g., community health deficit)	Indicators of health ill-being of countries (e.g., country health deficit)

(continued)

Table 6.1 (continued)

Indicators of ill-being	Domain	Individual level	Community level	Societal level
	Environmental ill-being	Formative indicators of environmental ill-being of individuals (e.g., exposure to pollution at home—air, water, noise, and other toxins in the immediate neighborhood)	Aggregation of environmental ill-being scores of community members	Aggregation of individual or community level scores of environmental ill-being of a given country
		Indicators of environmental ill-being of individuals (e.g., dilapidated neighborhood)	Indicators of environmental ill-being of communities (e.g., measures of environmental pollution of an entire community, deterioration of community infrastructure, population density and over crowdedness)	Indicators of environmental ill-being of countries (e.g., country level of environmental pollution—air, water, land, noise, etc.; level of environmental degradation through deforestation)
	Residential ill-being	Formative indicators of residential ill-being of individuals (e.g., housing deficit, adequate shelter, neighborhood crime, personal victimization, racial/ethnic strife in the neighborhood, environmental toxins in home—interior and exterior)	Aggregation of residential ill-being scores of community members	Aggregation of individual or community level scores of residential ill-being of a given country
		Indicators of residential ill-being of individuals (e.g., dilapidated residential living)	Indicators of residential ill-being of communities (e.g., measures of homelessness, community housing deficits)	Indicators of residential ill-being of countries (e.g., country level of housing shortage)

(continued)

Table 6.1 (continued)

Indicators of ill-being	Domain	Individual level	Community level	Societal level
Whole (capturing ill-being holistically)	**Overall ill-being**	Indicators of personal ill-being (e.g., the suffering life, the tolerable life, life of subsistence)	Aggregation of personal ill-being scores of community members	Aggregation of individual or community level scores of overall ill-being of a given country
			Indicators of community ill-being (e.g., community disintegration and dysfunction)	Indicators of national ill-being (e.g., failed states, rogue states, failing states)

Notes:
Formative indicators are essentially constructs composed of several conceptual dimensions. For example, life satisfaction can be construed as a formative construct made up of satisfaction in various life domains (composite of satisfaction scores in family life, social life, work life, leisure life, cultural life, material life, etc.)
The community-level analysis signals not only a geographic community (i.e., community residents) but also other types of demographic groups (e.g., specific age group, specific gender group, specific marital status group, specific income group, and so on)
Societal-level analysis focuses on country-level indicators

Table 6.2 Outcome indicators of well-being at various levels of analysis

Indicators of well-being	Domain	Individual level	Community level	Societal level
Parts (capturing specific dimensions of well-being)	**Social well-being**	Formative indicators of social well-being of individuals (e.g., personal sociability and friendships, personal membership or affiliation with reference groups)	Aggregation of individual level social well-being scores of community members	Aggregation of individual or community level social well-being scores for a given country
		Indicators of social well-being of individuals (e.g., social capital of individuals)	Indicators of social well-being of communities (e.g., community cohesion, community esprit de corps, community solidarity)	Indicators of social well-being of countries (e.g., national identity and patriotism)

(continued)

Table 6.2 (continued)

Indicators of well-being	Domain	Individual level	Community level	Societal level
	Leisure well-being	Formative indicators of leisure well-being of individuals (e.g., level of personal engagement in leisure, sports, and recreational activities)	Aggregation of individual level leisure well-being scores of community members	Aggregation of individual or community level leisure well-being scores for a given country
		Indicators of leisure well-being of individuals (e.g., personal leisure capital)	Indicators of leisure well-being of communities (e.g., community's leisure capacity)	Indicators of leisure well-being of countries (e.g., the country's leisure capacity)
	Work well-being	Formative indicators of work-well-being of individuals (e.g., personal occupational status and prestige, personal educational attainment, personal engagement in professional development, personal engagement in intellectual activities)	Aggregation of work well-being scores of community members	Aggregation of individual or community level scores of work well-being for a given country
		Indicators of work well-being of individuals (e.g., work efficacy)	Indicators of work well-being of communities (e.g., work productivity of a given community)	Indicators of work well-being of countries (e.g., national productivity and work readiness)

(continued)

Table 6.2 (continued)

Indicators of well-being	Domain	Individual level	Community level	Societal level
	Culture well-being	Formative indicators of culture well-being of individuals (e.g., personal engagement in cultural activities and the arts)	Aggregation of cultural well-being scores of community members	Aggregation of individual or community level scores of culture well-being for a given country
		Indicators of culture well-being of individuals (e.g., personal "culturedeness")	Indicators of culture well-being of communities (e.g., community "culturedeness")	Indicators of culture well-being of countries (e.g., national "culturedness")
	Spiritual well-being	Formative indicators of spiritual well-being of individuals (e.g., personal engagement in spiritual and charitable activities)	Aggregation of spiritual well-being scores of community members	Aggregation ofindividual or community level scores of spiritual well-being for a given country
		Indicators of spiritual well-being of individuals (e.g., moral sensitivity)	Indicators of spiritual well-being of communities (e.g., community spirituality)	Indicators of spiritual well-being of countries (e.g., country spirituality)
	Financial well-being	Formative indicators of financial well-being of individuals (e.g., personal wealth)	Aggregation of financial well-being scores of community members	Aggregation of individual or community level scores of financial well-being for a given country
		Indicators of financial well-being of individuals (e.g., personal wealth and affluence)	Indicators of financial well-being of communities (e.g., community wealth and affluence)	Indicators of financial well-being of countries (e.g., country wealth and affluence)

(continued)

Table 6.2 (continued)

Indicators of well-being	Domain	Individual level	Community level	Societal level
	Shopping well-being	Formative indicators of shopping well-being of individuals (e.g., personal access to shopping and acquisition of discretionary goods and services)	Aggregation of shopping well-being scores of community members	Aggregation of individual or community level scores of shopping well-being for a given country
		Indicators of shopping well-being of individuals (e.g., affluent shopping)	Indicators of shopping well-being of communities (e.g., affluent community shopping)	Indicators of shopping well-being of countries (e.g., national shopping affluence)
	Health well-being	Formative indicators of health well-being of individuals (e.g., vigor, vitality, optimism, extraversion, self-esteem, conscientiousness)	Aggregation of health well-being scores of community members	Aggregation of individual or community level scores of health well-being for a given country
		Indicators of health well-being of individuals (e.g., personal longevity, successful aging, resilience)	Indicators of health well-being of communities (e.g., community health)	Indicators of health well-being of countries (e.g., national health and well-being)
	Environmental well-being	Formative indicators of environmental well-being of individuals (e.g., beauty and aesthetics of housing landscape—interior and exterior; neighborhood landscape, architecture and aesthetics of the environment at work)	Aggregation of environmental well-being scores of community members	Aggregation of individual or community level scores of environmental well-being for a given country

(continued)

Table 6.2 (continued)

Indicators of well-being	Domain	Individual level	Community level	Societal level
		Indicators of environmental well-being of individuals (e.g., sense of beauty of the environment at large)	Indicators of environmental well-being of communities (e.g., measures of beauty of neighborhood landscape)	Indicators of environmental well-being of countries (e.g., national measures of landscape aesthetics, national forests, wildlife preserves)
	Residential well-being	Formative indicators of residential well-being of individuals (e.g., housing aesthetics, neighborhood crime, personal victimization, racial/ethnic strife in the neighborhood, environmental toxins in home—interior and exterior)	Aggregation of residential well-being scores of community members	Aggregation of individual or community level scores of for a given country
		Indicators of residential well-being of individuals (e.g., quality residential living)	Indicators of residential well-being of communities (e.g., measures of community living)	Indicators of residential well-being of countries (e.g., national pride in relation to the country's housing infrastructure)
Whole (capturing well-being holistically)	**Overall well-being**	Indicators of personal well-being (e.g., personal happiness)	Aggregation of personal well-being scores of community members	Aggregation of individual or community level scores of overall ill-being of a given country
			Indicators of community well-being (e.g., community cohesion and growth)	Indicators of national well-being (e.g., national pride)

(continued)

Table 6.2 (continued)

Notes:
Formative indicators are essentially constructs composed of several conceptual dimensions. For example, life satisfaction can be construed as a formative construct made up of satisfaction in various life domains (composite of satisfaction scores in family life, social life, work life, leisure life, cultural life, material life, etc.)
The community-level analysis signals not only a geographic community (i.e., community residents) but also other types of demographic groups (e.g., specific age group, specific gender group, specific marital status group, specific income group, and so on)
Societal-level analysis focuses on country-level indicators

As shown in Tables 6.1 and 6.2, all outcome indicators are categorized in terms of life domains. These are social life, leisure life, work life, culture life, spiritual life, financial life, shopping life, health life, environmental life, and residential life. Table 6.1 shows indicators of ill-being across these life domains, whereas Table 6.2 focuses on indicators of well-being across the same domains. Domain indicators of both ill-being and well-being are considered "part" indicators, to be contrasted with "whole" indicators. Whole indicators of both ill-being and well-being capture the unit of analysis (individual, community, and country) holistically. In other words, whole indicators capture the phenomena of ill-being and well-being at an emergent level (i.e., a meta-level). In contrast, parts indicators are essentially formative constructs involving several dimensions.

Specifically and with respect to *social ill-being*, indicators can be identified at three levels of analysis, namely the individual level, the community level, and societal level. Individual level indicators of social ill-being focus on pain and suffering experienced as a result of social isolation, social disengagement, social avoidance, social shyness, and personal victimization. One can view the factors that can lead to social well-being at the individual level to be dimensions of social ill-being. Hence, a composite index can be developed that reflect the totality of social ill-being through a formative construct involving the aforementioned drivers. These drivers become the dimensions of the formative construct, and a composite score can reflect social ill-being accordingly. This composite index of social ill-being is to be contrasted with a meta version of the same construct such as loneliness (see Table 6.1). Loneliness can be argued to be a construct that captures social ill-being in a holistic sense (see Table 6.1). Furthermore, social ill-being can also be captured at both community and country levels. The reader should now turn to Table 6.2 and contrast indicators of social ill-being with social well-being. Social well-being at the individual level can be captured using a formative construct involving drivers of social well-being such as personal sociability and friendships, personal membership or affiliation with reference groups such as clubs, churches, sports teams, and so on. In contrast, indicators of social well-being (as a reflective, not a formative construct) can be captured in the form of "social capital," a construct that has gained much traction in quality-of-life studies.

At the community level, we can compute a social ill-being score for a given community by simply aggregating individual-level scores of social ill-being. The aggregation of individual-level scores at the community level can be either based on the formative construct of social ill-being (i.e., composite score reflective of several dimensions such as social isolation, social disengagement, social avoidance, social shyness, and personal victimization) or the reflective construct of social ill-being (e.g., loneliness) (see Table 6.1). Furthermore, a community-level score of social ill-being can be formulated based on a community-level construct of community social-ill-being (the focus here is on the community as a whole, not individuals who make up that community). An example of such community-level constructs may include community strife and community crime (see Table 6.1). Note that my definition of community is broad. It denotes residents of a specific geographic area (such as a neighborhood, town, or city) or it could be a specific demographic segment such as people over 60 years of age, of middle income people, or people who a specific disease such as diabetes. Now the reader should turn to Table 6.2 to contrast community indicators of social ill-being with social well-being. Constructs of social well-being that focus on the community as a whole (not the sum of its parts) can be captured in terms of "community cohesion," "community esprit de corps," or "community solidarity."

A similar formulation can be applied at the societal level. That is, one can develop an index of social ill-being of a specific country or state by aggregating individual level scores (those individuals considered residing within the focal state) or community level scores (those communities considered to be part of the focal state). In contrast, one can develop a country-level social ill-being index using a meta construct that reflects the characteristics of an emergent phenomenon such as national strife, national corruption, etc. (see Table 6.1). Table 6.2 shows indicators of social well-being at the societal level that can be contrasted with social ill-being. Meta-constructs of social well-being at the societal level can include concepts such as national identity, national patriotism, etc.

Table 6.1 shows my conception of ill-being indicators for all other domains: leisure ill-being, work ill-being, culture ill-being, spiritual ill-being, financial ill-being, shopping ill-being, health ill-being, environmental ill-being, and residential ill-being. Table 6.2 shows indicators of well-being corresponding to the same life domains. The logic I used to develop social ill-being and well-being indicators at the three levels of analysis (individual, community, and societal) equally applies to the development of ill-being and well-being indicators in the other domains. Furthermore, a comparable logic is used to characterize indicators of *overall* ill-being and well-being at the three levels of analysis (see "Whole/Capturing Ill-Being Holistically" in Table 6.1 and "Whole/Capturing Well-Being Holistically" in Table 6.2). That is, one can capture overall personal ill-being at the individual level through meta-indicators of personal ill-being with constructs such as the "suffering life," the "tolerable life," or the "life of subsistence." In contrast, overall personal well-being at the individual level can be captured using meta-indicators such as "personal happiness." Similarly, at the community level, one can capture overall community ill-being of a specific community using two approaches, namely the aggregation approach and the meta-construct approach. The aggregation approach involves aggregating scores of overall personal ill-being of individuals residing in the target community. The second approach (meta construct) involves the formulation of community-level constructs of community overall ill-being. Examples of such constructs may include "community disintegration," community dysfunction," "failing communities," etc. (see Table 6.1). Contrast these meta-indicators of social ill-being of a community with meta-indicators of social well-being: "community cohesion and growth" (see Table 6.2). At the societal level, the pertinent meta constructs may include "failed states," "rogue states," "failing states," etc. (see Table 6.1). The corresponding constructs of social well-being at the societal level may include "national pride" (see Table 6.2).

Action Indicators

Some well-being/ill-being indicators focus on factors that concurrently affect the objective *and* subjective states of the totality of life at the individual level. Such indicators, also called action indicators, are one step removed from outcomes. They are essentially factors in *the social, cultural, political, technological,* and *physical environments* that impact the quality of life of individuals who comprise a specific demographic segment (e.g., children, adolescents, young adults, mature adults, elderly) or a geographic segment (e.g., a specific neighborhood, community, state/province, or country). For example, consider health indicators as action indicators. Health outcomes (as captured by physical and mental health indicators) are affected by factors such as institutional and medical care activities and programs in a given city or town. Action health indicators related to institutional dynamics may include the number of primary care physicians per capita, the cost of health care, financial access to health care, and access to mental health services. Information about medical care may include data about immunization rates, early prenatal care, health education, and prevention and early treatment.

Now focus on action indicators that directly correspond to the outcome indicators of both ill-being and well-being highlighted in Tables 6.1 and 6.2. Focus specifically on action indicators related to health ill-being and well-being. At the most micro level, we have individual-level indicators of health ill-being such as disease incidence, physical frailty, disability, pain sensation, physical injury, and psychopathology. Action to reduce health well-being can be taken by individuals and institutions. Individual action (and their indicators) may involve physical exercise, regular medical checkups, eating right, avoiding stressful events, avoiding risky behaviors, meditation, among others. Quality-of-life researchers capture these individual efforts to reduce health ill-being using corresponding constructs and measuring instruments. In addition to individual efforts there are institutional efforts too. That is, action to reduce health ill-being can be initiated and managed by healthcare institutions (such as family medical clinics, specialty medical clinics, and hospitals), the insurance industry and health insurers, as well as a host of other institutions such as employers, government agencies overseeing aspects of health for different population groups (e.g., children, elderly, disabled, etc.), NGOs that promote a health agenda (e.g., immunization to reduce infant mortality), among others. At the community level, action indicators designed to reduce well-being are also directly related to a variety of institutions (government, business, and NGOs). Traditionally, quality-of-life researchers have focused on action indicators such as number of physicians per 1000 community residents and the number of hospitals per 50,000 people, These are examples of community indicators that reflect "action" to reduce health ill-being within a community. At the societal level, quality-of-life researchers tend to focus on economic resources devoted to healthcare. Allocation of resources seems to be a very common indicator of action taken to reduce health ill-being at the societal level.

In contrast, action indicators related to health well-being are very different from action indicators related to health ill-being. Consider outcome indicators of health well-being at the individual level may include personal longevity, successful aging, and resilience. Individual as well as institutional efforts are directed to increase personal longevity, successful aging, and resilience. Examples may include efforts to increase sociability given that much research has shown that such a state play an important role in these health well-being outcomes. One can also document institutional efforts designed to enhance personal longevity, successful aging, and resilience. For example, employers may have work-life balance programs that incentivize employees to "have a social life." They host social events, fund social travel, and provide time off work to allow employees to spend more time with their families and friends. These institutional programs can be documented as they reflect action indicators of health well-being. Action indicators that reflect resource expenditures related to preventative healthcare can be considered as action indicators of health well-being at the societal level. It is beyond the scope of this chapter to document all the action indicators at the three levels of analysis because they are so many and so varied.

Conclusion

I believe that the public policy implications to the indicator distinctions I made here are significant. First, the distinction between indicators of well-being and ill-being should guide public policy makers to consider both sets of indicators in policy formulation. In many instances, public policy officials focus on ill-being, not much on well-being. Making this distinction clear should prompt decision makers to realize that achieving a maximal level of quality of life of an individual, a community, or a country means that policies should address the entire spectrum of human development needs, both basic needs and growth needs *al la* Maslow. That is, public policy should be formulated to reduce ill-being (by meeting basic needs) and increase well-being (by meeting growth needs).

Second, the distinction between outcome and action indicators should prompt policy makers to examine both action and outcome indicators of well-being and ill-being. Action indicators are those that are proximal to programs and policies designed to impact well-being/ill-being outcomes. Public policy officials should also monitor the extent to which action indicators contribute to changes in outcome indicators. If changes in certain action indicators do not lead to anticipated changes in the corresponding outcome indicators then those policies related to the action indicators should be revisited.

Third, the distinction among the three levels of analysis (individual, community, and societal level) signals should inform indicators researchers that there is much overlap commonality between ill-being/well-being indicators at these three levels. That is, indicators of ill-being/well-being at the individual level can be applied to capture communities and states. However, it should be noted that there are emergent constructs that are truly distinct at higher levels of analysis (community and societal levels). Perhaps in many situations public policy at the community (or societal) level should be guided by indicators that are based on an emergent level rather than the individual level.

In sum, this chapter accomplished several goals. First, the chapter highlighted the concept of ill-being (or human suffering) to the quality-of-life research literature in juxtaposing indicators of ill-being with indicators of well-being. Second, the chapter brought to light the notion that human suffering can be construed not only at the individual level but also at the community and societal levels. Third, the chapter brought to the forefront the notion that ill-being indicators (as well as well-being indicators) are further distinguished in terms of outcome versus action. The public policy implications of this distinction is very important given that policies are based on action indicators with the hope that these policies would impact outcome indicators. Fourth, the chapter noted a further distinction between ill-being/well-being composite indices (designed to capture ill-being/well-being for target communities and states by aggregating individual-level scores of the target communities and states) and meta-level constructs of community and state ill-being/well-being. Fifth, the chapter emphasized the fact that the vast majority of indicators of ill-being and well-being can be classified in terms of life domains: social, leisure, work, culture, spiritual, financial, shopping, health, environment, and residential life. In contrast to domain-level constructs, ill-being and well-being can be captured holistically. As such, the chapter made the distinction between indicators capturing the "whole" of ill-being (and well-being) at the individual/community/societal levels and indicators that focus on "parts" or specific life domains.

References

Anderson, R. E. (2014). *Human suffering and quality of life: Conceptualizing stories and statistics*. Dordrecht: Springer.

Anderson, R. E. (2015). Implications of world suffering for human progress. In E. E. Anderson (Ed.), *World suffering and quality of life* (pp. 3–30). Dordrecht: Springer.

Andrews, F. M., & Withey, S. B. (1976). *Social indicators of well-being: Americans' perceptions of life quality*. New York: Plenum Press.

Argyle, M. (1996). Subjective well-being. In A. Offer (Ed.), *In pursuit of the quality of life* (pp. 18–45). New York: Oxford University Press.

Bradburn, N. M. (1969). *The structure of psychological well-being*. Chicago: Aldine.

Campbell, A., Converse, P. E., & Rodgers, W. L. (1975). *The quality of American life: Perceptions, evaluations, and satisfactions*. New York: Russell Sage Foundation.

Chaaban, J., Irani, A., & Khoury, A. (2016). The Composite Global Well-Being Index (CGWBI): A new multi-dimensional measure of human development. *Social Indicators Research, 129*, 465–487.

Diener, E. (1984). Subjective well-being. *Psychological Bulletin, 95*, 542–575.

Hagerty, M., Vogel, J., & Møeller, V. (Eds.). (2002). Assessing quality of life and living conditions: The state of the art. [Special issue]. *Social Indicators Research, 58*, 1–440.

Headey, B., Holmstrom, E., & Wearing, A. (1984). Well-being and ill-being: Different dimensions. *Social Indicators Research, 14*, 115–139.

Land, K. C., Lamb, V. L., & Fu, Q. (2015). Child well-being and child suffering. In E. E. Anderson (Ed.), *World suffering and quality of life* (pp. 173–186). Dordrecht: Springer.

Lee, W-S., & Oguzoglu, U. (2004). *Well-being and ill-being: A bivariate panel data analysis* (A discussion paper). http://papers.ssrn.com/sol3/papers.cfm?abstract_id=1029914

Lloyd, K. M., & Auld, C. J. (2002). The role of leisure in determining quality of life: Issues of content and measurement. *Social Indicators Research, 57*, 43–71.

Maslow, A. H. (1954). *Motivation and personality*. New York: Harper.

Michalos, A. C. (Ed.). (2014). *Encyclopedia of quality of life and well-being research*. Dordrecht: Springer.

Michalos, A. C., & Zumbo, B. D. (2003). Leisure activities, health and the quality of life. In A. C. Michalos (Ed.), *Essays on the quality of life* (pp. 217–238). Dordrecht: Kluwer Academic Publishers.

Sirgy, M. J. (2011). Theoretical perspectives guiding QOL indicator projects. *Social Indicators Research, 103*, 1–22.

Sirgy, M. J. (2012). *The psychology of quality of life: Hedonic well-being, life satisfaction, and eudaimonia* (2nd ed.). Dordrechet: Springer.

Veenhoven, R. (1988). The utility of happiness? *Social Indicators Research, 20*, 334–354.

Veenhoven, R. (1991). Is happiness relative? *Social Indicators Research, 24*, 1–34.

Chapter 7
Alleviating Mental Suffering in Rural Bangladesh: Evidence from a Survey of Three Villages

Muhammad Faress Bhuiyan

Introduction: Mental Suffering and Quality of Life

Economists have a long tradition of studying income per capita and economic growth (Malthus 1872; Solow 1956; Romer 1986; Acemoglu et al. 2000) but the investigation of subjective well-being measures is a relatively recent addition.[1] Easterlin (1974) pioneered the study of subjective well-being among economists when he pointed out that while the income per capita of the United States and Western Europe tripled over three decades following the Second World War, the average self-reported happiness did not increase. It saw the invention of "happiness economics." The discipline now recognizes that certain cognitive experiences (e.g., happiness, emotional state, feeling persecuted, etc.) are not only important quality of life constituents but are most effectively measured through self-reported responses.

One quality of life constituent highlighted in the 2013 World Happiness Report (Helliwell et al. 2013) is mental health. It is usually measured using responses to a series of questions about the responder's experienced emotional states. Often classified as negative or positive affect, these questions ask the respondents to report on a 3- to 10-point Cantril ladder, how often they felt certain emotions such as enjoyment, sadness, and anxiety yesterday. They are self-reported responses to the question of how often the respondent felt worried and depressed yesterday on a 5-point scale ranging from "not at all" to "all day." Negative affect can be thought of as a type

[1] The prominence of the former is primarily based on (a) the traditional assumption that income is an adequate proxy for quality of life and (b) objectively measured variables are superior to self-reported ones. Consequently, economists prefer using measures based on revealed preferences (i.e. voluntarily chosen actions) and objective criteria (such as per capita income) for conducting empirical analyses.

M.F. Bhuiyan (✉)
Faculty of Economics, Carleton College, 1 North College Street, Northfield, MN 55057, USA
e-mail: fbhuiyan@carleton.edu

R.E. Anderson (ed.), *Alleviating World Suffering*, Social Indicators Research Series 67, DOI 10.1007/978-3-319-51391-1_7

of mental suffering. Anderson (2015) classifies mental suffering as one of the three broad categories of suffering (the other two being physical and social suffering), defining it as a "distress perceived as originating in one's cognitive or affective self-identity." I study two types of mental suffering similar to what Kahneman and Deaton (2010) call the "blues affect." For the rest of the paper, I will refer to feeling depressed or worried as mental suffering or suffering. The term is not perfect since the two measures may also have social suffering components. For instance, an individual may be depressed because they feel relatively deprived in the presence of their neighbors' relative affluence. This is an example of social suffering i.e. suffering whose sources are social collectives and or social institutions (Anderson 2015).

The primary objective of this paper is to explore what policies are most likely to alleviate mental suffering in the context of rural communities in a developing country. To this end, I begin by analyzing data from a census of three contiguous villages in the Tangail district of Bangladesh to identify the statistically significant correlates of mental suffering. In particular, I examine how suffering is affected by demographic variables (age, gender, and marital status), human development variables (living standards, health, and education), and perceptions of economic position relative to different reference groups (neighbors and siblings). Based on this analyses, I am able to (a) identify which demographic group suffers most and hence should be targeted by policymakers, (b) ascertain whether current policies aimed at improving living standards, health, and education will also alleviate mental suffering, and (c) discover additional policies that can be adopted to affect the correlates in a way that will reduce suffering.

This chapter makes two additional contributions. First, it adds to the scant literature on the alleviation of mental suffering, particularly in the context of a developing country. Second, it explores the effect of economic position relative to different reference groups on suffering. The next section provides some context about Bangladesh, Tangail and the villages that are being studied here.

Quality of Life in Bangladesh: The Tangail Survey

On the heels of a decade of robust economic growth, an unprecedented expansion of the textile industry, and the proliferation of microfinance institutions, Bangladesh is transitioning from a low-income to a lower-middle-income country.[2] According to the 2015 Millennium Development Goals Progress Report, Bangladesh has been quite successful in achieving several milestones (e.g. reducing incidence of poverty, attaining gender parity in primary and secondary level education, etc.).

The spread of microfinance and the textile industry in rural and urban areas, respectively, has lead to a significant increase of female participation in market

[2] This is based on World Bank's classification of countries into four groups based on their per capita income – low-income, lower-middle income, upper-middle income, and high-income. Up until 2015, Bangladesh fell into the low-income category.

Table 7.1 Selected national indexes and Bangladesh's rank in the world

Dimension	Instrument	Source, Year	Rank
Income per capita	Gross domestic product (GDP) per capita (Atlas method)	World Bank, 2014	181/213
Human development index	A weighted average of a country's gross national product per capita, life expectancy at birth, mean years of schooling and expected years of schooling	United Nations, 2014	142/188
Corruption perception index	Perceived levels of corruption as determined by expert assessments and opinion surveys	Transparency International, 2014	145/174
Subjective life evaluation	Average of responses to a Cantril ladder question asking respondents to value their lives today on a scale of 0 ("worst possible life") to 10 ("best possible life")	World Happiness Report, 2015	109/158
Change in life evaluation	Change in Average Life Evaluation Between 2005–2007 to 2012–2014	World Happiness Report, 2015	46/125
Negative experience index	Fraction of respondents who report yes to four out of five questions about whether the respondent felt a lot of physical pain, worry, sadness, stress, and/or anger yesterday	Gallup, 2013	87/138

activities. Nonetheless, males are still considered the primary breadwinners and the society remains mostly patriarchal. Despite all the successes, Bangladesh continues to grapple with a high level of poverty, underemployment of youth, violations of women and children's rights, political instability, natural calamities (associated mainly with flooding and sea level rise), unplanned urbanization, widespread corruption, and a high population density. Low income, widespread poverty, and a general lack of government-sponsored safety nets make financial security and the future prospects of the youth a major source of worry for most households. Table 7.1 reports Bangladesh's rank in the world in terms of several socioeconomic and demographic national statistics. Compared to the country's rank in human development index, income per capita, and corruption, Bangladesh ranks much better in the level (and growth) of average life evaluation and the negative experience index. It is quite interesting that Bangladesh reports a lower negative experience index than the United States and is in the company of countries such as France and Germany. Figure 7.1 illustrates that the relatively good rank in average life evaluation of Bangladesh is accompanied by a downward trend in the negative experience index in recent years.

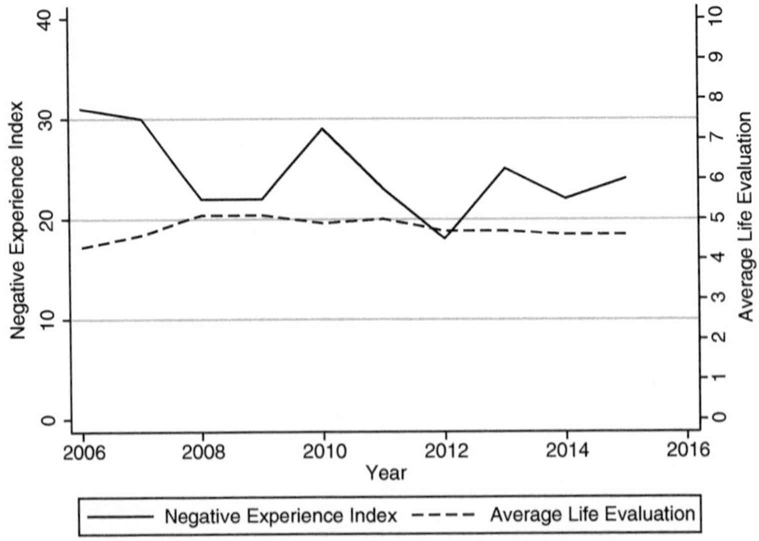

Fig. 7.1 Trends in negative experience index and average life evaluation for Bangladesh – Gallup World Poll data

The Tangail Survey: Context

Conducted during the summer of 2013, the Tangail Survey (TS) is a census of roughly 1400 households from three contiguous villages of the Tangail district of Dhaka Division, Bangladesh (Bhuiyan and Szulga 2013).[3] The respondents were mostly household heads with the exception of a few cases discussed in section "Living standards, health, and education". Table 7.2 provides some district level socioeconomic statistics of Tangail compared to Bangladesh as a whole. Overall, women in Tangail tend to marry early. There is no indication that the average living standard of Tangail is any different from the rest of the country. Educational achievements, measured by the fraction of children and adults getting primary and secondary education, is slightly higher than the national average. Child mortality is higher and maternal services are worse in Tangail. In the three villages covered by the TS, 58% of the households have electricity while the number of households that own or have access to a television is 29%. The former is very similar to the country average while the latter is lower. The difference in television ownership may be due to the fact that villages tend to have lower television ownership compared to urban areas.

There is no comprehensive district level data available on suffering with which to compare the TS data. The closest thing is the national survey conducted by Gallup. According to the Gallup survey, during 2012 and 2013 the percentage of Bangladeshis who noted experiencing "a lot of worry yesterday" is 23% and 34%,

[3] Roughly 1042 of the observations have non-missing values for the mental suffering variables.

Table 7.2 Socioeconomic and demographic characteristics of Tangail and Bangladesh

Variable	Tangail	Bangladesh
Total fertility rate	2.19	2.52
Proportion married among women aged 15–19 yrs.	51.5	41.3
Use of contraception (%)	63.3	62.6
Household with electricity (%)	59.5	54.7
Household owning a radio (%)	11.2	11.7
Household owning a television (%)	36.1	35.9
Households in the lowest wealth quintile (%)	20.5	21.7
Girls aged 12–15 who completed primary educ. (%)	69.1	67.2
Boys aged 12–15 who completed primary educ. (%)	61.4	57.3
Girls aged 15–19 who completed primary educ. (%)	81.1	80.5
Boys aged 15–19 who completed primary educ. (%)	73.8	72.0
Girls aged 18–24 who completed second. Educ. (%)	16.9	17.0
Boys aged 18–24 who completed second. Educ. (%)	26.8	22.7
Under 5 mortality	50	56
Antenatal care visits (at least once) (%)	69.4	71.2
Delivery attended by qualified doctor, nurse, midwife, paramedic, etc. (%)	25.2	26.5

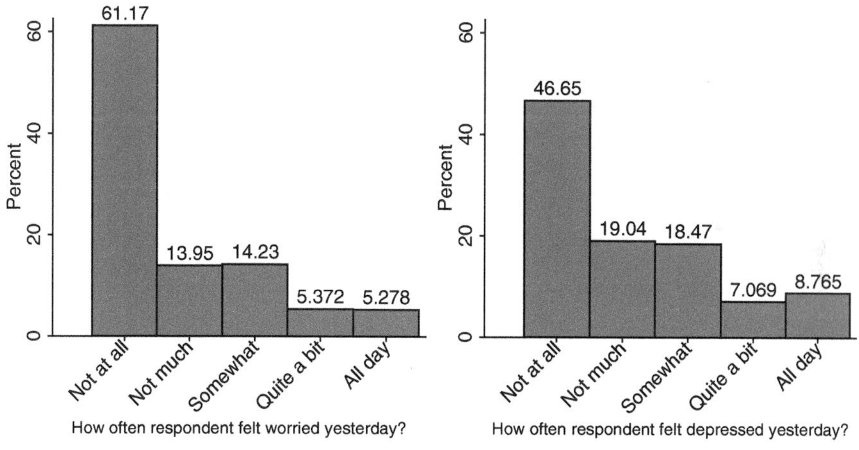

Fig. 7.2 Distribution of mental suffering in the Tangail survey

respectively. The TS asks a similar question on "how often the respondents felt worried yesterday."

Figure 7.2 shows the distribution of the responses. Roughly 18% of the respondents were worried "quite a bit" or more while 34% were at least "somewhat" worried. A quarter of the individuals reported feeling "somewhat" or "more" depressed yesterday. Conditional on feeling depressed, roughly 80% of the respondents show qualitatively a similar experience of feeling worried. For instance, 81% of all respondents who reported feeling "somewhat" depressed yesterday also reported feeling “somewhat” worried yesterday. The reverse conditional relationship is less predictive. Overall, the respondents suffer from feeling worried less than feeling depressed.

Correlates of Mental Suffering

Before addressing the question of how to best alleviate mental suffering, it is important to identify the statistically significant correlates of mental suffering. The findings in this section will inform the policy recommendations in sections “Discussion” and “Policy implications and future research”. Although a substantial number of studies explore the correlates of life satisfaction (e.g. Clark and Oswald 1996), mental suffering remains relatively understudied in economics. There is some evidence that the correlates of life satisfaction and suffering are different (e.g. Kahneman and Deaton 2010). In this section, I analyze three groups of potential correlates of mental suffering.

The first group includes demographic variables such as age, gender, and marital status. Using 355,334 interviews in the United States, Stone et al. (2010) find that individuals’ self-reported level of worry stays elevated between the ages of 18 and 50 years before falling, while sadness remains mostly flat with a very slight inverted U-shape. The authors speculate that the fall in worry and sadness after 50 years is “generally consistent with Baltes’ theory of increased “wisdom” and emotional intelligence with age (at least through middle age), wherein decreased negative affective states could be a result of increasing wisdom, and with Carstensen *et al.*’s socioemotional selectivity theory, wherein older people have an increased ability to self-regulate their emotions and view their situations positively.”[4] They also find no difference in suffering among males and females. Based on these studies, policies aimed at alleviating mental suffering in the United States should target individuals between the ages of 18 and 50 without making any gender-wise distinctions.

The second group of correlates includes arguably the three most important dimensions of human development as operationalized by policymakers—living standards, health, and educational attainment.[5] Living standards are usually measured by income or consumption at a household level. There is extensive literature on the effect of higher income on life satisfaction. One camp spearheaded by Easterlin (1974) provides evidence that at a national level, higher income does not buy happiness. On the other hand, several recent studies (e.g. Stevenson and Wolfers 2008, 2013) find that not only does higher income improve life satisfaction but also

---

[4]As far as life satisfaction goes there is some evidence of a U-shaped relationship with age. In particular, life satisfaction reaches a minimum between 35 and 45 years (Lelkes 2006; Blanchflower and Oswald 2008; Bhuiyan and Szulga 2017). However, Frijters and Beatton (2012) do not find this relationship to be robust while Mroczek and Spiro (2005) find evidence of an opposite relationship.

[5]These three dimensions form the basis of United Nation’s Human Development Index.

there is no satiation point for this effect. Neither do Kahneman and Deaton (2010) find evidence of a satiation point for life satisfaction in the United States. However, they find a cut-off income of about $75,000 after which sadness and worry is not reduced any further. They also find that education is not a significant correlate while better health significantly reduces mental suffering. Thus, in the United States improving living standards will alleviate mental suffering up to a point while improving physical health will reduce worry and depression considerably.

The third group of correlates is based on relative income measures. There are numerous empirical studies that find preferences to be interdependent and affecting life satisfaction (McGuire et al. 1993; Van de Stadt et al. 1985; Blanchflower and Oswald 2004; Clark and Oswald 1996; Stutzer 2004; Easterlin 1995; Easterlin 2001; Duncan 1975; Diener et al. 1999; Dynan and Ravina 2007; Bhuiyan 2012; Luttmer 2004; and Solnick and Hemenway 1998). However, there is not much work, if any, done on the effect of relative economic position on mental suffering. Higher relative economic position is often found to increase life satisfaction when the reference group is defined as some combination of those with similar age, gender, educational qualifications, residential address, etc. These empirical relationships are usually viewed by the literature as evidence for the theories of interdependent preferences driven by envy, status concerns, evolutionary needs, or an aspiration to keep up with the reference group (Duesenberry 1949; Frank 1985a,b; Rayo and Becker 2007). Some studies also find the reverse relationship whereby individuals enjoy increases in the economic well-being of their reference groups such as neighbors (Hirschman and Rothschild 1973; Senik 2004; Kingdon and Knight 2007).[6]

It should be noted that most of the studies on suffering and even life satisfaction discussed above are based on developed countries and thus it is not clear if the findings from these nations will hold in the context of a developing country like Bangladesh. The next four sections explore the relationship between suffering and the three groups of correlates in the TS.

Gender, Age, and Marital Status

Due to missing data, I used roughly 1042 observations out of the possible 1430 observations available in the TS. By design 94% of the respondents in the TS are household heads. The remaining 6% are spouses of the household heads.[7] Figure 7.3

---

[6] This type of relationship may be attributed to altruistic feelings towards one's neighbors (Kingdon and Knight 2007) and the "tunnel effect" (Hirschman and Rothschild 1973; Senik 2004). Tunnel effect here refers to individuals using the current change in the economic fortune of some relevant reference groups (e.g. neighbors) as a predictor of their own future economic conditions.

[7] Only two of the respondents are the household head's brothers. After repeated attempts if it was not possible to interview the household head, the TS interviewers were instructed to survey the spouse of the respondent.

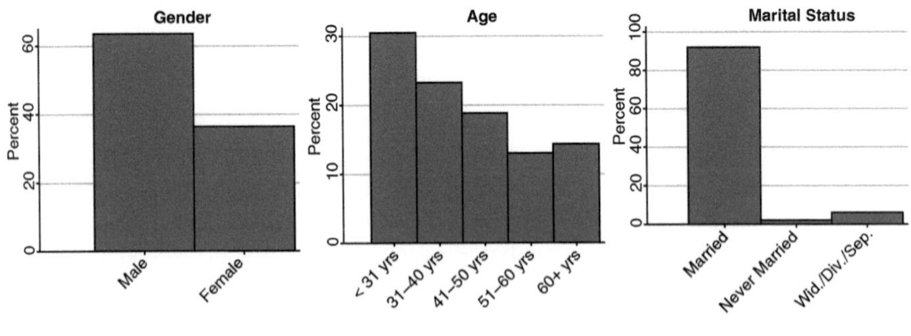

Fig. 7.3 Tangail survey—distribution of demographic variables

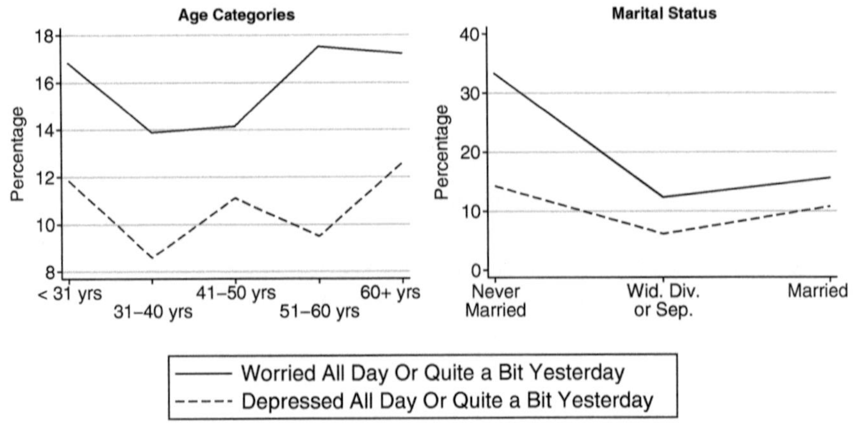

Fig. 7.4 Correlates of mental suffering: demographic variables in Tangail survey

shows the distribution of some demographic characteristics of the respondents. The majority of respondents are married (92%) with a mean age of 43 years.

I found no obvious gender-wise trend with respect to how frequently individuals worry. Focusing on the fraction of respondents who did not worry much or did not worry at all (67% of males to 63% of females), males suffered slightly less. However, if the fraction of respondents who worried quite a bit or more is considered, females do slightly better (a difference of less than 1%). In terms of feeling depressed, males are better off although the difference is mostly driven by those who reported not feeling depressed much or at all. The lack of a significant relationship between gender and suffering is similar to that reported by Stone et al. (2010). There is a slight increase in the fraction of respondents feeling worried all day for the age group 51 to 60 years (Fig. 7.4).[8] Those aged 31 to 40 years reported the least amount of worry

[8] Note that Fig. 7.4 and later Figs. 7.5 and 7.7 illustrate the percentage of individuals who report feeling worried/depressed "all day" or "quite a bit" yesterday. The other three categories that individual reported are "somewhat," "not much," and "not at all." This grouping of categories used in the aforementioned figures of sections "Gender, age, and marital status", "Living standards, health,

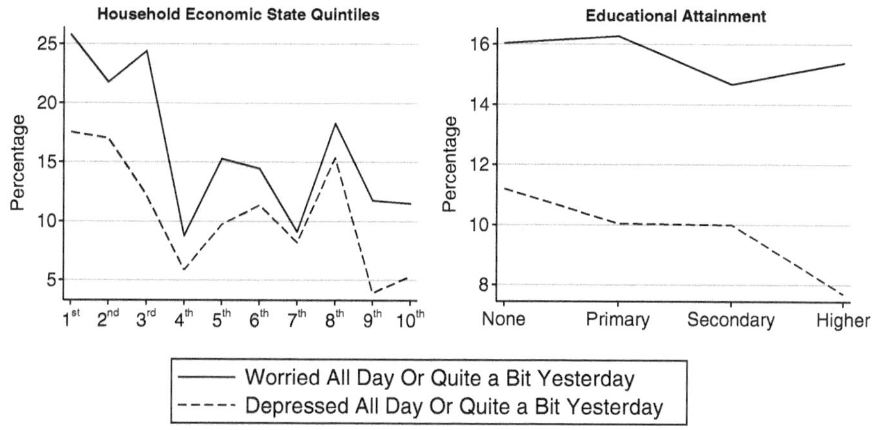

Fig. 7.5 Correlates of Mental Suffering: Living Standards and Education

or feeling depressed all day. Overall, respondents' age and suffering does not seem to be related. The absence of a relationship between age and feeling depressed matches the findings of Stone et al. (2010). There was, however, no indication of a fall in the level of worry for individuals after reaching a particular age.

Individuals who have never been married reported being more depressed and worried than those who are married, divorced, widowed or separated. It is important to note that these singles constitute about 2% of those surveyed (21 out of 1042 individuals). Of these 21 individuals, only 6 individuals are over the age of 30 years. Culturally, it is very odd for individuals to remain unmarried at this age. Also, these individuals are all household heads. This implies for some reason or other, 15 unmarried individuals under the age of 30 years are household heads. Becoming the household head at such an early age is not very usual in a setting where extended families are the norm and the average age of household heads is 43 years. Hence, while the single household heads seemed to be the most worried and depressed, this trend was based on a small fraction of individuals who are culturally playing the unexpected role of being a household head. Being married did not seem to uniformly increase or decrease suffering compared to being widowed, divorced, or separated.

and education", and "Relative economic position: siblings and neighbors" are for expositional convenience. The multivariate analysis that follows (section "Formal multivariate modeling") exploits the variation from all five categories of these variables.

Living Standards, Health, and Education

Measuring household income or consumption accurately in developing countries is difficult. Monthly consumption and income data in the TS are very noisy and unreliable. Hence, I employed principal-component factor analysis with orthogonal varimax rotation to generate a composite index of living standards from the more reliable objective measures of living conditions, household assets, and landholdings. Four of the eight components are binary variables that record whether the household owns a cell phone, television, refrigerator and land. The other four variables are (a) the residence construction material (non-brick/concrete, some brick-concrete, and only brick-concrete), (b) the number of rooms in the household, (c) whether the household has electricity and (d) whether the household has any international migrants.[9] The predicted composite index, the household economic state, was then normalized between 0 and 100.

I used information on whether the "respondent was seriously ill last year or not" as a measure of physical health. About one-fifth of the respondents reported being seriously ill last year. Most of the respondents have very little to no education. I categorized educational achievements into four groups: no education, primary education, secondary education and higher than secondary education. Sixty-two percent of the respondents have no education while 20%, 14% and 4% have primary, secondary and higher than secondary education, respectively.

Twenty-four percent of the individuals reporting a serious illness last year report feeling worried quite a bit or more compared to 13% of those who were not ill. Illness also tends to increase feeling depressed from 10% to 14%. It seemed physical suffering increases mental suffering. Based on the definition of household economic state, respondents living in richer households tend to suffer less. The trend is a bit choppy; nonetheless, when comparing the poorest to the richest households, the latter enjoys less depressive feelings. The relationship between household economic state and suffering became less pronounced for those enjoying a higher living standard. The relationship between educational achievements and suffering did not seem to follow a meaningful trend. Thus, in terms of alleviating mental suffering, improving physical health amenities should provide the most bang for the buck. Large increases in living standards are necessary to alleviate feelings of depression and worry.

Relative Economic Position: Siblings and Neighbors

The TS includes several questions that ask the respondents to report how their financial condition compares to different reference groups on a five-point scale of "much lower," "lower," "same," "higher," and "much higher." I used responses associated

[9] Factor analysis indicates that there is only one underlying factor with an eigenvalue greater than 1 explaining about 37% of the total variance of these eight factors. All eight components are positively correlated with the composite index with household type, number of rooms, ownership of television and ownership of fridge being the most important components.

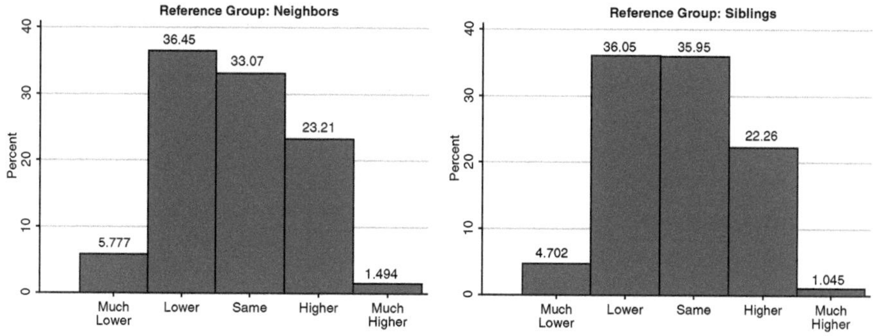

Fig. 7.6 Tangail survey – distribution of perceptions of relative economic position

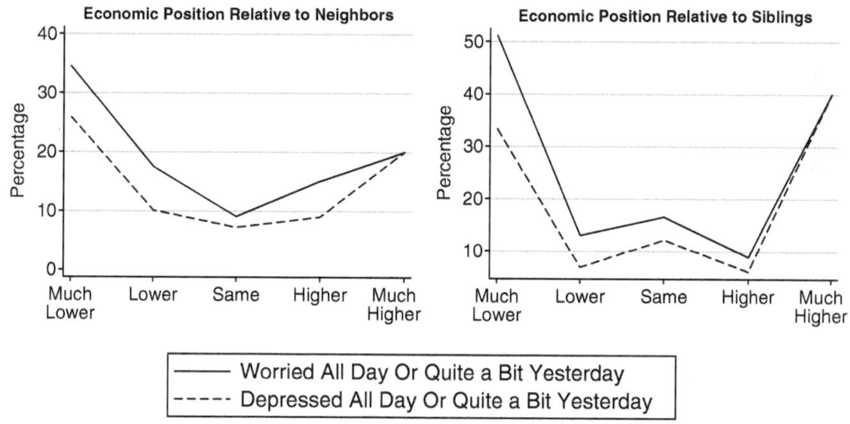

Fig. 7.7 Correlates of mental suffering: perceptions of relative economic position – Tangail survey

with two reference groups of neighbors and siblings. Figure 7.6 shows the distribution of the responses. These perception measures of relative economic position are similar to those used by Mayraz et al. (2009). The relationship between relative position and suffering was quite strong (Fig. 7.7).

In particular, there is a U-shaped relationship between suffering and economic position relative to neighbors and siblings. Those who are doing much better or much worse financially compared to their siblings or neighbors tend to feel more worried and depressed. A roughly similar relationship holds for economic position relative to neighbors.[10] This is a very interesting result because it indicates the

[10] Due to lack of observations and potential selection bias issues, I am not presenting the results associated with relative economic state compared to others in the same profession. The lack of observations for this variable may be attributed to the fact that a number of individuals were not employed and hence had no profession-based reference group to compare to. For those interested in the trends based on the smaller sample, suffering seems to generally decrease with higher relative economic position compared to colleagues although there is some evidence of a U-shaped relationship as well.

possibility that making monetary transfers from the rich to the poor may alleviate suffering for both. It is analogous to reducing inequality in the society. I discuss this result in more details in sections "Discussion" and "Policy implications and future research".

Formal Multivariate Modeling

In this section, I present results from ordered logit regressions to check for the statistical significance and robustness of the trends discussed in the previous three sections. Ordered logit is a type of discrete response regression model that is used to analyze categorical dependent variables that have a natural ordering. Since the measures of suffering used here are categorical and ordered, the ordered logit is an appropriate model for carrying out multivariate analyses.[11]

The ethnic, religious, and cultural homogeneity of the respondents in the TS sample is expected to reduce omitted variable biases and econometric complications. Additionally, the TS provides information not only on mental suffering but also on perceptions of economic position compared to different reference groups. For each type of suffering (feeling depressed or worried), I ran five separate ordered logits. The first model, the baseline model, in Table 7.3 presents ordered logit estimates from regressing "feeling worried" on marital status, age, gender, logarithm of household economic state, education, an indicator of whether the respondent was seriously ill within the past year, and village level dummies.

The second and third regressions are identical to the baseline model except relative economic position compared to neighbors was introduced using a linear and a quadratic functional specification, respectively. The fourth and fifth regressions are similar to the second and third ones, but the siblings-based measure of relative economic position was used instead of the neighbor-based measure. Table 7.4 presents ordered logit estimates similar to those in Table 7.3 but uses "feeling depressed" as the dependent variable. Robust standard errors clustered by interviewers and villages were used for all the regressions.

The numbers of correlates that are statistically significant are strikingly low. For instance, household economic state fails to be a statistically significant predictor of suffering in all the regression specifications. Relative economic position and physical health are the only variables that are consistently statistically significant. Better physical health alleviates both types of suffering. The relationship between each of the two types of relative economic position and feeling depressed or worried follows a U-shape i.e. individuals with a lower and higher relative economic position tend to feel more depressed.

[11] For a discussion of ordered logits and discrete response models consult Wooldridge (chapter IV, 2010).

Table 7.3 Ordered logit estimates – correlates of feeling worried yesterday

		Including relative economic position to the baseline model			
Regression specification	Baseline model	Neighbor (Linear)	Neighbor (Quadratic)	Sibling (Linear)	Sibling (Quadratic)
Logarithm of household economic state	0.902	0.938	0.945	0.954	0.951
	(0.139)	(0.384)	(0.440)	(0.527)	(0.494)
Rel. Economic position: neighbor		0.864*	0.267***		
		(0.056)	(0.001)		
Rel. Economic position: neighbor squared			1.229***		
			(0.004)		
Rel. Economic position: sibling				0.844**	0.230***
				(0.022)	(0.001)
Rel. Economic position: sibling squared					1.260***
					(0.002)
Seriously ill (last year)	1.689***	1.592***	1.593***	1.581***	1.508**
	(0.001)	(0.004)	(0.004)	(0.006)	(0.014)
Never married	2.943**	2.607*	2.713*	1.480	1.540
	(0.049)	(0.076)	(0.058)	(0.512)	(0.470)
Divorced, widowed, or separated	0.902	0.898	0.899	1.010	0.999
	(0.673)	(0.688)	(0.696)	(0.973)	(0.998)
Female	1.217	1.230	1.249	1.157	1.208
	(0.144)	(0.140)	(0.114)	(0.299)	(0.184)
Age	1.045**	1.051***	1.056***	1.035*	1.040**
	(0.016)	(0.009)	(0.004)	(0.075)	(0.037)
Age squared	1.000**	1.000**	1.000***	1.000	1.000*
	(0.028)	(0.020)	(0.008)	(0.149)	(0.073)
Education: some/ completed Primary	1.182	1.138	1.183	1.066	1.086
	(0.267)	(0.413)	(0.288)	(0.693)	(0.607)
Education: some/ completed secondary	1.033	0.980	0.991	1.011	0.987
	(0.860)	(0.916)	(0.960)	(0.955)	(0.946)
Education: higher than secondary	0.925	0.984	0.974	0.792	0.779
	(0.829)	(0.965)	(0.943)	(0.553)	(0.520)
Observations	1042	985	985	940	940

Note: The reported coefficients are odds ratios. Robust p-values in parentheses. *** p<0.01, ** p<0.05, * p<0.1

Village fixed effect dummies included in all regressions. Standard errors are robust and clustered by village and interviewers. The base groups for age, marital status, gender, and education are 31–40 years, married, males, and no education, respectively. The dependent variable is a response to the question "how often you felt worried yesterday?" and is measured using the 5-point scale: 1 – "Not At All", 2 – "Not Much", 3 – "Somewhat". 4 – "Quite a Bit", 5 – "All day"

Table 7.4 Ordered logit estimates – correlates of feeling depressed yesterday

Regression specification	Baseline model	Including relative economic position to the baseline model: Neighbor (Linear)	Neighbor (Quadratic)	Sibling (Linear)	Sibling (Quadratic)
Logarithm of household economic state	0.931	0.972	0.979	0.932	0.932
	(0.329)	(0.713)	(0.781)	(0.369)	(0.373)
Rel. Economic position: neighbor		0.903	0.156***		
		(0.210)	(0.000)		
Rel. Economic position: neighbor squared			1.364***		
			(0.000)		
Rel. Economic position: sibling				0.893	0.203***
				(0.170)	(0.000)
Rel. Economic position: sibling squared					1.302***
					(0.001)
Seriously Ill (last year)	1.555***	1.497**	1.491**	1.514**	1.442**
	(0.004)	(0.011)	(0.013)	(0.011)	(0.026)
Never married	2.043	1.807	1.864	0.987	1.007
	(0.116)	(0.181)	(0.150)	(0.981)	(0.990)
Divorced, widowed, or separated	0.972	0.915	0.932	1.037	1.033
	(0.909)	(0.741)	(0.800)	(0.899)	(0.912)
Female	1.107	1.158	1.184	1.022	1.067
	(0.471)	(0.319)	(0.260)	(0.883)	(0.667)
Age	1.033*	1.040*	1.045**	1.030	1.036*
	(0.096)	(0.050)	(0.029)	(0.150)	(0.086)
Age squared	1.000*	1.000**	1.000**	1.000	1.000
	(0.079)	(0.045)	(0.024)	(0.200)	(0.104)
Education: some/completed primary	0.970	0.942	0.993	0.926	0.941
	(0.846)	(0.720)	(0.964)	(0.655)	(0.718)
Education: come/ completed secondary	0.837	0.749	0.734	0.821	0.772
	(0.419)	(0.211)	(0.180)	(0.404)	(0.275)
Education: higher than secondary	1.024	1.107	1.105	1.023	0.985
	(0.943)	(0.760)	(0.776)	(0.950)	(0.967)
Observations	1042	985	985	940	940

Note: The reported coefficients are odds ratios. Robust p-values in parentheses. *** p<0.01, ** p<0.05, * p<0.1

Village fixed effect dummies included in all regressions. Standard errors are robust and clustered by village and interviewers. The base groups for age, marital status, gender, and education are 31–40 years, married, males, and no education, respectively. The dependent variable is a response to the question "how often you felt depressed yesterday?" and is measured using the 5-point scale: 1 – "Not At All," 2 – "Not Much," 3 – "Somewhat," 4 – "Quite a Bit," 5 – "All day"

Marital status and age are the only other correlates that are statistically significant in at least a few of the regressions. There is some indication that individuals who have never been married worry more compared to married individuals. However, this is statistically significant at a 5% significance level in only one of the five regressions with feeling worried as the dependent variable. It fails to be significant when the dependent variable is feeling depressed. Age exhibits a statistically significant but slightly inverted U-shaped relationship with feeling worried in some of the regressions. Middle-aged individuals around 50 years of age tend to worry the most. A similar trend holds for age and feeling depressed. However, it is mostly not statistically significant at a 5% significance level.

Robustness Checks, Limitations, and Extreme Suffering

The findings in the previous section are robust to the inclusion of a number of other controls, functional transformation of the correlates, and to different types of regression models. The primary results did not change if least squares or ordered probits were used instead of ordered logits (Wooldridge 2010). I checked for the sensitivity of the results to different functional transformations of age, relative economic state, and household economic state. Running separate regressions for the three villages reduced the statistical significance of the correlates without changing the main results.

The results are robust to including household economic state without taking the natural log or introducing it in the quintile form. Including age as a categorical variable by defining cohort dummies (e.g. <30 years, 30–49 years, 50–59 years, etc.) made age an insignificant variable. I tried a number of ways of defining the cohort dummies and choosing different base groups (to exclude in the regressions) but the limited statistical significance of age is replaced by no statistical significance. Introducing the 5-point scale relative economic state variable as four binary dummy variables did not change the findings in a meaningful way.

I repeated the analyses by including a number of additional controls one at a time. These controls included variables indicating whether the household had any microfinance members, if the household had an international or domestic migrant, the number of children under the age of 5 living in the household, and the employment status of the respondent (classified as employed, unemployed or self-employed). None of these variables were statistically significant, and the main results in Tables 7.3 and 7.4 were robust to the inclusion of these controls. One control that was statistically significant in a few regressions when feeling worried is the dependent variable is self-reported level of religiosity with the more religious worrying more. It had no statistically significant affect on feeling depressed.

It is possible that the lack of statistical significance may be due to multicolinearity between the various regressors. However, the variance inflation factor for all regressors in the different specification of Tables 7.3 and 7.4 were below 2, with the exception of the quadratic variables (e.g., age and age-squared).[12] Thus, lack of significance could be ruled out as stemming from multicolinearity. However, as is the case with most analyses, it is difficult to rule out omitted variable bias. Also, the findings apply to household heads. It is possible that for the general population in these villages, the inclusion of non-household head members in the sample would change the results.

To check and see if the statistically significant correlates of extreme worry and depression are similar to those of general worry and depression, I recoded the 5-point scale feeling worried and depressed variable into a binary variable. Extreme worry was thus coded as 1 if the respondent felt worried "all day" or "quite a bit" yesterday, and 0 otherwise. Similarly, a binary measure of extreme depression was constructed. Using these extreme measures of depression and worry as the dependent variable, I re-ran the analyses in Table 7.3 and 7.4.[13] The results did not change much except the physical illness variable stopped being a statistically significant predictor of depression. The relative income measures continued exhibiting a U-shaped relationship with the extreme measures of worry and depression.

Discussion

Based on the results of the exploratory empirical analyses presented in section "Correlates of Mental Suffering", there are several main findings. First, the unhealthy, middle-aged, and the unmarried suffer the most among household heads. Thus, policies aimed at alleviating mental suffering should target these individuals. There seems to be no need to make any distinction based on gender or level of education achieved. The findings that education and gender does not affect suffering while physical health does, corroborate the findings of similar studies conducted in developed countries (Kahneman and Deaton 2010; Stone et al. 2010). It is surprising that household economic state does not affect suffering.[14] Satiation can most certainly be ruled out here since the living standards of the sampled households are very low (the average monthly expenditure is roughly $100).

Second, older individuals tend to suffer more in developing countries compared with those in developed countries, and hence require more attention. The drop in worry for individuals reaching the age of 50 found by Stone et al. (2010) is not as pronounced or statistically significant in the TS. There are two possible contextual forces at play here. On one hand, since retirement benefits such as pension are mostly absent in rural Bangladesh, older individuals tend to become financial liabilities for the families they live with as they age. They also face a considerable amount of uncertainty with respect to future income. Such a marginalized position within the

[12] This is not surprising.

[13] This time I ran logit regressions instead of ordered logits since the dependent variable is binary.

[14] Multicolinearity with the controls used can be ruled out since the variance inflation factor of the household economic state variable is less than 2. I also checked for a quadratic relationship.

household and uncertainty of their economic future is expected to increase suffering thus countering the wisdom and emotional experience channel mentioned earlier. However, the respondents of the TS are household heads, which implies that these older individuals hold a certain amount of authority within the household. The financial insecurity for older individuals is expected to be less severe in the context of developed countries. This may explain why there is not as pronounced a drop in suffering after the age of 50 in the TS dataset when compared to the United States. If the respondents were not predominantly household heads, the suffering of the older individuals may have been higher.[15] Thus, in the context of developing countries relative to developed countries, effective strategies for alleviating mental suffering should target older individuals, i.e. those over the age of 50.

Third, a very small fraction of the variation in individuals feeling worried or depressed can be explained by the correlates used here. The pseudo r-squared, a measure of goodness-of-fit, is no more than 0.04. This implies about 4 percent of the variation of the dependent variables (feeling depressed or worried) from its mean value can be explained by the correlates explored here. Changing the dependent variable to life satisfaction in the TS analyses increases the pseudo r-squared to about 11 percent. There are multiple potential reasons for such a low goodness of fit measure. It may be the case that the dependent variables used here are very noisy. Note that the question asks individuals about how they felt "yesterday" which is different than the typical question about life satisfaction that asks individuals to note "in general" how satisfied they are with their life. Kahneman and Krueger (2006) propose better measures of suffering, such as using day reconstruction methods, that are less likely to suffer from temporal cognitive biases and noise. However, their criticism is also levied against the aforementioned measure of life satisfaction. Another possibility is that the regressors in the TS suffer from too much measurement errors. While it is difficult to argue that the data used here do not have measurement errors, it does not explain the difference in the goodness-of-fit between regressions using life satisfaction and suffering as the dependent variable. Thus, much more research needs to be conducted on mental suffering to identify other channels and sources that may be exploited to alleviate suffering.

The most interesting finding here is that relative economic state affects mental suffering. In particular, the U-shaped relationship between relative economic position (for neighbors and siblings) and suffering is quite remarkable. Higher reported suffering for those whose perceived relative economic position is much lower than their siblings, neighbors and colleagues can be explained by theories of envy and relative deprivation. However, it is not clear why individuals who perceive themselves to be doing better than their siblings or neighbors tend to worry and feel depressed more often. One possible explanation is that richer siblings tend to be financially responsible for their poorer siblings. Since formal credit (and insurance) markets are limited, households are generally poor, and family ties remain strong in rural Bangladesh, it is likely that the richest siblings, especially the household head,

[15] It is also possible that the older household heads are predominantly poor. However, this is not case in the TS.

act as caretakers of their extended families. They tend to be the person of last resort when a member of the family faces major difficulties. This added responsibility is expected to increase their suffering. The same argument can be made for neighbors who are often extended family members. Thus, it would appear that the rural Bangladeshi families and communities studied had higher social solidarity than those of typical Western societies.

From the perspective of alleviating mental suffering, the above finding implies that a more egalitarian or unequal society may alleviate suffering for both the rich and the poor. For instance, if we transfer some income from the relatively rich to the relatively poor, it will reduce the worry and feelings of depression for both types of individuals. Based on the discussion of possible reasons for the U-shape above, the reason for the reduction in suffering associated with the transfer is different for the rich and poor. For the poor, it reduces their sense of relative deprivation and increases their financial security. For the rich, the transfer would reduce their responsibilities of taking care of their poor siblings, neighbors or extended family members. This is true not only because a reduction of income makes the rich less likely to be viewed as the person of last resort but the simultaneous increase in the income of the poor will make them less dependent on the rich. This type of redistribution is analogous to a government that taxes the rich and provides a safety net for the poor. Instead of making policies more complicated, interdependent preferences here allow for a situation that is a win-win for both the rich and the poor. It is important to recognize that the strong familial and social ties and a sense of responsibility toward the community makes income equality an effective device for alleviating suffering. This may not hold for societies where such familial and social relationships are weak (e.g. urban areas).

Policy Implications and Future Research

The findings here shed light on those who are suffering and whether the current developmental policies aimed at improving human development are expected to alleviate mental suffering as well. The analyses indicate that middle-aged, unmarried, and unhealthy household heads who are financially doing much better or much worse than their siblings and neighbors, tend to suffer the most. Thus, these are individuals who should be targeted by policymakers interested in alleviating mental suffering. These findings should not be misconstrued as opposing the view that women, children, and elders are marginalized in rural developing countries such as Bangladesh. Instead, it is being pointed out that when considering "household heads" and self-reported mental suffering, there are no gender-wise differences, and the older individuals do not necessarily suffer more. Given that the study only looks at household heads, I am unable to comment on the mental suffering of children. In the context of rural Bangladesh, the household heads usually make the most important decisions for the family (and often the extended families), so reducing their suffering may lead to more optimal decision making.

Improving health services is the most effective tool for alleviating suffering among the three human development tools that get the most attention (the other two being standard of living and education). Given the low level of household income in these communities, small increases in living standards will most likely not reduce mental suffering by much. Based on the findings here, however, there is a strong case to be made for alleviating suffering by promoting a more egalitarian society. Instead of depending on external sources of funding such as the national government, it may be prudent for the local governments or other formal institutions in these villages to offer safety nets (or cash transfers) to the poor who are funded by taxing the rich within the villages. This will reduce inequality and alleviate the mental suffering of both the rich and the poor.

Further research needs to be conducted to identify other correlates of mental suffering and clarify factors that alleviate mental suffering in specific social contexts. It is also important that social scientists focus on improving methods of measuring suffering so as to make them reliable and comparable across countries. Most importantly, mental suffering remains an understudied topic in the contexts of developing countries and should be explored exhaustively. The socioeconomic and cultural contexts of these developing countries are very diverse, and the mental suffering most likely functions differently as well. Most worthy of further comparative research is the finding of this study that economic equality rather than inequality in the community alleviates mental suffering, specifically worrying and/or feeling depressed daily.

References

Acemoglu, D., Johnson, S., & Robinson, J. A. (2000). *The colonial origins of comparative development: An empirical investigation, No. w7771*. Cambridge, MA: National Bureau of Economic Research.

Anderson, R. E. (2015). *World suffering and quality of life* (Vol. 56). Dordrecht: Springer.

Bhuiyan, M. F. (2012). Relative consumption: A model of peers, status, and labor supply. *American Journal of Agricultural Economics, 95*(2), 368–375.

Bhuiyan, M. F., & Szulga, R. (2013). The *Tangail Survey: Household Level Census of Subjective Well-Being, Perceptions of Relative Economic Position, and International Migration: 2013 [Tangail, Bangladesh]*. Ann Arbor: Inter-university Consortium for Political and Social Research [distributor], 2016–03-23. http://doi.org/10.3886/E61146V1

Bhuiyan, M. F., & Szulga, R. (2017). Extreme bounds of subjective well-being: Economic development and micro determinants of life satisfaction. *Applied Economics, 49*(14), 1351–1378.

Blanchflower, D. G., & Oswald, A. J. (2004). Well-being over time in Britain and the USA. *Journal of Public Economics, 88*(7), 1359–1386.

Blanchflower, D. G., & Oswald, A. J. (2008). Is well-being U-shaped over the life cycle? *Social Science & Medicine, 66*(8), 1733–1749.

Clark, A. E., & Oswald, A. J. (1996). Satisfaction and comparison income. *Journal of Public Economics, 61*(3), 359–381.

Diener, E., Suh, E., Lucas, R. E., & Smith, H. L. (1999). Subjective well-being: Three decades of progress. *Psychological Bulletin, 125*(2), 276–302.

Duesenberry, J. S. (1949). *Income, saving, and the theory of consumer behavior*. Cambridge: Harvard University Press.

Duncan, O. D. (1975). Does money buy satisfaction? *Social Indicators Research, 2*(3), 267–274.
Dynan, K. E., & Ravina, E. (2007). Increasing income inequality, external habits, and self-reported happiness. *American Economic Review, 97*(2), 226–231.
Easterlin, R. A. (1974). Does economic growth improve the human lot? Some empirical evidence. *Nations and Households in Economic Growth, 89*, 89–125.
Easterlin, R. A. (1995). Will raising the incomes of all increase the happiness of all? *Journal of Economic Behavior & Organization, 27*(1), 35–47.
Easterlin, R. A. (2001). Income and happiness: Towards a unified theory. *The Economic Journal, 111*(473), 465–484.
Frank, R. H. (1985a). *Choosing the right pond: Human behavior and the quest for status*. Oxford: Oxford University Press.
Frank, R. H. (1985b). The demand for unobservable and other non-positional goods. *The American Economic Review, 75*(1), 101–116.
Frijters, P., & Beatton, T. (2012). The mystery of the U-shaped relationship between happiness and age. *Journal of Economic Behavior & Organization, 82*(2), 525–542.
Helliwell, J. F., Layard, R., & Sachs, J. (2013). World happiness report.
Hirschman, A. O., & Rothschild, M. (1973). The changing tolerance for income inequality in the course of economic development. *The Quarterly Journal of Economics, 87*, 544–566.
Kahneman, D., & Deaton, A. (2010). High income improves evaluation of life but not emotional well-being. *Proceedings of the National Academy of Sciences, 107*(38), 16489–16493.
Kahneman, D., & Krueger, A. B. (2006). Developments in the measurement of subjective well-being. *The Journal of Economic Perspectives, 20*(1), 3–24.
Kingdon, G. G., & Knight, J. (2007). Community, comparisons and subjective well-being in a divided society. *Journal of Economic Behavior & Organization, 64*(1), 69–90.
Lelkes, O. (2006). Tasting freedom: Happiness, religion and economic transition. *Journal of Economic Behavior & Organization, 59*(2), 173–194.
Luttmer, E. F. (2004). *Neighbors as negatives: Relative earnings and well-being, No. w10667*. Cambridge: National Bureau of Economic Research.
Malthus, T. R.. (1872). An essay on the principle of population or a view of its past and present effects on human happiness, an inquiry into our prospects respecting the future removal or mitigation of the evils which it occasions by Rev. TR Malthus. Reeves and Turner.
Mayraz, G., Wagner, G. G., & Schupp, J. (2009). Life satisfaction and relative income-perceptions and evidence.
McGuire, M. T., Fairbanks, L. A., & Raleigh, M. J. (1993). Life-history strategies, adaptation variations, and behaviour-physiologic interventions: the sociophysiology of Vervet monkeys.
Mroczek, D. K., & Spiro, A., III. (2005). Change in life satisfaction during adulthood: Findings from the veterans affairs normative aging study. *Journal of Personality and Social Psychology, 88*(1), 189.
Rayo, L., & Becker, G. S. (2007). Evolutionary efficiency and happiness. *Journal of Political Economy, 115*(2), 302–337.
Romer, P. M. (1986). Increasing returns and long-run growth. *The Journal of Political Economy*, 1002–1037.
Senik, C. (2004). When information dominates comparison: Learning from Russian subjective panel data. *Journal of Public Economics, 88*(9), 2099–2123.
Solnick, S. J., & Hemenway, D. (1998). Is more always better?: A survey on positional concerns. *Journal of Economic Behavior & Organization, 37*(3), 373–383.
Solow, R. M. (1956). A contribution to the theory of economic growth. *The Quarterly Journal of Economics*, 65–94.
Stevenson, B., & Wolfers, J. (2008). *Economic growth and subjective well-being: Reassessing the Easterlin paradox, No. w14282*. Cambridge: National Bureau of Economic Research.
Stevenson, B., & Wolfers, J. (2013). *Subjective well-being and income: Is there any evidence of satiation? No. w18992*. Cambridge: National Bureau of Economic Research.

Stone, A. A., Schwartz, J. E., Broderick, J. E., & Deaton, A. (2010). A snapshot of the age distribution of psychological well-being in the United States. *Proceedings of the National Academy of Sciences of the United States of America, 107*(22), 9985–9990.

Stutzer, A. (2004). The role of income aspirations in individual happiness. *Journal of Economic Behavior & Organization, 54*(1), 89–109.

Van de Stadt, H., Kapteyn, A., & Van de Geer, S. (1985). The relativity of utility: Evidence from panel data. *The Review of Economics and Statistics*, 179–187.

Wooldridge, J. M. (2010). *Econometric analysis of cross section and panel data*. Cambridge: MIT Press.

Chapter 8
Emotions, the Inner Lives of Those Who Work Toward Suffering Relief

Caitlin O. Mahoney and Laura M. Harder

Introduction

The alleviation of world suffering requires action on the part of individuals, including both person-to-person efforts toward immediate relief and those enacted to drive long range prevention, involving institutional and social change (Anderson 2014). Many theorists consider emotion to be an integral component of such social change. Yet, aside from the motivational energy that propels collective movements, emotions are integral to the 'interior' lives of activists themselves (Brown and Pickerill 2009). The very act of facing suffering and/or injustice tends to provoke strong emotion that is almost invariably negative in valence. Such aversive reactions are highly functional, as they draw our attention to situations that require change and offer motivational energy toward the work involved to enact transformation (Mahoney and Harder 2015). Yet, evidence suggests that awareness of suffering and the act of caring itself may encumber costs for the advocate that diminish their own well-being and that add to total suffering worldwide. How can caregivers maintain intensity and endurance in the pursuit of the large-scale alleviation of suffering, without undermining their own health or the efficacy of their labors?

In this chapter, our primary focus is that of caregivers (those that work directly with people across contexts), activists (people who protest failure to follow a given policy) and advocates (those that publically represent a particular idea or entity). In all three approaches our end concern is the alleviation of suffering of various types. We address the experience of those that might be assumed to care, already, about the

C.O. Mahoney (✉)
Faculty of Psychology, Metropolitan State University, St. Paul, MN 55106, USA
e-mail: Caitlin.Mahoney@metrostate.edu

L.M. Harder
Faculty of Psychology, Metropolitan State University, St. Paul, MN 55106, USA
e-mail: Laura.Harder@metrostate.edu

R.E. Anderson (ed.), *Alleviating World Suffering*, Social Indicators Research Series 67, DOI 10.1007/978-3-319-51391-1_8

suffering of others and that might be expected to know something about it (as compared with many potential helpers addressed in the chapter by Rosenblatt). As the quality of life of caregivers depreciates, so too does their ability to tend to others in ways that are personally and socially sustainable. These costs seem especially keen against the felt sense of stagnated systemic social change.

Rosenblatt (2017) has argued that, "if the vast amount of suffering worldwide is to be alleviated, ideally as many people as possible must step up and act. But in the absence of that, perhaps those who are able and willing to act might ideally be given as much support for their efforts as possible and as much help at being as good as they can be about what they do."Thus, it is our intention to offer practical recommendations regarding the development of the personal and social resources necessary to respond to suffering effectively without multiplying it. Our capacities for attention and awareness, connection, acceptance, and conscious reappraisal seem to be at the core of our responses to suffering (Hölzel et al. 2011). Thus, privately, caregivers, advocates and activists might learn to deliberately recognize and direct these capacities toward more effective responses. Moreover, our sense of self and our communities play a part in how we manage our experience of emotions and our beliefs about social change. In particular, communal norms that construct advocacy as necessarily onerous may fail to acknowledge the limitations of caregivers and advocates, while supportive communities that prioritize connection and celebration may alleviate helping stress. Sustainable social change will require an awareness of the ways in which these individual beliefs and behaviors, institutional policies, and cultural rhetoric in the advocacy field may hamper the alleviation of suffering. We attempt to build a picture of a more conscious engagement for 'helpers' by integrating thinking that may be useful in constructing the emotional experience of caring and of advocacy in ways that are less harmful, more sustainable, and more impactful.

Empathy & Emotion

To understand how best to engage and sustain individuals in work aimed at the alleviation of suffering, we must first understand the ways in which suffering 'out there' is filtered through the lens of personal experience on the part of the observer. Batson (1990), Wiseman (1996), Pinker (2011) and others have proposed that the primary pathway by which we attend to another's suffering is that of empathy. Those others may be close to us (e.g. kin) or they may be quite far away (e.g. victims of natural disasters), but the processes by which we make sense of their experience are quite similar. The principal phases of empathy include recognition of emotion, emotional resonance, self-regulation of emotion, and role-taking. Taken together, these components have the potential to incite compassion and altruistic action. All of these processes occur within the contexts of mental abilities, valued cognitions and social settings. Thus, emotion is not the sole determinate of desires or attempts to reduce suffering, nor is empathy the sole component of the experience of suffering; But rather both emotion and empathy play major roles in the choice to reduce suffering. In particular, they can help to clarify the personal value of relieving suffering as a principal source of meaning in life. As we relate to the experience of another and recognize the emotional responses it ignites, we are granted the opportunity to reflect on our internal signals of what is important to us and what response would best reflect our values.

Empathy, defined more as a process rather than as emotion, is the key component to understanding how emotions lead to prosocial behavior. According to Eisenberg, empathy is "an affective response that stems from the apprehension or comprehension of another's emotional state" (2002, pp. 135). In other words, empathy is role taking or vicarious enactment of another's experience. Empathy may be engaged in both immediate interpersonal healing and long-term efforts toward structural changes in cultures and institutions. In the former instance empathy may help us to connect directly with our target: accurately perceiving another's internal frame of reference, emotional experience and meanings as if we were the person ourselves, but "without ever losing the 'as if' condition" (Rogers, 1975). The 'as if' condition is an important component to our empathic approach, as it prevents us from imposing our own values or beliefs about what actions would be helpful on the experience of another. Batson (1990) argued that empathy sustains our attention, engagement and drive to help when escape from a situation is possible. Thus, empathy is what keeps us in the trenches when we have the option to exit a situation to protect ourselves (our time, our energy, our resources). In the instance of social suffering, empathy may be leveraged to engage the support of wider collectives: to ignite and grow awareness of suffering, to motivate behaviors aimed at helping (monetary donations, political activism, and changes in habits of daily living), to generate and sustain the energy of social protest, or to shift the boundaries of personal identities.

Within the empathic process, environmental events serve as triggers that lead to emotional arousal. When the external events are persons exhibiting signs of suffering, the empathic arousal is called emotional reactivity or, more often, emotional resonance. These terms refer to the extent to which someone's emotions are ignited as his or her own experiences absorb the new external information. Reactivity or resonance in such contexts of suffering are more often linked to negative emotions of the sufferer. As the form of emotional response may differ depending on the perceiver, so too may the threshold of arousal needed to generate emotional resonance differ across external stimuli and person to person. Someone who is particularly reactive will experience stronger emotions than someone who demonstrates lower emotional resonance. As one's ability to regulate these responses is strengthened, the intensity of the response will also differ (Carlo et al. 2012).

Self-regulation is the monitoring and control process that begins in infancy and allows us to moderate our reactions (Geangu 2011). It is intimately linked to our emotional reactivity. Habits of emotional responding emerge from genetic predispositions and social learning. To the extent that emotions become consistent ways of responding, they may be more difficult to regulate (Lerner and Keltner 2001). As we will see, these patterns of emotional responding have a great deal to do with one's physical and mental well-being and professional efficacy. As Carlo et al. (2012) explain, "To engage in caring actions toward others requires effective regulation of one's own emotions." Consider what occurs when we engage in too little or too much regulation.

If someone is highly regulatory they might constrain their emotions and behaviors to such an extent that they do not engage at all with someone who is suffering. Studies have shown this type of response when people are faced with needs of large populations. They see the need as enormous and regulate themselves to prevent an overwhelming emotional response (Cameron and Payne 2011). The counterpart to this notion is the effect of failing to regulate emotions enough. A person with low self-regulation may fail to control their emotions, leading to personal distress. Personal distress, as defined by Eisenberg, is the "aversive, self-focused reaction to others in need or distress" (Eisenberg 2000, pp. 668). So, low levels of self-regulation lead to personal distress, which leads to a focus on the self. If we are focusing on our own experience, we are unable to effectively tend to the needs of others. Consequently, personal distress and low levels of self-regulation have been shown to decrease helping behaviors (Eisenberg, 2000).

Empathy and self-regulation can help us to understand how emotions lead us to alleviate the suffering of others. The importance of equilibrium in these processes is compartively important to understand. In order to be most effective in tending to the needs of others, we must be able to see their perspective and feel for them emotionally, but also regulate these reactions to maintain a healthy boundary between our own experience and theirs. Only then will we be able to be truly effective in our attempt to help.

The Costs of Caring

Framed positively, empathic pain felt in response to the suffering of others, is a route to understanding and an opportunity to leverage the information gleaned from "feeling into" another's distress (Lipps 1903a, b as cited in Zabinski and Valsiner, 2004) to respond in ways that promote healing and may ultimately lead to flourishing. Yet, in either the personal/social or the structural domain, its consequences may also be harmful. Unmoderated empathy may detract from the quality of life of helpers and obstruct the pursuit and efficacy of their labors.

Helpers of all types are at risk for burnout, the "mental and physical exhaustion" (Maslach et al. 2001) implicit in work that fails to provide consistent rewards, a sense of control, identifiable achievements or a felt sense of competence. Though burnout has been connected to a variety of causes, at its core, burnout consists of a sense of emotional exhaustion (feeling overwhelmed by the emotional demands of a job), depersonalization (feelings of disconnection with others, clients or otherwise), and a decreased sense of personal accomplishment (Maslach et al. 1986).

Professionals who work with those who are suffering experience occupational hazards surrounding mental health at disproportionately higher rates than their counterparts. In the field of nursing, experiential rates of compassion fatigue can reach 79% (Conrad and Kellar-Guenther 2006). Similarly, a Canadian study demonstrated that 80% of nurses have utilized the Employee Assistance Program services provided by their employer – a rate of more than double those employed in non-helping fields (Statistics Canada 2005). These effects are seen across the professional helping spectrum – from child protection workers (Conrad and Kellar-Guenther 2006) and clergy members (Jackson-Jordan 2013) to police officers (Russell et al. 2014) and domestic violence attorneys (Levin and Greisberg 2003).

Professionals of all types crave rewards for hard work and feelings of control over outcomes and milestones. A specialized form of learned helplessness occurs in professions like advocacy that see repetitive cases or little progress toward systemic change (Harder 2014). These individuals may frequently experience the sense that they have "taken two steps forward, one step back," that is, small victories may be immediately followed by an ever growing to-do list. As the demands seem to be insurmountable, an understandable response to such work is to try harder - even at the cost of one's mental and physical well-being.

Bobel (2007) has demonstrated that activism, in particular, calls forth associations of *rigor*, as defined by "relentless dedication" and "unyielding sacrifice," such that those who earn the title of 'activist' are believed to "(work) very hard and at great personal cost over a long period of time." The standards of rigor pose several challenges. First, non-activists may perceive activists to be arrogant or haughty, potentially alienating the target audience. Second, such harsh and demanding behavioral criterion may render the work itself an unachievable standard. Third, those that might be inclined to pursue the activist identity, even so rigorously defined, are at risk of glorifying the experience of burnout and undervaluing or demonizing the work of self-care. So too, changemakers of all types may come to punish colleagues that fail to comply with the social norms implied by the standards of rigor. In studies of group membership status, normative members are "upgraded" while deviant members are "derogated." Such "derogation of deviant ingroup members (is) associated with a socializing and a punishing intention toward new members and full members, respectively" (Pinto et al. 2010). As such, advocates may learn to police and shame each other for failure to uphold the relentless and self-sacrificial pursuit of social justice, and such disparagement may prevent the orientation and self-care that would make their efforts more durable.

Other forms of emotional weight are implicit in the ways in which individuals and groups construct social change itself. Sometimes individuals suffer the emotional maelstrom of the felt discrepancy between things as they are, things as we believe they should be, and things as they might be in our ideal future. These perceived discrepancies drain the motivational power that we might otherwise harness to drive change (Higgins et al. 1986). Movements also suffer when they do not have a common vision toward which to strive (Boulding 1988). Gilbert (1988) has noted that one of the psychological factors inhibiting activism is a perceived "maze of objectives." While there may be consensus that the widespread relief of suffering is valuable, various groups operationalize goals toward that end quite differently. Hopelessness may be a natural response to situations where goals are unclear, individuals lack a sense of agency or control in their efforts, and/or lack trust that they have the knowledge and resources necessary to traverse barriers they might encounter on the road to change (Snyder 2002). Finally, social movements invariably face the resistance of status quo actors and institutions and the contrary and system justifying belief systems of potential allies (Mahoney et al. 2015). Against these challenges, advocates and activists risk alienation (Bashir et al. 2013), cynicism (Maslach et al. 2001), and despair (Macy 1983).

Evidence points to these costs of caring affecting those with the highest capacities for empathy (Figley 1995) and also suggests that caring for oneself can provide relief from the effects of helping others (Salloum et al. 2015). Interestingly, as helpers often experience guilt relating to perceived inequality (Van Dierendonck et al. 2001), traditional approaches to self-care such as exercise, therapy and taking time off may not only be ineffective, but could potentially increase one's suffering by compounding already manifested guilt. Thus, in many ways, even as they try to care for themselves, helpers come to add to total suffering by making others' pain their own, or by creating new suffering implicit in their reactions to the work itself.

The emotional experience of caregivers and activists stretches past the individual into the lives of those for whom they advocate. For instance, certain types of psychological pain seem to prime one toward defensiveness against impending threat. Hawkley et al. (2003) found that the pain of loneliness is associated with "higher stress appraisals and poorer social interactions," including a tendency to be less understanding and more distrustful. So, to the extent that one is enmeshed in one's own pain, he or she may be less likely to notice the pain of others and/or less able to understand it.

Our pain may not only prevent us from noticing or understanding the suffering of others, it may actually alter our perception of another's experience. Those experiencing elevated stress at work, for example, are more likely to remember and record negative aspects of a client's case than positive (Harder and Mahoney 2015). We know that interventions that focus on well-being can create a cognitive-affective shift from negativity to positivity (Seligman et al. 2005), which can in turn lead to positive outcomes relating to improved health and decreased stress (Kabat-Zinn 1990). As building on the positive factors in a client's life leads to better outcomes than focusing on negatives, sustainable change begins with the emotional experience of the advocate. Self-care becomes collective care where it prevents our own suffering from being compounded onto others.

As our personal suffering seems to be an inevitable risk with dire consequences on our efficacy, it behooves us to consider how to mitigate the suffering of those that do the hard work of social change. As we strive toward the realization of socially just ends and in pursuit of wide scale human flourishing, advocates will make a greater impact by first recognizing and addressing their own pain in such demanding work.

Reframing Our Orientation Toward Suffering

If we did not have an aversive reaction to suffering, we would not be motivated to relieve it. That we feel for those who are suffering is a testament to our shared humanity. This response need not be a source of added suffering itself, as long as we also tend to how we are engaging with those feelings. McGonigal (2013, 2016) has suggested that how we think about and act in stressful circumstances transforms the bodily and physiological experience of stress. Those who consider stressful circumstances to be unhealthy experience stress-induced health complications at much higher rates than those who frame the stress response as an embodied means of rising to a challenge. Similarly, those who report high levels of stress found resilience and immunity from stress related health problems by simply connecting and helping others. It is possible that changing our orientation toward the experience of suffering (i.e. how we feel about our feelings) may also alter the physical and social consequences of suffering felt vicariously. We can put this into practice using a variety of different techniques.

One means of transforming our experience of stress, or suffering more generally, is to bring our response within the realm of conscious awareness. Such awareness is a precondition for mindful engagement with the cognitive and emotional structures that lock us into very specific, and often toxic, performances of caring and/or advocacy. And while we may not be able to choose our immediate emotional reactions, we can learn to better regulate them and in some sense to choose how we feel about and respond to those reactions themselves. Finally, we may transform our experience of stress by consciously engaging systems of social support. These interpersonal relationships may buffer stress in several ways. Combined with the creation of institutional policies which frame advocacy with more attention to the humanity of the advocate, communities of support may help us to approach the dishabituation of both our internal and systemic reactions to suffering.

Generating and Working with Awareness

Research on the nature and utility of mindfulness has surged in the past 30 years. Anchored in Buddhist psychology, the construct has been defined differently by various western psychologists (most notably, Kabat-Zinn 1990; Langer 2014; Brown and Ryan 2003). Implicit in each of these definitions is a focus on mindfulness as a particular orientation of conscious experience, including our capacities for attention and awareness. Brown et al. (2007) regard awareness as the "conscious registration of stimuli." Attention to an object or event is only held when the stimulus is strong enough. After attention is ignited, automatic cognitive and emotional processes of appraisal are engaged (identifying features as 'good' or 'bad', etc.). Our perception of objects and events in the world are habitually focused and filtered through expectations anchored in past experience. A mindful mode of being is one by which our processes of awareness and attention are limited to only what we personally observe in that moment, while our reactions to these observations (thoughts, feelings, memories, judgments, etc.) may themselves be made the object of awareness. As with many definitions of mindfulness, this form of being conscious is described as "being present to reality," an orientation that is contrasted with "react(ing) to (reality) or habitually processing it through conceptual filters." Brown et al. (2007) argue that this orientation infuses "clarity" and allows, "more flexible, more objectively informed psychological and behavioral responses."

Mindfulness, per se, is not an emotion, but rather a means of recognizing and regulating emotion. Interventions aimed at growing and leveraging mindfulness for enhanced well-being often focus on practices of meditation, but many theorists (Langer 2014) and practitioners (e.g. Hahn 1992) have emphasized that *any* activity might be pursued mindfully and utilized as a means of practicing and growing the attention and awareness implicit in a mindful way of being.

Kabat-Zinn (1990) and his associates claim that, through mindfulness meditative practices, we can learn to attend humanely to our own suffering and grow our capacity to trust others. Training in mindfulness meditation centers largely on enhancing one's attention and awareness, grounding one in present experience (rather than the past or future) without attempting to flee or to change it. Such an orientation enables us to work to shift our relationship to our stressors and reactions. In addition to better noticing, regulating, and responding to our own experiences, these practices have important implications for how we relate to others. As mindfulness training has been shown to ground us in awareness and understanding of our own bodily experience, it secondarily grows our capacity to understand others (Decety and Jackson 2004), increases our empathic engagement (Dekeyser et al. 2008), and enhances inclination to take compassionate action on behalf of others (Condon et al. 2013).

It's perhaps also important to note that while mindfulness is often presented as a positively valued construct, Langer (2014) has argued that sometimes mindlessness may actually prove the more effective strategy. That is to say, some tasks and experiences benefit from being done mindfully, while others are more effective when done mindlessly (consider, for example, the act of typing - when we call attention to those processes that have become automatized, our pace and accuracy actually diminish). So perhaps, individuals working toward social change might also consider ways in which mindlessness might be leveraged to automate processes and habits to serve socially just ends. By taking time to mindlessly engage in a monotonous task (for example, organizing a donation closet or filing papers alphabetically), one can regain the mental capacity for other job requirements that call for mindfulness (like meeting one on one with clients or debriefing with co-workers). Mindlessness, while psychologically protective in some regards, might best be engaged mindfully. We must be able to recognize when we need time away from mindful engagement with those who are suffering and call upon a change in behavior to ease the vicarious stress that can result.

Mindfulness alone is insufficient to better manage our reactions to suffering; as to create emotional shifts more is required than just awareness. To practice mindfulness meditation without applying it in the contexts of everyday life may not alter our relationship to suffering. Jim Doty, clinical professor of neurosurgery at Stanford University and founder and director of the Center for Compassion and Altruism Research and Education (CCARE), has also argued that mindfulness, without compassion, can be used to focus performance, but may simultaneously spur competitive cycles that further tax our resources and generates more suffering (in an interview with Newman 2016, June 9). Some research has demonstrated the added importance of non-reactivity and non-judgmental acceptance in moderating the effects of awareness on emotional symptoms (Van Dam et al. 2009; Baer et al. 2006). As, to be mindful in trying times can call our attention to great pain. Applying mindfulness in these contexts is about a deeper application of "being in the moment." As we sit in the company of another who is suffering, mindfulness serves as a key to a true connection with their experience. Mindfulness, though, can also be a tool in providing relief from the distress that can occur in these situations.

Rather than passively responding to cues in our environments, we might learn to actively choose/construct elements of our contexts with attention to their variability (Langer 2014). Through intention in our actions, we can practice nearly any act mindfully. In advocacy work, mindfully attending to our emotional responses to the experiences of others may infuse psychological space between our suffering and theirs. After we connect with another's suffering, awareness allows us to acknowledge its effect. Once we become aware of how connecting with their experience feels in our mind and body, we can mindfully clarify to ourselves, "This is not my suffering. I feel this way because they are suffering and I care about them. But their suffering is not my suffering." That is, while connecting to the present moment can indeed lead us to suffer vicariously through the experiences of others, mindfulness can also connect us to the following moment: the moment past the suffering. A domestic violence advocate may at one moment be connecting with a client on the phone, hearing a gut-wrenching story of violence, but in the moment that follows her hanging up the phone, the advocate has a choice. In choosing to take that moment to connect with the vicarious suffering she experiences from her empathic nature, to sit and feel this pain, she can readjust the perception she holds of her own arousal. She can remind herself that this response is out of empathy and that she can choose to move her focused attention on to something else.

Emotion regulation assists with addressing suffering by providing us with the key ability to protect ourselves from overreaching our emotional threshold. While emotion regulation is clearly imperative in alleviating our own experience of suffering, the psychological flexibility grown through mindful practices goes beyond this notion, as it entails the choice of whether or not to enter a situation at all. Thus, it is predicated on the ability to notice contextual boundaries around an experience. By recognizing situations that may leave us emotionally vulnerable as they occur, we provide ourselves with the opportunity for protection from suffering that may result. Of course, such present moment awareness may be uncomfortable. Psychotherapeutically we know that discomfort is often the first spark toward change and being drawn out of complacency. Thus, it is not our intent to suggest that we should notice that we are (or might be) in pain and disengage, but rather that we should enter the discomfort consciously and manage our engagement strategically. It is by reflecting on this discomfort that we foster the capacity to manage our vulnerability.

Communities of Support

While certainly the regulation of emotion is a task of the individual, our emotions are also incited and regulated in part by those around us (Lewis et al. 2007). Those who value independence may believe that they should be able to carry and manage the weight of suffering, whether their own or the weight of the world, alone. They may believe that to fold under its weight or to ask for help in its management is a weakness, in the face of the standards of rigor. Or they may simply struggle to shake the perceptual filter that leads us to believe that we, alone, are responsible for the management of our own emotions. Yet our history of evolution and the manifestations of our biological responses, including the experience of loneliness or the impulse to care about others at all, suggest that humans have evolved systems that require the attention of others for their survival (Cacioppo and Patrick, 2008).

Communities of support help us to meet our basic needs, so that we can devote more time to other pursuits (Maslow 1970). They lend emotional (McGuire 2007), instrumental, informational, and spiritual support (Uchino 2004). Thus, their buffering effect (Cohen 2004) may prevent us from suffering stress or burnout in the first place or they may quell the repercussions of trying to do too much for too long. Empathic communities may also assist in the cognitive work of processing and reframing our own approach to suffering: reminding us that things may change, that change takes time, and that we are secure and supported along the way. Similarly, communities may aid in humbling our ambitions of alleviating the suffering of others. By serving as a sort of barometer for what expectations are realistic, community can keep our desires in check and help us achieve what is in fact possible. They help us cope with the concept of incremental progress and remind us that we are sowing seeds whose fruit we may not see but, that we are pursuing essential work, all the same, to lay the groundwork of progress toward achieving an ultimate goal. Communities, too, can take the burden off of individual members for what they hope to accomplish by distributing responsibilities between all members. That is, communities cannot only buffer us from our own suffering, but also from the effects of helping others who are suffering. If nothing else, the act of witness is a tremendous and underestimated component of human community. Carl Roger's (1975) argued that, "simply listening attentively is an important way of being helpful." It follows that the experience of being seen may quell some of the pain of existential angst that is implicit in working towards a more just and equitable world. Caregivers may need to learn to allow themselves to be listened to and to witness to each other as much as those whom they serve.

Brown and Pickerill (2009) have suggested that social movements rarely blend activists and advocates across generations and that there might be value in passing on what has been learned, about emotion management in particular, from one generation to the next. Though having "been there" does not always increase empathy (Ruttan et al. 2015). There is a danger that emotional memory for suffering fades while the realization that a situation may be lived through remains, leaving survivors callous toward those currently in the throes of suffering. These dynamics may be less acute for those who recall having failed themselves, or for those encouraged to consider how they were helped by others during difficult times.

It is imperative to note that sharing such difficult work with others is not without its consequences. Social workers who report perceived burnout in their coworkers display higher symptoms of helping stress themselves (Gonzalez-Morales et al. 2012). This idea of collective burnout sheds light on how, once we are a part of an empathic community, we open ourselves and our own stress to more people who already experience high levels of stress and suffering. The concept of "sliming" our coworkers with stories of suffering is used in compassion fatigue literature to describe situations of inadvertently harming others. It refers to our impulse to share our suffering with those closest to us before lending them the opportunity to ask for space or time to prepare mentally (Mathieu, 2012). When we jump into sharing our experience without first providing this opportunity for space, we rob the other of the option to protect themselves from vicariously taking on our stress. Mindful engagement with suffering can help us to not only moderate our response to other's suffering, but also be cognizant of the effect our suffering has on others. By reflecting on how sharing our suffering with someone else impacts them, we can prevent the adverse effects of sharing these stories can sometimes have on those whom we care about.

Similarly, the ways in which leaders and organizations support their staff have the capacity to alleviate or compound stress and suffering. To create positive, sustainable change, we must construct empathic communities that provide the safety and emotional climate necessary to muddle through the hard realities of social justice work together. Leadership can provide a strong foundation for such a community. We need to select and grow leaders who can give constructive feedback while balancing the challenge to achieve more with kindness and appreciation. Leaders need the emotional intelligence to sit with their employees' discomfort, with the weight of the work, and their own reactions to both. Such leaders may also serve as powerful role models who themselves are open to critique and compliment, who set and hold boundaries on their own self care, and who construct the experience of advocacy more mindfully. They can challenge the way things have been so that self-care becomes the status quo, rather than a sign of weakness or shame.

Though reflective engagement with our experience may open us to the potential for pain, it also thrusts open access to all experiences, including positive ones. Communities may help us to notice, savor and share the joys of success as well as cradle us through perceived failure. Singularly focused on a fixed and distant guidepost, advocates and activists may not take time to celebrate victories, however small. Yet the fires of activism may be fueled by the mutual joy of connecting with others who share one's values and vision (Brown and Pickerill, 2009). As positive emotional experiences may liberate our energies to continue work toward a difficult task, activism as a whole will benefit by prioritizing celebration of progress. Celebrations provide a means of sharing and affirming identity (Green and Chalip 1998), of socializing values, and can offer perspective on how far we've come [one element of a strategy referred to as Positive Mental Time Travel (Quoidbach et al. 2010)]. In short, celebrations fuel human connection, camaraderie and hope.

Conclusions

The relief of suffering requires the efforts of individuals, both in response to their own suffering and that of others. Whereas an aversion to suffering may be innate, the desire to end specific oppressive systems may require socialization (Anderson 2014). While there is value in clarifying the personal and social utility of relieving suffering of all types, individual commitment and action is at the epicenter of sustainable change. As we continue to grow communities that value humanitarian ethos, we might devote more attention to supporting those who are already engaged in personal, social and systemic relief of suffering. This focus allows us to relieve the suffering of helpers and to prevent their future suffering while facilitating their ability to tend to the relief and prevention of the suffering of others.

The human empathic response is one that induces automatic arousal within us. Empathizing with another is essentially what sparks our emotional reaction toward suffering of others, while emotional resonance and regulation dictates not only our personal experience of suffering, but also whether or not we will engage with it. We've outlined how individuals may work to enhance their awareness and attention around their engagement with suffering, including noticing and regulating their emotional experiences and working to shift their habitual reactions toward the realm of conscious choice. Such psychological flexibility allows one to choose when and in what ways engaging with suffering will be effective. Yet, we acknowledge that the work of individuals is nested within larger ecologies and within a cultural rhetoric around caring and advocacy. Thus, we may need to slowly transform cultures of all types, including organizations, communities and nations. Within these environments we might strive to enshrine more modest normative approaches to work by establishing "reasonable goals regarding our capacity to give" and setting and maintaining realistic boundaries around individual efforts and availability (Doty as interviewed by Newman 2016, June 9). Further, a cultural shift in the value of interdependence over our more isolating and paradigmatic independent frames (Cacioppo and Patrick 2008) might be useful in two ways. First, to shift the ways in which changemakers access systems of social support themselves and second, to frame the large scale alleviation of suffering as a social and cultural imperative.

References

Anderson, R. E. (2014). *Human suffering and quality of life: Conceptualizing stories and statistics*. New York: Springer Science & Business Media.
Baer, R. A., Smith, G. T., Hopkins, J., Krietemeyer, J., & Toney, L. (2006). Using self-report assessment methods to explore facets of mindfulness. *Assessment, 13*(1), 27–45.
Bashir, N. Y., Lockwood, P., Chasteen, A. L., Nadolny, D., & Noyes, I. (2013). The ironic impact of activists: Negative stereotypes reduce social change influence. *European Journal of Social Psychology, 43*(7), 614–626.
Batson, C. D. (1990). How social an animal: The human capacity for caring. *American Psychologist, 45*(3), 336–346.
Bobel, C. (2007). 'I'm not an activist, though I've done a lot of it': Doing activism, being activist and the 'Perfect Standard' in a contemporary movement. *Social Movement Studies, 6*(2), 147–159.
Boulding, E. (1988). Image and action in peace building. *Journal of Social Issues, 44*(2), 17–37.
Brown, G., & Pickerill, J. (2009). Space for emotion in the spaces of activism. *Emotion, Space and Society, 2*(1), 24–35.
Brown, K. W., & Ryan, R. M. (2003). The benefits of being present: mindfulness and its role in psychological well-being. *Journal of Personality and Social Psychology, 84*(4), 822.
Brown, K. W., Ryan, R. M., & Creswell, J. D. (2007). Mindfulness: Theoretical foundations and evidence for its salutary effects. *Psychological Inquiry, 18*(4), 211–237.
Cacioppo, J. T., & Patrick, W. (2008). *Loneliness: Human nature and the need for social connection*. New York: WW Norton & Company.
Cameron, D. C., & Payne, B. K. (2011). Escaping affect: How motivated emotion regulation creates insensitivity to mass suffering. *Attitudes and Social Cognition, 100*(1), 1–15.
Carlo, G., Crockett, L. J., Wolff, J. M., & Beal, S. J. (2012). The role of emotional reactivity, self-regulation, and puberty in adolescents' prosocial behaviors. *Social Development, 21*(4), 667–685.
Cohen, S. (2004). Social relationships and health. *American Psychologist, 59*, 676–684.
Condon, P., Desbordes, G., Miller, W. B., & DeSteno, D. (2013). Meditation increases compassionate responses to suffering. *Psychological Science, 24*(10), 2125–2127.
Conrad, D., & Kellar-Guenther, Y. (2006). Compassion fatigue, burnout, and compassion satisfaction among Colorado child protection workers. *Child Abuse and Neglect, 30*(10), 1071–1080.
Decety, J., & Jackson, P. L. (2004). The functional architecture of human empathy. *Behavioral and Cognitive Neuroscience Reviews, 3*, 71–100.
Dekeyser, M., Raes, F., Leijssen, M., Leysen, S., & Dewulf, D. (2008). Mindfulness skills and interpersonal behavior. *Personality and Individual Differences, 44*, 1235–1245.
Eisenberg, N. (2000). Emotion, regulation, and moral development. *Annual Review of Psychology, 51*, 665–697.
Eisenberg, N. (2002). Empathy related emotional responses, altruism, and their socialization. In R. J. Davidson & A. Harrington (Eds.), *Visions of compassion* (pp. 131–164). Oxford: Oxford University Press.
Figley, C. R. (Ed.). (1995). *Compassion fatigue: Coping with secondary traumatic stress disorder in those who treat the traumatized*. New York: Brunner/Mazel.
Geangu, E. (2011). Individual differences in infant's emotional resonance to a peer in distress: Self-other awareness and emotion regulation. *Social Development, 20*(3), 450–470. doi:10.1111/j.1467–9507.2010.00596.x.
Gilbert, R. K. (1988). The dynamics of inaction: Psychological factors inhibiting arms control activism. *American Psychologist, 43*(10), 755.
Gonzalez-Morales, M. G., Peiro, J. M., Rodriguez, I., & Bliese, P. D. (2012). Perceived collective burnout: A multilevel explanation of burnout. *Anxiety Stress and Coping, 25*(1), 43–61.
Green, B. C., & Chalip, L. (1998). Sport tourism as the celebration of subculture. *Annals of Tourism Research, 25*(2), 275–291.

Hahn, T. N. (1992). *Peace is every step*. New York: Bantam Books.
Harder, L. (2014). *The revolving door effect: Learned helplessness and burnout in human services* (Unpublished master's thesis). Metropolitan State University, Saint Paul.
Harder, L.M., & Mahoney, C.O. (2015, February). *Keeping it positive: An experimental study on how burnout impacts the counselor-client relationship*. Poster presented at the 16th Annual Meeting of the Society for Personality and Social Psychology (SPSP), Long Beach, CA
Hawkley, L. C., Burleson, M. H., Berntson, G. G., & Cacioppo, J. T. (2003). Loneliness in everyday life: Cardiovascular activity, psychosocial context, and health behaviors. *Journal of Personality and Social Psychology, 85*(1), 105.
Higgins, E. T., et al. (1986). Self-discrepancies and emotional vulnerability: How magnitude, accessibility, and type of discrepancy influence affect. *Journal of Personality and Social Psychology, 51*(1), 5–15.
Hölzel, B. K., Lazar, S. W., Gard, T., Schuman-Olivier, Z., Vago, D. R., & Ott, U. (2011). How does mindfulness meditation work? Proposing mechanisms of action from a conceptual and neural perspective. *Perspectives on Psychological Science, 6*(6), 537–559.
Jackson-Jordan, E. A. (2013). Clergy burnout and resilience: A review of the literature. *Journal of Pastoral Care and Counseling, 61*(1), 1–5.
Kabat-Zinn, J. (1990). *Full catastrophe living*. New York: Bantam Dell.
Langer, E. (2014). Mindfulness: 25th Anniversary Edition. Addison-Wesley/Addison Wesley Longman.
Lerner & Keltner. (2001). Fear, anger, and risk. *Journal of Personality and Social Psychology, 81*(1), 146–159.
Levin, A. P., & Greisberg, S. (2003). Vicarious trauma in attorneys. *Pace L. Review, 24*(1), 245–246.
Lewis, T., Amini, F., & Lannon, R. (2007). *A general theory of love*. New York: Vintage.
Lipps, T. (1903a). *Grundlegung der Aesthetik*. Bamburg und Leipzig: W. Englemann.
Lipps, T. (1903b). Einfülung, innere nachahmung und organenempfindung. *Archiv. Für die gesamte. Psyychologie, I,* part 2 Leipzig: W. Engelmann.
Macy, J. (1983). *Despair and personal power in the nuclear age*. Philadelphia: New Society Publishers.
Mahoney, C. O., & Harder, L. M. (2015). Emotions, empathy, and the choice to alleviate suffering. In*World suffering and quality of life* (pp. 413–425). Dordrecht: Springer.
Mahoney, C. O., Weiner, E., & Loskota, T. (2015). Social norms and social change. In A. Dost-Gozkan & D. Sonmez Keith (Eds.), *Norms, group, conflict, and social change: Rediscovering Muzafer Sherif's psychology*. Piscataway: Transaction Publishers.
Maslach, C., Jackson, S. E., Leiter, M. P., Schaufeli, W. B., & Schwab, R. L. (1986). *Maslach burnout inventory manual and non-reproducible instrument and scoring guide*. Menlo Park: Mind Garden.
Maslach, C., Schaufeli, W. B., & Leiter, M. P. (2001). Job burnout. *Annual Review of Psychology, 52*(1), 397–422.
Maslow, A. (1970). *Motivation and personality* (Rev. ed.). New York: Harper & Row.
Mathieu, F. (2012). *The compassion fatigue workbook: Creative tools for transforming compassion fatigue and vicarious traumatization*. New York: Routledge.
McGonigal, K. (2013). How to make stress your friend. *Ted Global, Edinburgh, Scotland, 6*, 13.
McGonigal, K. (2016). *The upside of stress: Why stress is good for you, and how to get good at it*. New York: Penguin.
McGuire, G. M. (2007). Intimate work a typology of the social support that workers provide to their network members. *Work and Occupations, 34*(2), 125–147.
Newman, K.M. (2016, June 9). *What mindfulness is missing [Interview]*. Retrieved from: http://greatergood.berkeley.edu/article/item/what_mindfulness_is_missing
Pinker, S. (2011). *Better angels of our nature: Why violence has declined*. New York: Penguin Books.

Pinto, I. R., Marques, J. M., Levine, J. M., & Abrams, D. (2010). Membership status and subjective group dynamics: Who triggers the black sheep effect? *Journal of Personality and Social Psychology, 99*(1), 107–119. doi:10.1037/a0018187.
Quoidbach, J., Berry, E. V., Hansenne, M., & Mikolajczak, M. (2010). Positive emotion regulation and well-being: Comparing the impact of eight savoring and dampening strategies. *Personality and Individual Differences, 49*(5), 368–373.
Rogers, C. R. (1975). Empathic: An unappreciated way of being. *The Counseling Psychologist, 5*(2), 2–10.
Rosenblatt, P. C. (2017). Why people might be reluctant to alleviate the suffering of others. In R. E. Anderson (Ed.), *Alleviating world suffering: The challenge of negative quality of life*. New York: Springer.
Russell, L. M., Cole, B. M., & Jones III, R. J. (2014). High-risk occupations: How leadership, stress, and ability to cope influence burnout in law enforcement. *Journal of Leadership, Accountability and Ethics, 11*(3), 49–69.
Ruttan, R. L., McDonnell, M. H., & Nordgren, L. F. (2015). Having "been there" doesn't mean I care: When prior experience reduces compassion for emotional distress. *Journal of Personality and Social Psychology, 108*(4), 610.
Salloum, A., Kondrat, D. C., Johnco, C., & Olson, K. R. (2015). The role of self-care on compassion satisfaction, burnout and secondary trauma among child welfare workers. *Children and Youth Services Review, 49*(2015), 54–61.
Seligman, M. E. P., Steen, T., Park, N., & Peterson, C. (2005). Positive psychology progress: Empirical validation of interventions. *American Psychologist, 60*(5), 410–421.
Snyder, C. R. (2002). Hope theory: Rainbows in the mind. *Psychological Inquiry, 13*(4), 249–275.
Statistics Canada. (2005). *National survey of the work and health of nurses*. www.statcan.gc.ca (March 10, 2016).
Uchino, B. N. (2004). *Social support and physical health: Understanding the health consequences of relationships*. New Haven: Yale University Press.
Van Dam, N. T., Earleywine, M., & Danoff-Burg, S. (2009). Differential item function across meditators and non-meditators on the Five Facet Mindfulness Questionnaire. *Personality and Individual Differences, 47*(5), 516–521.
Van Dierendonck, D., Schaufeli, W. B., & Buunk, B. P. (2001). Burnout and inequity among human service professionals: A longitudinal study. *Journal of Occupational Health Psychology, 6*(1), 43–52.
Wiseman, T. (1996). A concept analysis of empathy. *Journal of Advanced Nursing, 23, 1162–1167.*
Zabinski, B. & Valsiner, J. (2004). *Affective synthesis of the other through the self: A new look at empathy*. Paper presented at the 3rd International conference on dialogical self, August, 28, Warsaw, Poland.

Chapter 9
Altruistic Values of Self and In-Groups and Implications for Suffering Alleviation

Hye Won Kwon and Rengin B. Firat

Introduction

Altruism is often defined as selfless behavior that accepts costs to the self for the good of others (Anderson 2014; Johnston 2015; Schopenhauer 2004). By sacrificing personal benefits, some people pursue "an ultimate goal of increasing another's welfare" (Batson and Shaw 1991:108) and help alleviate others' suffering. While altruism is defined as "selflessness," people who engage in altruistic behavior are far from lacking a consistent representation of their self and identity. One of the primary prerequisites for a need and desire to help ease the pain of those who suffer is a personal identity disposition that values altruistic behavior (Finkelstein et al. 2005; Piliavin and Callero 1991). Researchers have documented that self-sacrificing people have altruistic motives and values evoking helping behaviors that reduce others' suffering (Stocks et al. 2009). Personal identities are a strong predictor of prosocial and altruistic behavior and orientations (e.g., volunteer identity, blood donations) (Hitlin 2003; Lee et al. 1999). However, personal identities do not develop in a vacuum; as has been echoed as early as Cooley (1902) in his concept of "the looking-glass self" and Mead (1934) in his notion of "me," self and identity develop through social interactions and self-reflective perceptions of others (Stryker 2008). Yet very little work explores altruistic personal identities as they relate to social identities, and almost no work investigates the implications of altruistic value obligations like benevolence and caring for the community.

H.W. Kwon (✉)
Department of Sociology, University of Iowa, Iowa City, IA 52242, USA
e-mail: hyewon-kwon@uiowa.edu

R.B. Firat
Global Studies Institute, Department of Sociology and Neuroscience Institute, Georgia State University, Atlanta, GA 30302, USA
e-mail: rfirat@gsu.edu

R.E. Anderson (ed.), *Alleviating World Suffering*, Social Indicators Research Series 67, DOI 10.1007/978-3-319-51391-1_9

This chapter attempts to address this gap by establishing the linkages between an altruistic personal identity operationalized as holding altruistic value orientations and social identities measured by identifying with in-groups that promote these values. We argue that a stable, motivational basis that places the expansion of attention and heed from the individual or self to the social or collective as an end goal is a key driver of an altruistic personal identity. Therefore, in order to capture this motivational component, we specifically focus on value orientations that people prioritize and attribute to others. Values are desirable goals that provide guiding principles to people by motivating behavior (Rokeach 1973; Schwartz 1994). They are shaped by various cultural and socio-structural factors such as social class and occupations (Kohn and Schooler 1969; Pearlin and Kohn 1966), religion (Alwin 1986), as well as socio-economic development and historical heritage (Inglehart and Baker 2000). Values are core to the self and personal identities; personal identities are constructed through personal value commitments (Hitlin 2003). Furthermore, values push behavior toward desired outcomes (Hitlin 2003, 2007). Previous research also demonstrated the importance of values for social behavior by linking them to collective outcomes like interpersonal trust (Putnam 2001) and to social involvement and political activism (Schwartz 2007b).

We draw on a widely used cross-cultural theory of values, Schwartz's value orientations theory (Schwartz 1994), which identifies ten basic, universal values as desirable, trans-situational goals that are culturally or individually assigned with varying degrees of importance (Schwartz 1992, 1994, 2012). We specifically investigate two altruistic values among Schwartz's ten basic values: benevolence and universalism, which are categorized under the self-transcendence higher-order value domain (Schwartz and Bardi 2001; Schwartz and Boehnke 2004). They are related to transcending beyond oneself to preserving and promoting the welfare of others (Radkiewicz et al. 2008), while also being theoretically opposed to the self-enhancement values focused on self-interest (Schwartz 1992), thus making them ideally situated to capture the selflessness and self-sacrificing aspects of the altruistic domain. While benevolence values revolve around caring for the welfare of close others with whom people frequently interact (i.e., family and friends), universalism emphasizes caring about others beyond the immediate social circle, such as being concerned with social equality and diversity that can benefit members of the society in general (Schwartz 2007a). These two altruistic values are consistently ranked as two of the most important values throughout the world (Schwartz 2012).

The main premise of this chapter is that an altruistic social identity measured with identifying with groups that value benevolence and caring for others can contribute to the development of an altruistic personal identity that prioritizes benevolence and caring, potentially contributing to the relief of others' suffering. Since the groups that people feel they belong to (i.e., in-groups) are an important source of social identity and provide cognitive schema (Stryker 2008), people tend to build attitudes, values, and behaviors in concert with an in-group with which they identify (Stets and Burke 2000). We test the relationship between value attribution to the in-group and individual's disposition to relieve the suffering of others by analyzing data from a new cross-cultural survey, the Moral Schemas, Cultural Conflict, and

Socio-Political Action Survey (2015) that provides national data collected from the United States, France, Turkey, and South Korea using a novel measurement technique of values attributed to in-group members.

Altruistic Identity and Implications for Alleviating Suffering

Altruistic Personal and Social Identities

Even though contemporary Western ideas assume that relieving suffering is a "widely accepted human value" (Anderson 2015:430), not everyone values this cause equally. When confronted with various types of suffering, some people tend to care more about others' well-being (Anderson 2014; Williams 2008). By perceiving moral sensibilities and responsibilities for alleviating others' suffering and pain, some people see helping others as a life mission or purpose (Anderson 2014). Thus, researchers have proposed that a strong belief in benevolence and compassion can lead to reduction of suffering (Sznaider 2015). We suggest that by focusing on altruistic personal identities and the factors facilitating and nourishing them, we can obtain a better understanding of what leads to the propensity to relieve others' suffering.

We define altruistic personal identity as a fluid yet also stable entity of emotional and cognitive self-relevant meanings, subsuming internalized social positions with motivation to sacrifice one's self interests and accept personal costs to advance the welfare of others. Personal identity is developed through meaning making, it is reflexive (it can be its own object) and it is a process continuously constructed through social interactions (Becker and Strauss 1956). Yet personal identity is also stable and structured, reflecting patterned relationships, which allow drawing links among social hierarchies, roles, and status differences and the self (Stets 2006). As elaborated by Identity Theory (McCall 2003; Stryker 2000), on one hand identity strives to be stable by reducing uncertainty through self-verification processes confirming consistent information about one's self (Burke 1991, 2004). On the other hand, identity is also reflexive and is continuously reproduced in social interactions with other people. While this conceptualization is in line with the concept of moral identity from previous research suggesting that people pursue goal-directed action verifying their moral identities (Stets 2010; Stets and Carter 2011, 2012), we diverge from previous research by focusing on the linkages between social and personal altruistic identities by also incorporating the motivation for goal-directed action through operationalizing values.

Our theoretical framework emphasizes that social identities people use to categorize themselves and other people into in-groups and out-groups are important for increasing in-group altruism, coherence and cooperation and also providing positive evaluations for oneself through identifying with valued others (Tajfel and Turner 1979; Turner 1975, 1985). Figure 9.1 visualizes our theory and operationalization to

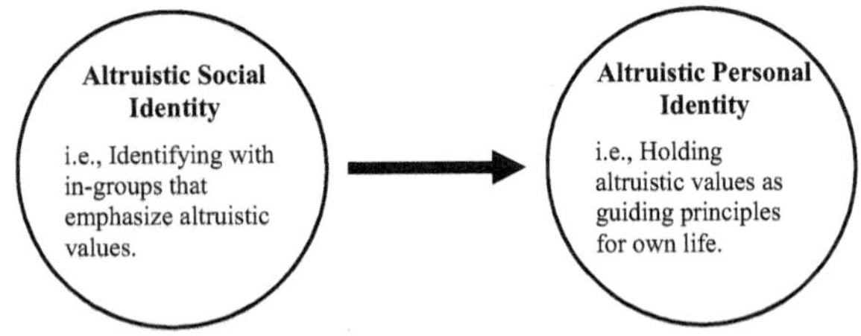

Fig. 9.1 The relationship between altruistic personal and social identities

understand the relationship between altruistic personal identity and social identity. Specifically, we propose that altruistic personal identity is captured by whether a person holds altruistic values as a guiding principle of one's own life while altruistic social identity is captured by whether a person identifies with an in-group that values altruistic dispositions. We argue that altruistic social identity contributes to building an altruistic personal identity and seek to empirically test this relationship.

Social Values as a Guiding Principle for Individuals

We argue that the relationship between personal and social identities can best be captured by examining value orientations. Values are an important part of the process whereby culturally important goals and motivations enter into individual decisions shaping interactions and attitudes giving way to an altruistic, social self. Values are abstract, cognitive systems that push behavior toward desirable outcomes (Howard 1995; Rokeach 1973; Schwartz 1992, 1994). Studying values to understand identities and self is especially important for three reasons: first, values provide cognitive maps to guide behavior; therefore, examination of behavioral changes requires articulation of the value changes of individuals. Second, studying value orientations provides a starting point for the examination of differences among groups (such as age groups, ethnic groups, or countries) because people sharing commonalities (such as political identities, language, etc.) also share value orientations. And finally, studying values enables us to draw links between individual, social-structural, and cultural levels, since they operate at all of these levels (Hitlin and Piliavin 2004).

Schwartz defines values as desirable, trans-situational goals—varying in importance—that serve as guiding principles in people's lives (Bardi and Schwartz 2003; Schwartz 1992; Schwartz and Bardi 2001). Accordingly, there are ten fundamental human values constituting four general value domains: self-enhancement (power and achievement), conservation (security, tradition, and conformity), openness to change (self-direction, stimulation, and hedonism), and self-transcendence (benevolence and universalism) according to the motivation that underlies each of them

(Schwartz 1992). In this chapter, we focus on the benevolence and universalism values, which reflect the pro-social domain that expresses the motivation to promote social interaction and the welfare of others by transcending self-interest (Schwartz 1992; Schwartz and Bilsky 1987). Cross-culturally, universalism and benevolence value orientations are also ranked as the most important value orientations (Schwartz et al. 2001). Previous research has indicated that values focused on benevolence and universalism—being concerned with the welfare of others—are closely associated with both social trust and civic outcomes (Karp 1996; Schwartz 2010; Stern 1992). However, the "socialness" or the "collective essence" of these values so far has only been measured by solely aggregating individual values to the cultural or country level. We offer an alternative theoretical and empirical tool that helps capture the group-level value attributions and discuss its implications in personal inclination to help suffering others.

We suggest that prioritizing benevolence and universalism values indicates an altruistic disposition or personal identity. While benevolence value is potentially associated with caring for close others with mild to extreme suffering, the value of social diversity and equality is linked to eradicating the main components of social suffering such as discrimination, social exclusion and stigma. However, altruistic personal identity is incubated and promoted through social interactions with others who also emphasize these values. Therefore, identifying with benevolent and universalistic or caring others is also crucial for developing an altruistic personal identity. We argue that the altruistic personal and social identities are linked to each other through an identity verification process suggested by the Identity Control Theory (or cybernetic control theory) (Burke 1991; Stets 2006). Accordingly, we propose that if and when people receive information from their in-group members indicating their altruism levels, they compare this against their personal altruistic motives and, in the end, through conscious and implicit mechanisms, verify their personal identities by either adjusting their inclinations of altruism (if there is a mismatch) or just maintaining their current dispositions. Through this step-wise relationship between altruistic personal and social identities, an altruistic self that is motivated to contribute to the alleviation of the suffering of others flourishes.

Data

Data for this study are from the 2015 Moral Schemas, Cultural Conflict, and Socio-Political Action Survey, a new survey of moral values and identities. Data have been collected in the U.S., France, Turkey, and South Korea through an online panel survey company (See Table 9.1 for descriptive statistics and sample sizes). The sampling for this study was carried out using quota sampling on gender and age groups to ensure their representativeness in each country.

Table 9.1 Descriptive statistics

Variable	U.S.A. (N = 437)				France (N = 448)				Turkey (N = 420)				South Korea (N = 449)			
	Mean	Std. Dev.	Min	Max	Mean	Std. Dev.	Min	Max	Mean	Std. Dev.	Min	Max	Mean	Std. Dev.	Min	Max
Age	46.09	17.09	18	83	46.24	16.15	18	99	34.22	12.28	18	98	42.80	13.92	18	73
Male	0.50	0.50	0	1	0.50	0.50	0	1	0.55	0.50	0	1	0.48	0.50	0	1
Racial majority (White/Turkish)	0.80	0.40	0	1	0.86	0.35	0	1	0.85	0.36	0	1				
College or above	0.42	0.49	0	1	0.52	0.50	0	1	0.67	0.47	0	1	0.64	0.48	0	1
Household income	5.61	3.37	1	11	4.93	2.79	1	10	8.48	3.08	1	12	5.62	2.86	1	11
Married	0.48	0.50	0	1	0.38	0.48	0	1	0.49	0.50	0	1	0.60	0.49	0	1
Religiosity	5.52	3.39	0	10	4.13	3.31	0	10	5.64	2.79	0	10	3.94	3.18	0	10
Political ideology	5.64	2.50	0	10	5.05	2.81	0	10	4.74	2.93	0	10	4.87	2.38	0	10
In-group types																
Occupation	0.15	0.36	0	1	0.21	0.40	0	1	0.15	0.36	0	1	0.25	0.43	0	1
Gender	0.08	0.28	0	1	0.14	0.35	0	1	0.06	0.24	0	1	0.05	0.22	0	1
Age	0.06	0.25	0	1	0.09	0.28	0	1	0.04	0.20	0	1	0.07	0.26	0	1
Religion	0.14	0.35	0	1	0.03	0.18	0	1	0.18	0.38	0	1	0.06	0.23	0	1
Political party	0.02	0.13	0	1	0.01	0.08	0	1	0.02	0.14	0	1	0.01	0.09	0	1
Nationality	0.03	0.17	0	1	0.10	0.30	0	1	0.06	0.25	0	1	0.02	0.12	0	1
Family status	0.38	0.49	0	1	0.29	0.45	0	1	0.35	0.48	0	1	0.42	0.49	0	1
Social class	0.02	0.13	0	1	0.05	0.21	0	1	0.05	0.21	0	1	0.07	0.26	0	1
Part of country	0.05	0.21	0	1	0.04	0.20	0	1	0.04	0.19	0	1	0.02	0.13	0	1
Race/Ethnicity	0.06	0.25	0	1	0.05	0.22	0	1	0.04	0.20	0	1	0.04	0.19	0	1
Values																
Personal benevolence	4.74	0.99	1	6	4.58	0.99	1	6	4.82	1.06	1	6	4.10	1.02	1	6
Personal universalism	4.52	1.12	1	6	4.53	1.07	1	6	4.84	1.06	1	6	4.27	0.97	1.5	6
In-group benevolence	0.38	0.49	0	1	0.17	0.38	0	1	0.35	0.48	0	1	0.27	0.45	0	1
In-group universalism	0.27	0.44	0	1	0.43	0.50	0	1	0.39	0.49	0	1	0.44	0.50	0	1

Measures

In-Group Identification

This variable is measured with the following question taken from the International Social Survey Program 2003 (ISSP Research Group 2003): "We are all part of different groups. Some are more important to us than others when we think of ourselves. In general, which in the following list is most important to you in describing who you are?" The respondents were provided with ten categories to choose from: occupation, race, gender, age, religion, political party, nationality, family status, social class, and the part of America/France/Turkey/Korea they live in.

Attributing Altruistic Values to the Self and In-Group Members

Individual Values We used two values that fell under self-transcendence value domain from the 21-item Portrait Values Questionnaire (PVQ) (Schwartz et al. 2001) to measure two altruistic values: benevolence and universalism. The PVQ includes verbal portraits of 21 different people, gender-matched with the respondent. Respondents indicate how much that person is like them on a six-item scale ranging from "very much like me" to "not like me at all." An individual's scores for benevolence values are the average of two items: (1) It's very important to her/him to help the people around her/him. She/he wants to care for their wellbeing. (2) It is important to her/him to be loyal to her/his friends. She/he wants to devote herself/himself to people close to her/him. For universalism values, the following two items were used: (1) She/he thinks it is important that every person in the world be treated equally. She/he believes everyone should have equal opportunities in life. (2) It is important to her/him to listen to people who are different from her/him. Even when she/he disagrees with them, she/he still wants to understand them.

In-Group Values We present a novel measurement of identifying the most and the least important values attributed to in-group members (See Fig. 9.2). We asked people to (a) select valued in-groups ("in-group identification"), then to (b) report the values that they think members of those groups hold as most important from the diagram in Fig. 9.2. In our analysis, we focus on values that respondents chose as most important. In original survey we have 10 Schwartz value labels, and our measure for altruistic values only includes two Schwartz values: benevolence and universalism (1 = selected, 0 = not selected).

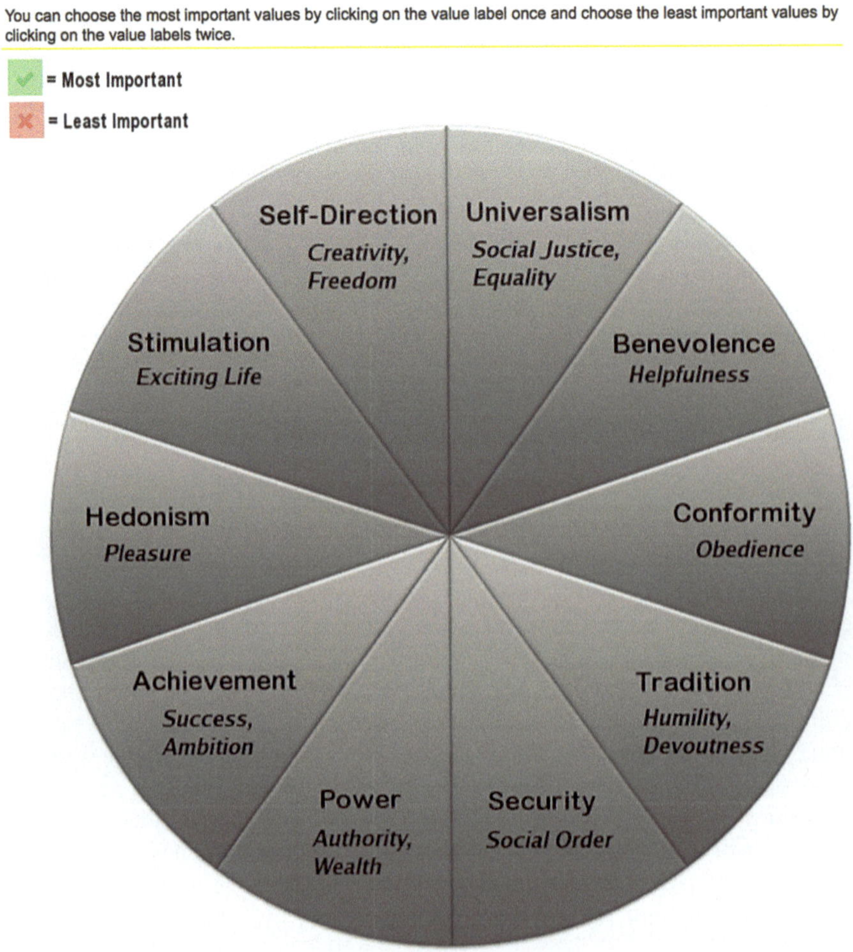

Fig. 9.2 Measurement of group values – clicking on a section turns it to the color of a tiny box in the *upper left corner*

Demographics

We control for several demographic variables that were shown to be related to personal values by previous research including age, gender (1 = male, 0 = female), racial/ethnic majority (1 = white in the U.S. and France; Turkish in Turkey, 0 = non-white in the U.S. and France; non-Turkish in Turkey), highest degree of education completed, household income, marital status (1 = married, 0 = not married), religiosity and political ideology. Education was included as a dummy variable (1 = college or above). Religiosity is measured with an 11-point Likert scale ranging from 0 "not at all religious" to 10 "very religious." Political ideology is measured with an 11-point Likert scale (higher values indicate right-wing orientation).

Results

Demographic characteristics of each country are summarized in Table 9.1 below. As can be seen from this table, average age in the United States and France is quite similar (46), while in South Korea age is slightly lower (43) and in Turkey quite a bit younger (34). These age distributions are relatively similar to the age distributions in respective country populations as according to the CIA World Factbook 2016 estimates. Overall samples from all countries are highly educated. While in the United States, college completion rate of 42% compared similarly to the population average of 44%; other countries ranked well above population averages with French sample ranking 20%, Turkish sample ranking 50% and Korean sample ranking 19% above the population rates (source for population education rates: OECD 2016). This educational discrepancy, which is especially visible in Turkey, is probably due to the higher access of younger and educated people to the internet.

With regard to in-group identifications, family status and occupation are reported as the most valued in-groups across our four nation samples. When we turn our attention to altruistic values, we see that personal benevolence and universalism were ranked equally high in all samples. The highest percentage of attributing benevolence to in-groups was observed in the United States and Turkey (38% and 35% respectively), followed by Korea (27%) and France (17%). For attributing universalism to the in-groups on the other hand, France, Turkey, and Korea ranked relatively similar (43%, 39% and 44% respectively), while the United States scored relatively lower—27%.

Tables 9.2 and 9.3 present OLS regression results on the effects of social benevolent and universalistic dispositions, respectively.

Table 9.2 shows that in the United States, France, and Korea, those who identify with benevolent in-groups are more likely to value the welfare of close friends and family members in their own lives, suggesting a linkage between a benevolent social identity and a benevolent personal identity. The effect of in-group benevolence is statistically significant in these three countries on benevolent value dispositions ($p < .05$), even after controlling for the types of in-group with which a respondent identifies. In Turkey, whether a person believes her/his in-group is benevolent or helpful is not statistically associated with personal disposition of caring about the welfare of close others. Instead, which group a person identifies with matters for the personal inclination of valuing benevolence among Turks: if a person identifies with the family status, people with the same religion, the same occupation, or the same nationality, the person tends to care for close other's welfare than those who chose other in-group types in Turkey. These results partially support our assertion that identifying with an in-group that prioritizes altruistic values such as benevolence (an altruistic social identity) will contribute to the development of an altruistic personal identity.

Table 9.3 presents OLS regression results on the effects of social universalistic disposition on personal universalism. We find supporting evidence across the United States, France and Turkey, where identifying with an in-group that values social

Table 9.2 OLS regression on personal benevolence

Variable	U.S.A. (N=437)	Variable	France (N=448)	Variable	Turkey (N=420)	Variable	Korea (N=449)
Group value and types							
In-group benevolence	0.212* (0.098)	In-group benevolence	0.309* (0.122)	In-group benevolence	0.080 (0.116)	In-group benevolence	0.571*** (0.107)
In-group types (ref=other groups		*In-group types (ref=other groups)*		*In-group types (ref=other groups*		*In-group types (ref=other groups)*	
Family	0.480*** (0.123)	Family	0.178 (0.128)	Family	0.382** (0.136)	Family	0.098 (0.131)
Occupation	0.235 (0.154)	Occupation	−0.012 (0.136)	Religion	0.540** (0.171)	Occupation	0.026 (0.143)
Religion	0.473** (0.167)	Gender	0.134 (0.154)	Occupation	0.431** (0.166)	Age	0.211 (0.201)
Gender	0.107 (0.182)	Nationality	−0.024 (0.171)	Nationality	0.820*** (0.228)	Social Class	−0.104 (0.205)
Socio-demographics							
Age	0.000 (0.003)	Age	−0.004 (0.003)	Age	−0.004 (0.005)	Age	0.011** (0.004)
Gender (1=Male)	−0.330*** (0.096)	Gender (1=Male)	−0.218* (0.096)	Gender (1=Male)	0.039 (0.106)	Gender (1=Male)	0.096 (0.093)
Racial majority (1=White)	−0.050 (0.118)	Racial majority (1=White)	−0.034 (0.140)	Racial majority (1=Turkish)	−0.188 (0.144)		
College	0.016 (0.102)	College	−0.018 (0.098)	College	0.048 (0.118)	College	0.032 (0.101)

Income	0.023 (0.017)	Income	0.019 (0.018)	Income	0.051** (0.019)	Income	0.045* (0.017)
Marital status (1 = Married)	−0.049 (0.110)	Marital status (1 = Married)	0.073 (0.106)	Marital status (1 = Married)	0.081 (0.118)	Marital status (1 = Married)	−0.102 (0.115)
Religiosity	0.012 (0.016)	Religiosity	0.028 (0.015)	Religiosity	0.015 (0.021)	Religiosity	0.040* (0.016)
Political ideology (Right-wing)	−0.020 (0.020)	Political ideology (Right-wing)	−0.060*** (0.017)	Political ideology (Right-wing)	0.004 (0.021)	Political ideology (Right-wing)	0.001 (0.020)
Constant	4.508*** (0.212)	Constant	4.873*** (0.225)	Constant	4.120*** (0.253)	Constant	2.989*** (0.214)
Adj. R^2	0.0959	Adj. R^2	0.0574	Adj. R^2	0.0505	Adj. R^2	0.1185

* $p < .05$, ** $p < .01$, *** $p < .001$

Table 9.3 OLS regression on personal universalism

Variable	U.S.A. (N=437)	Variable	France (N=448)	Variable	Turkey (N=420)	Variable	Korea (N=449)
Group Value and Types							
In-Group	0.462***	In-Group	0.226*	In-Group	0.212*	In-Group	0.059
Universalism	(0.123)	Universalism	(0.101)	Universalism	(0.106)	Universalism	(0.095)
In-Group Types (ref=other groups)		*In-Group Types (ref=other groups)*		*In-Group Types (ref=other groups)*		*In-Group Types (ref=other groups)*	
Family	0.252	Family	0.171	Family	0.558***	Family	0.130
	(0.141)		(0.136)		(0.134)		(0.131)
Occupation	0.220	Occupation	0.124	Religion	0.123	Occupation	0.032
	(0.177)		(0.144)		(0.165)		(0.143)
Religion	0.390*	Gender	0.097	Occupation	0.506**	Age	0.039
	(0.191)		(0.163)		(0.164)		(0.202)
Gender	0.246	Nationality	0.209	Nationality	0.646**	Social Class	−0.026
	(0.210)		(0.181)		(0.223)		(0.205)
Socio-demographics							
Age	−0.002	Age	−0.006	Age	−0.010*	Age	0.004
	(0.003)		(0.003)		(0.005)		(0.004)
Gender	−0.210	Gender	−0.207*	Gender	0.012	Gender	−0.098
(1=Male)	(0.110)	(1=Male)	(0.102)	(1=Male)	(0.104)	(1=Male)	(0.094)
Racial Majority	−0.156	Racial Majority	−0.095	Racial Majority	0.174		
(1=White)	(0.135)	(1=White)	(0.147)	(1=Turkish)	(0.142)		
College	0.033	College	0.088	College	−0.017	College	0.067
	(0.117)		(0.103)		(0.116)		(0.101)

Income	0.016	Income	−0.000	Income	0.057**	Income	−0.026
	(0.019)		(0.019)		(0.018)		(0.018)
Marital Status	−0.144	Marital Status	−0.022	Marital Status	−0.062	Marital Status	0.026
(1 = Married)	(0.127)	(1 = Married)	(0.112)	(1 = Married)	(0.116)	(1 = Married)	(0.116)
Religiosity	−0.012	Religiosity	0.008	Religiosity	−0.007	Religiosity	0.018
	(0.019)		(0.015)		(0.021)		(0.016)
Political Ideology	−0.050*	Political Ideology	−0.088***	Political Ideology	−0.018	Political Ideology	−0.054**
(Right-wing)	(0.024)	(Right-wing)	(0.018)	(Right-wing)	(0.021)	(Right-wing)	(0.020)
Constant	4.845***	Constant	5.169***	Constant	4.285***	Constant	4.347***
	(0.253)		(0.249)		(0.254)		(0.212)
Adj. R^2	0.0686	Adj. R^2	0.0838	Adj. R^2	0.0654	Adj. R^2	0.0068

* $p<.05$, ** $p<.01$, *** $p<.001$

equality and diversity (i.e., holding the caring social identity) is predictive of personal value orientations of emphasizing the value of social equality and diversity in one's own life ($p < .05$). However, in Korea neither in-group universalism value nor other in-group types show statistically significant effects on personal inclination of valuing equality and social diversity.

Conclusion and Discussion

In this chapter, we find support for our proposition that an altruistic social identity embedded in benevolent and universalistic value orientations implies a disposition to help or relieve the suffering of others. Previous empirical studies have documented the implications of holding altruistic value orientations for alleviating suffering. Possessing benevolent values is often linked to actions that might contribute to the welfare of immediate others or the community with which one identifies while holding universalistic values is associated with behaviors promoting equality and social diversity in an attempt to reduce major causes of social suffering such as social exclusion and discrimination.

Our empirical results from cross-cultural data showed that identifying with in-groups that prioritize altruistic values is closely linked to holding altruistic personal identities. This result supports our hypothesis that identifying with groups that value benevolence and caring has implications for the development of an altruistic personal identity. However, we also found interesting cross-cultural differences in the linkage between the altruistic social identity and personal identity. While the American and French regression results support the relationship between holding an altruistic social identity and exhibiting an altruistic personal identity for both benevolence and universalism, this relationship is only partially supported in Turkey and South Korea. In Turkey, identifying with universalistic in-groups shows a statistically significant influence on self-universalism, while identifying with benevolent in-groups does not have any significant effects on self-benevolence. Instead, the type of in-group that a person identifies with seems more important in predicting one's benevolent and caring personal identities in Turkey. These results might be partly due to the high traditionalist and religious context of the Turkish society (see for example Inglehart and Baker 2000 for a cross-national comparison of ethno-religious cultures) in which mere belonging (and conformity) to social groups becomes more important for personal development than reflecting on the group characteristics. In contrast, in South Korea identifying with benevolent in-groups is strongly associated with having a benevolent identity, while identifying with universalistic in-group is not statistically associated with a caring identity. Given the explanatory power of the regression on universalistic value orientation in the Korean sample is quite low, it seems like the model that helps us construe the sources of altruistic personal identities in the other three countries is not helpful to understand the universalistic personal identity in the Korean context. This could be partly understood in line with the collectivistic context of Korean society. The in-group culture may exert more powerful influence on the development of a person's benevolent personal identity in South Korea where social connectedness and harmony within in-groups is highly valued (Hofstede 2001). In contrast, the universalistic values that are not exclusively associated with one's important in-groups may provide relatively less influence on constructing a universalistic personal identity in the collectivistic Korean society.

Our findings suggest that encouraging people to affiliate with the groups that value altruism (i.e. developing altruistic social identity) would be an important step for fostering altruistic personal identity that potentially leads to altruistic behaviors. One possible way to achieve this could be implementing educational interventions that aim to promote people's development of altruistic social and personal identities by promoting their affiliation with altruistic social groups such as volunteer or humanitarian community organizations. Individuals are motivated to verify the identity standards (the perceived group values in our case) they receive from their important in-groups (Burke 1991; Stets 2006), and this process is particularly vital in the development of self at early ages (e.g. Mead 1934). For example, classroom is an important place of socialization to encourage the development of altruistic social and personal identities of children: teachers can develop activities that increase student's awareness of the concept of altruism and the importance of identifying with benevolent, caring groups, or that help students solve problems by caring (Robinson and Curry 2005). By building altruistic, caring culture in classrooms that encourages affiliation with altruistic social groups, students will be exposed to the value of altruism and develop altruistic social and personal identities as they grow up.

Second, emphasizing family values such as caring and nurturing could be another significant way to foster altruistic social identity. Family is the very first and important source of social identity. Family formation and the relationship between parents and children for the most part rely on the value of caring and nurturing (Nelson et al. 2011; Openshaw et al. 1984). In our samples, family status is chosen as the most important source of our respondents' social identities across four nations (38% of the American respondents, 29% of French respondents, 35% of Turkish respondents, and 42% of Korean respondents are identified with family). Given this, reinforcement of family values and participation would be helpful for promoting the development of altruistic social identity. Despite this importance of family and family values as a source of one's altruistic personal and social identities, previous research documented that parents in many countries have hardly invested enough time in their family because of managing their careers (Aycan 2011; Greenhaus and Beutell 1985). Thus, we argue that implementing policies that help keep a balance between work and family is not only helpful for our generation's well-being, but also helpful for alleviating the suffering of others in the next generation as it helps revive the role of family and promotes altruistic values.

There are several future implications of the current work. First, while we have examined the effects of social identities on personal identities, it is also possible that the causality of the relationship goes in the opposite direction such that social identity may be a product of personal identity. For example, people who hold altruistic personal identity may be more likely to identify with altruistic in-groups. Future research should investigate this issue of causality. Second, while our chapter demonstrated the links between altruistic personal and social identities, the effects of these altruistic dispositions on self-sacrificing or benevolent behavior to alleviate suffering were not explored. As previous work has articulated, there are three main categories of suffering: physical suffering (pain such as soreness and discomfort), mental suffering (emotional and cognitive pain including distress, depression and frustration) and social suffering (suffering caused by social institutions or social forces, e.g., social exclusion and discrimination) (Anderson 2014; Kleinman et al. 1997). Future research can shed light on what types of altruistic self and value dispositions, in the context of different situations, lead to different types of suffering alleviation.

Acknowledments This material is based upon work supported by the U. S. Department of Defense Minerva Initiative (2013), the U. S. Army Research Laboratory and the U. S. Army Research Office under contract/grant number W911NF1310342.

References

Alwin, D. F. (1986). Religion and parental child-rearing orientations: Evidence of a catholic-protestant convergence. *American Journal of Sociology, 92*(2), 412–440.

Anderson, R. E. (2014). Conceptualizing human pain and suffering. In R. E. Anderson (Ed.), *Human suffering and quality of life* (pp. 1–16). Dordrecht: Springer.

Anderson, R. E. (2015). How suffering challenges our future. In R. E. Anderson (Ed.), *World suffering and quality of life* (pp. 427–439). Dordrecht: Springer.

Aycan, Z. (2011). Cross-cultural approaches to work-family. In K. Korabik & D. Lero (Eds.), *Handbook of work-family conflict: Research, theory, and best practices* (pp. 359–371). London: Cambridge University Press.

Bardi, A., & Schwartz, S. H. (2003). Values and behavior: Strength and structure of relations. *Personality and Social Psychology Bulletin, 29*(10), 1207–1220.

Batson, C. D., & Shaw, L. L. (1991). Evidence for altruism: Toward a pluralism of prosocial motives. *Psychological Inquiry, 2*(2), 107–122.

Becker, H. S., & Strauss, A. L. (1956). Careers, personality, and adult socialization. *American Journal of Sociology, 62*(3), 253–263.

Burke, P. J. (1991). Identity processes and social stress. *American Sociological Review, 56*, 836–849.

Burke, P. J. (2004). Identities and social structure: The 2003 Cooley-Mead award address. *Social Psychology Quarterly, 67*(1), 5–15.

Cooley, C. H. (1902). *Human nature and the social order*. New York: Scribner's.

Finkelstein, M. A., Penner, L. A., & Brannick, M. T. (2005). Motive, role identity, and prosocial personality as predictors of volunteer activity. *Social Behavior and Personality: An International Journal, 33*(4), 403–418.

Greenhaus, J. H., & Beutell, N. J. (1985). Sources of conflict between work and family roles. *Academy of Management Review, 10*(1), 76–88.

Hitlin, S. (2003). Values as the core of personal identity: Drawing links between two theories of self. *Social Psychology Quarterly, 66*(2), 118–137.

Hitlin, S. (2007). Doing good, feeling good: Values and the self's moral center. *The Journal of Positive Psychology, 2*(4), 249–259.

Hitlin, S., & Piliavin, J. A. (2004). Values: Reviving a dormant concept. *Annual Review of Sociology, 30*, 359–393.
Hofstede, G. (2001). *Culture's consequences: Comparing values, behaviors, institutions and organizations across nations*. Thousand Oaks: Sage.
Howard, J. A. (1995). Attitudes, beliefs and behavior. In K. S. Cook, G. A. Fine, & J. S. House (Eds.), *Sociological perspectives on social psychology* (pp. 90–117). Boston: Allyn and Bacon.
Inglehart, R., & Baker, W. E. (2000). Modernization, cultural change, and the persistence of traditional values. *American Sociological Review, 65*(1), 19–51.
ISSP Research Group. (2003). *International social survey programme: National identity II*. Cologne: ISSP Research Group.
Johnston, N. E. (2015). Healing suffering: The evolution of caring practices. In E. A. Ronald (Ed.), *World suffering and quality of life* (pp. 101–113). Dordrecht: Springer.
Karp, D. G. (1996). Values and their effect on pro-environmental behavior. *Environment and Behavior, 28*(1), 111–133.
Kleinman, A., Das, V., & Lock, M. M. (1997). *Social suffering*. Berkeley: University of California Press.
Kohn, M. L., & Schooler, C. (1969). Class, occupation, and orientation. *American Sociological Review, 34*(5), 659–678.
Lee, L., Piliavin, J. A., & Call, V. R. A. (1999). Giving time, money, and blood: Similarities and differences. *Social Psychology Quarterly, 62*(3), 276–290.
McCall, G. J. (2003). The me and the not-me: Positive and negative poles of identity. In P. J. Burke, T. J. Owens, R. T. Serpe, & P. A. Thoits (Eds.), *Advances in identity theory and research* (pp. 11–25). New York: Kluwer Academic/Plenum.
Mead, G. H. (1934). Mind, self, and society: From the perspective of a social behaviorist. In C. W. Morris (Ed.), *Introduction*. Chicago: University of Chicago Press.
Mike Robinson, E. H., & Curry, J. R. (2005). Promoting altruism in the classroom. *Childhood Education, 82*(2), 68–73.
Nelson, L. J., Padilla-Walker, L. M., Christensen, K. J., Evans, C. A., & Carroll, J. S. (2011). Parenting in emerging adulthood: An examination of parenting clusters and correlates. *Journal of Youth and Adolescence, 40*(6), 730–743.
OECD Statistics. (2016). Educational attainment and labour-force status. http://stats.oecd.org/#
Openshaw, D. K., Thomas, D. L., & Rollins, B. C. (1984). Parental influences of adolescent self-esteem. *The Journal of Early Adolescence, 4*(3), 259–274.
Pearlin, L. I., & Kohn, M. L. (1966). Social class, occupation, and parental values: A cross-national study. *American Sociological Review, 31*(4), 466–479.
Piliavin, J. A., & Callero, P. L. (1991). *Giving blood: The development of an altruistic identity*. Johns Hopkins University Press.
Putnam, R. D. (2001). *Bowling alone: The collapse and revival of American community*. New York: Simon and Schuster.
Radkiewicz, P., De Zavala, A., & Skarżyńska, K. (2008). Pro-social basic human values and civic involvement. The moderating role of survival vs self-expression cultural context. *Polish Psychological Bulletin, 39*(4), 226–235.
Rokeach, M. (1973). *The nature of human values*. New York: Free Press.
Schopenhauer, A. (2004). *On the suffering of the world*. London: Penguin Great Ideas.
Schwartz, S. H. (1992). Universals in the content and structure of values: Theoretical advances and empirical tests in 20 countries. *Advances in Experimental Social Psychology, 25*(1), 1–65.
Schwartz, S. H. (1994). Are there universal aspects in the structure and contents of human values? *Journal of Social Issues, 50*(4), 19–45.
Schwartz, S. H. (2007a). Universalism values and the inclusiveness of our moral universe. *Journal of Cross-Cultural Psychology, 38*(6), 711–728.
Schwartz, S. H. (2007b). Value orientations: Measurement, antecedents and consequences across nations. In C. Roberts, R. Jowell, & R. Fitzgerald (Eds.), *Measuring attitudes cross-nationally: Lessons from the European social survey* (pp. 169–203). Los Angeles/London: Sage.

Schwartz, S. H. (2010). Basic values: How they motivate and inhibit prosocial behavior. In M. Mikulincer & P. R. Shaver (Eds.), *Prosocial motives, emotions, and behavior: The better angels of our nature* (pp. 221–241). Washington, DC: American Psychological Association.

Schwartz, S. H. (2012). An overview of the Schwartz theory of basic values. *Online Readings in Psychology and Culture, 2*(1), 11.

Schwartz, S. H., & Bardi, A. (2001). Value hierarchies across cultures taking a similarities perspective. *Journal of Cross-Cultural Psychology, 32*(3), 268–290.

Schwartz, S. H., & Bilsky, W. (1987). Toward a universal psychological structure of human values. *Journal of Personality and Social Psychology, 53*, 550–562.

Schwartz, S. H., & Boehnke, K. (2004). Evaluating the structure of human values with confirmatory factor analysis. *Journal of Research in Personality, 38*(3), 230–255.

Schwartz, S. H., Melech, G., Lehmann, A., Burgess, S., Harris, M., & Owens, V. (2001). Extending the cross-cultural validity of the theory of basic human values with a different method of measurement. *Journal of Cross-Cultural Psychology, 32*(5), 519–542.

Stern, P. C. (1992). Psychological dimensions of global environmental change. *Annual Review of Psychology, 43*(1), 269–302.

Stets, J. E. (2006). Identity theory. In P. Burke (Ed.), *Contemporary social psychological theories* (pp. 88–110). Stanford: Stanford University Press.

Stets, J. E. (2010). The social psychology of the moral identity. In *Handbook of the sociology of morality* (pp. 385–409). New York: Springer.

Stets, J. E., & Burke, P. J. (2000). Identity theory and social identity theory. *Social Psychology Quarterly, 63*(3), 224–237.

Stets, J. E., & Carter, M. J. (2011). The moral self applying identity theory. *Social Psychology Quarterly, 74*(2), 192–215.

Stets, J. E., & Carter, M. J. (2012). A theory of the self for the sociology of morality. *American Sociological Review, 77*(1), 120–140.

Stocks, E. L., Lishner, D. A., & Decker, S. K. (2009). Altruism or psychological escape: Why does empathy promote prosocial behavior? *European Journal of Social Psychology, 39*(5), 649–665.

Stryker, S. (2000). Identity competition: Key to differential social movement involvement. In S. Stryker, T. Owens, & R. White (Eds.), *Identity, self, and social movements* (pp. 21–40). Minneapolis: University of Minnesota Press.

Stryker, S. (2008). From Mead to a structural symbolic interactionism and beyond. *Annual Review of Sociology, 34*, 15–31.

Sznaider, N. (2015). Compassion, cruelty, and human rights. In R. E. Anderson (Ed.), *World suffering and quality of life* (pp. 55–64). Dordrecht: Springer.

Tajfel, H., & Turner, J. C. (1979). An integrative theory of intergroup conflict. In W. G. Austin & S. Worchel (Eds.), *The social psychology of intergroup relations* (pp. 33–47). Monterey: Brooks/Cole Pub. Co.

The World Factbook 2016–17. (2016). Washington, DC: Central Intelligence Agency. https://www.cia.gov/library/publications/the-world-factbook/index.html

Turner, J. C. (1975). Social comparison and social identity: Some prospects for intergroup behavior. *European Journal of Social Psychology, 5*, 5–34.

Turner, J. C. (1985). Social categorization and the self concept: A social cognitive theory of group behavior. In E. J. Lawler (Ed.), *Advances in group processes: Theory and research* (pp. 7–122). Greenwich: JAI Press.

Williams, C. R. (2008). Compassion, suffering and the self a moral psychology of social justice. *Current Sociology, 56*(1), 5–24.

Chapter 10
Grief Therapy as Intervening in Meaning: Principles and Practices

Robert A. Neimeyer

As a brilliant but troubled college student, Daniel had alternated between excelling in classes and succumbing to binges of drinking that challenged both his academic and social success. The decade that had followed college was similarly stormy, marked by lost jobs, a lost marriage and several rounds of treatment for substance abuse. Finally, in his early 30's, he moved back into his parents' home, stabilizing for a time before sliding back into the recurrent cycle of substance abuse.

It was in this context that Daniel arrived to his parents' home late one night, obviously inebriated, when his mother, Carol, met him. Exasperated, Carol broke off the ensuing confrontation between Daniel and his father about the son's behavior, suggesting that, "they all get to bed and return to the discussion in the morning." For Daniel, however, morning never came. As Carol began to worry about him as noon approached, she opened the door of his silent bedroom to a scene of horror instantly stamped in her mind: her son, tangled in the sheets, torso off the bed, the bedding awash in a swath of blood. Rushing to him as she screamed for her husband, she then attempted resuscitation as he called emergency services. Arriving to the scene within 20 min, the first responders hurried Daniel's unresponsive body to the hospital, where his death—apparently of drug overdose—was confirmed. Tormented by the horrific imagery of the death scene as well as her guilt for not having recognized his condition that fateful night, Carol sought therapy with me a few months later.

After inviting Carol to share photos of her son on her iPhone and hearing stories of both her pride and concern about his turbulent life, I was struck by the power of the death narrative to eclipse any sense of secure connection to her son "in spirit," though Carol was a religious person. I therefore introduced the possibility of doing a "slow motion replay" together of what she had seen, sensed, and suffered the

R.A. Neimeyer (✉)
Faculty of Psychology, University of Memphis,
400 Innovation Drive, Rm 202, Memphis, TN 38152-6400, USA
e-mail: neimeyer@memphis.edu

R.E. Anderson (ed.), *Alleviating World Suffering*, Social Indicators Research Series 67, DOI 10.1007/978-3-319-51391-1_10

morning she discovered her son's body, with the goal of helping her give voice to the silent story of the trauma, while being supported in managing the powerful emotions it triggered and in addressing the painful questions it posed. Bravely, Carol announced her readiness for this retelling, and we began with the events of the night before, the disturbed night of sleep for Carol that followed, and the careful unpacking in sensory detail of what unfolded as she, with increasing apprehension, opened her son's bedroom door. Braiding together the horrific images—the tangled body, the purple face, the splash of congealed red blood spilling from his mouth across the white sheets—with the associated feelings that welled up in her, we gradually walked through the experience, tracing its objective and subjective contours and the struggle to make sense of his death that ensued. Finally, as I asked what Carol would have done if she had been present to his dying, but unable to prevent it, she sobbed, "Just hold him, hold him... and tell him I loved him." Gently handing Carol a cushion, I watched as she spontaneously hugged it tightly to her chest and tearfully affirmed her love for her precious if imperfect child. After a few minutes, she set the pillow aside, dried her eyes, and noted how she felt "flooded with comfort" following the retelling, and less alone in a tragic story. As therapy continued, we then reflected on further healing steps that could be taken, including responsive engagement with the partly parallel, partly unique grief of her husband following a shared loss.

Introduction

As the historical Buddha recognized, the universality of suffering is the first of the "noble truths" of human existence, arising as it does from such root causes as poverty, old age, illness, and certainly the most ineluctable of all such causes, the inevitability of death itself. Indeed, in addition to anticipating and ultimately experiencing our own dying, nearly all people will contend across the course of their lifetimes with a litany of losses of others—parents and grandparents, friends and partners, siblings and too often children—and commonly will experience significant and sometimes sustained separation distress as a result. This existential condition of *being wired for attachment in a world of impermanence* gives rise to recurrent grief, and with it a risk of prolonged suffering that can for a substantial minority of the bereaved prove debilitating, and bring in its wake a cascade of other social and physical consequences that can be life limiting, and even life threatening (Neimeyer 2016a; Prigerson et al. 2009).

My goal in the present brief chapter is to build on my earlier discussion of research supporting a meaning-oriented perspective on grief-related suffering (Neimeyer 2015) by introducing and illustrating a selection of principles and practices to alleviate the anguish of loss, particularly in cases like Carol's, when the death is premature, violent, and in a word, traumatic. By highlighting the relevance of various evidence-informed models and methods and conveying them in clinical vignettes derived from my own work with clients, I hope to suggest something of the great range of therapeutic procedures that currently exist, which can be usefully organized within the frame of a meaning reconstruction model (Neimeyer 2016b).

Grief and the Quest for Meaning

Viewed in a constructivist perspective, grieving entails as a central process the *attempt to reaffirm or reconstruct a world of meaning that has been challenged by loss* (Neimeyer 2002). That is, a fundamental feature of human functioning is to seek order, pattern and significance in the events of our lives, and in the course of doing so to construct *a self-narrative*, a story of our life that we can make sense of, and that can make sense of us. The difficulty, of course, is that unwelcome change and loss repeatedly unsettle our best efforts to scaffold a story with consistent themes, goals and—perhaps most importantly—intimate others who give our lives meaning (Neimeyer and Young-Eisendrath 2015). The death of key attachment figures, especially under conditions that are premature, sudden, violent or unjust, therefore can massively challenge our assumptive world and its grounding in principles of predictability, beneficence and control (Janoff-Bulman and Berger 2000). Faced with an anguishing discrepancy between our core presuppositions and the reality of such loss, we are launched into a quest to reestablish or rebuild the meaning of our lives at practical, social, and often spiritual or existential levels.

Over the past decade a good deal of evidence has accumulated to support the propositions of this meaning reconstruction model (Neimeyer 2016b). For example, an inability to make sense of the loss has been associated with more intense symptoms of prolonged grief disorder in bereaved young adults (Holland et al. 2006). Likewise, in parents who have lost children, it accounts for as much as 15 times the variance in complicated grief symptomatology than does the passage of time (measured in weeks, months or years), the gender of the parent, or even whether the death was natural or violent (Keesee et al. 2008). In a cohort of older widowed persons, an unfulfilled struggle for meaning at 6 months after loss prospectively predicts higher levels of grief and depression a full 18 and 48 months later, whereas finding meaning early in bereavement predicts well-being and associated positive emotions 4 years after the death (Coleman and Neimeyer 2010). Similarly, mourners who across a period of months show greater capacity to make meaning of their experience also move toward lower levels of complicated grief (Holland et al. 2010), and such meaning making has "incremental validity" in predicting mental and physical health outcomes even after demographic characteristics, relationship to the deceased, manner of death and prolonged grief symptoms are taken into account (Holland et al. 2014). So powerful is the role of meaning making in predicting adjustment to bereavement that it accounts for essentially all of the difference between mourners who have lost loved ones to natural death, and those, like Carol, who have lost them to suicide, homicide and fatal accident (Currier et al. 2006). Likewise, in the palliative care context, a struggle to make sense of a loved one's pending death has proven to be a potent predictor of anticipatory grief, eclipsing the role of spiritual, relational, and demographic factors with which it also correlates (Burke et al. 2015). Just what such a search for meaning looks like in practical terms is conveyed in several of the actual clinical vignettes to follow, along with descriptions of the interventions that helped alleviate grief-related suffering through restoring some of the order and coherence of life stories that had been sundered by tragic loss.

A Narrative Frame for Pluralistic Practice

Just as classical (Kelly 1955) and contemporary constructivism (Neimeyer 2009) provide an integrative frame for psychotherapy in general, so too does a meaning reconstruction model of bereavement offer a flexible framework for addressing the specific goals of grief therapy. Viewed through a narrative constructivist lens, the pursuit of meaning making in loss concentrates on (1) *processing the "event story" of the death,* and its implications for our ongoing lives, and (2) *accessing the "back story" of our lives with the deceased loved one*, in a way that restores a measure of attachment security (Neimeyer and Thompson 2014). The former concentrates on integrating the story of the loss itself—what happened, how and why, including in many instances the complicated role of human or divine agency in bringing about the death. In contrast, the latter typically involves seeking to reconstruct rather than relinquish the emotional bond implied by the shared life story with the deceased, as well as the need to come to terms with its emotional "unfinished business." Each of these dialectics articulates with a range of contemporary bereavement theories and associated therapeutic practices, many of which are beginning to garner an evidence base that supports their efficacy.

Processing the Event Story of the Loss
When mourners struggle with making sense of the death and its implications for their lives, they may contend with questions like: *What is my role or responsibility in what has come to pass? What part, if any, did human intention or inattention have in causing the death? How do my religious or philosophic beliefs help me accommodate this experience, and how are they changed by it in turn? Who am I in light of this loss, now and in the future?* (Neimeyer and Thompson 2014). In other words, the "effort after meaning" can unfold on any scale from the focal (about a feature of the death itself or an internal feeling) to the global (about one's broader self-narrative or spiritual/existential concerns), as the mourner seeks to integrate the loss, and reconstruct his or her life. Two contemporary theories of grieving that dovetail with this perspective are Boelen and colleauges' (2006) cognitive-behavioral therapy (CBT) model and Stroebe and Schut's (1999, 2010) Dual Process Model of Coping with Bereavement.

From a CBT perspective, grief becomes complicated when mourners *fail to integrate the reality of the death into their autobiographical memory*, in effect, when they are unable to update their schemas to take in the painful circumstance of their loved one's absence (Boelen et al. 2006). This situation is often compounded by various forms of *experiential avoidance*, as when mourners attempt to mitigate intense grief by evading memories of the dying, or by no longer engaging in activities that were once associated strongly with the loved one.

A second conceptualization that conjoins with a meaning reconstruction approach is the Dual Process Model (DPM), which posits two fundamental orientations in coping with bereavement (Stroebe and Schut 1999, 2010). On the one hand, mourners engage the *loss orientation*, in which they reflect on the death, and attempt to modulate grief-related feelings, reorganize their bond to the deceased, and withdraw from the broader world to seek the support of a few trusted confidants. At other points, they engage in the *restoration orientation*, as they distract themselves from their grief by immersing themselves in work and other activities, step into new responsibilities, and ultimately explore new roles and goals required by their changed lives. Thus, according to the DPM, mourners *oscillate* between these two means of coping with the loss, though people differ in their degree of engagement with each as a function of personal disposition, family roles, gender and culture.

Common to these models is the view that complications in grieving arise when mourners are unable to "take in" the reality of the loss, and integrate its implications for their ongoing lives. Accordingly, a number of evidence-based procedures have been developed to promote doing so, which are featured in a variety of cognitive-behavioral, eclectic, and narrative constructivist therapies, as summarized below.

Restorative Retelling of the Event Story of the Death

Survivors of a difficult loss typically seek a context in which they can relate the story of their loved one's death, but rarely do they give voice to its most painful particulars, which live only as "silent stories" (Neimeyer 2006) in their own thoughts and nightmares, persisting as a haunting and unspoken subtext to the highly edited stories shared with others.

In *restorative retelling*, Rynearson and his colleagues (Rynearson 2006; Rynearson and Salloum 2011) first establish a safe relational "container" in the therapeutic relationship, by grounding the mourner in a more secure context (e.g., discussing what family members meant to one another before the loss, and what philosophic or religious beliefs they have relied on to deal with difficult times), before inviting a step-by-step recounting of the narrative of the dying. Like Shear's protocol for *situational revisiting* of the story of the death (Shear et al. 2011), This procedure encourages the mourner to "walk through" a slow-motion replay of the events of the dying, often repeating the process on multiple occasions as the person fills in details, modulates difficult emotions with the therapist's assistance, and gradually gains greater mastery of the painful narrative. In both cases the goal is to help the mourner integrate the story of the death in the presence of a compassionate witness, ultimately across several sessions being able to revisit the story with less avoidant coping, less emotional reactivity, and greater meaning. As such, this guided and evocative recounting of the story of the dying represents a direct attempt to alleviate suffering associated with a traumatizing loss by mastering its painful particulars, giving them voice in a supportive context, and seeking greater coherence and intelligibility in the process. Further procedures to enhance the power of retelling are available elsewhere (Neimeyer 2012c).

Data from an open trial on restorative retelling are encouraging in suggesting its efficacy in reducing traumatic arousal (Saindon et al. 2014), and Shear's Complicated Grief Therapy (CGT), in which revisiting the situation of the death is a cardinal procedure, has outperformed evidence-based therapy for depression in treating bereaved people in two major randomized clinical trials (Shear et al. 2005, 2014). Related cognitive-behavioral protocols featuring prolonged exposure to difficult details associated with the loss have also garnered support in RCTs (Boelen et al. 2007; Bryant et al. 2014).

An illustration of restorative retelling arose in the therapy of Luisa, who had struggled for several months to balance the needs of her 2-year-old son, her demanding work as an executive, and her husband Victor's treatment-resistant depression, which grew in severity with his drinking after several years of seemingly happy marriage. One fateful morning after taking their child to day care on her way to the office, she received a series of perturbing texts from Victor that she interpreted as a veiled suicide threat. Upon receiving no reply to her panicked phone calls to him, Luisa called the police and immediately rushed home to a silent house, the smell of gunpowder hanging in the air as she dashed through the back door. It was in the living room that Luisa discovered her husband's lifeless body slumped in his easy chair, the blood still trickling from one side of his head where the bullet had exited, with brain tissue splashed against the opposite wall. In the fog of anguish that followed, she somehow continued to function with the loving support of family and friends, but found it impossible to shake the haunting imagery of her husband's dying, and the equally troubling meaning of his suicidal choice.

After spending our initial sessions shoring up her coping and appreciatively reviewing photographs of her family in better times, we turned toward a detailed retelling of the event story of the death, beginning with the texts and continuing through her discovery of Victor's body, the arrival of the police and EMTs, and finally her cleaning up after the death scene with her brother's help. In the 40 min allotted to the retelling we specifically included the traumatic sensory particulars of the experience, as well as her inner landscape of emotion, and her desperate efforts to make sense of what had happened, pausing frequently to "breathe through" the most difficult parts, replaying them in her mind's eye and in her spoken narrative until she could recount them with less reactivity. In a subsequent session she brought in the sealed autopsy report from the coroner, sensing a need to review and take in its medical explanation of the context of the dying, but also terrified to do so alone. Slowly, across the course of the hour, I silently reviewed each section of the report, described its focus, and asked Luisa if she were ready to hear what each had to contribute to the narrative of the dying. Once again breathing through the painful details (e.g., the path of the bullet through various centers in Victor's brain, the great volume of alcohol in his internal organs), she gradually augmented her understanding of his mental and physical status at the time of his death. Ultimately she was able to begin to grasp the tragedy of his dying, but also imagine chapters in her own life story and that of her child that did not end with her husband's life.

Directed Journaling

Written as well as spoken narratives that bear on the loss experience can promote integration and meaning making, and have the advantage of being used either as self-help procedures as in Internet blogs or as therapist-assigned homework to augment the effectiveness of professional therapy. Two such forms of *directed journaling* foster *sense-making* and *benefit-finding*, respectively (Lichtenthal and Neimeyer 2012). In the former, clients who are some months or years into bereavement are encouraged to focus on questions about how and why the loss occurred, and what it portends for their lives. Prompts might include: *How did you make sense of the loss when it occurred? How do you interpret it now? How does this experience fit with your spiritual views about life, and how, if at all, have you changed those views in light of the loss? How has this loss shaped your life, and what meaning would you like it to have for you in the long run?* In contrast, benefit-finding journaling could be prompted by questions such as: *In your view, have you found any unsought gifts in grief? If so, what? How has this experience affected your sense of priorities? Your sense of yourself? What strengths in yourself or in others have you drawn on to get through this difficult transition? What lessons about living or about loving has this loss taught you? Has this experience deepened your gratitude for anything you've been given?* A randomized controlled trial of both forms of directed journaling compared to a standard expressive writing paradigm and a neutral control condition has established its efficacy and the maintenance of improvement over a 3-month follow up, with the impact of such writing being particularly impressive in the benefit-finding condition (Lichtenthal and Cruess 2010). Furthermore, a recent open trial of a Buddhist-inspired workshop for loss and unwelcome change integrated exercises in deep-listening, hearing one's loss story related to the group by a partner, brief interludes of mindfulness, and imaginative writing about themes of loss from a make-believe, self-distancing viewpoint to promote perspective taking (Neimeyer and Young-Eisendrath 2015). Group participants not only reported significantly relief from grief-related suffering, but also greater integration of the loss experience on a validated measure of meaning making (Holland et al. 2010).

Following the drowning death of her boyfriend when they were boating together on a summer holiday, Linda was tormented by memories of the event, as well as self-accusatory thoughts about what she hypothetically could have done to prevent the tragedy. Moreover, her keen separation distress was further fueled by her sense of the tragic incompleteness of their relationship, as they had just begun to talk about marriage and raising a family. As she tearfully poured out her "frozen grief" some 6 months after his death, Linda found that her loss of her partner was compounded by her loss of faith in God, though she considered herself a religious person. Angry and bitter, she had begun to lapse into cynicism about life in general, to the point of disengaging emotionally from the vulnerable patients to whom she attended in her work as a nurse. It was at this point that she recognized that, far from healing her wounds, the passage of time was simply deepening her loneliness, guilt and resentment, and that professional assistance was necessary.

In the course of restorative retelling of the traumatic loss in our therapy, Linda spontaneously began to keep a journal about the tragedy and what it meant to her. As she did so with my encouragement, she not only gave voice to her pain, but began also to understand "the gifts of grief," including her powerful recognition of how deeply she had been loved by her boyfriend and how loyal her closest friends and family had been throughout her challenging course of bereavement. Although she continued to harbor questions about God's intention in taking her lover from her, she found consolation in the sense that she had tenderly cared for him in life, and might one day be reunited with him in heaven. Ironically, she noted, even capturing the story in words was itself comforting, as this guaranteed that she "would never lose it," but instead could see it as a tragic chapter in a larger life story that continued to hold meaning going forward. In this, journaling helped her consolidate and find new meaning in the story of loss, which arose from her own deep engagement with its retelling, rather than relying on interpretations provided by the therapist.

Accessing the Back Story of the Relationship

In meaning reconstruction terms, bereaved people seek not only reaffirmation or rebuilding of a self-narrative challenged by loss, but also reconnection to the life narrative of their deceased loved one. In sharp distinction to the cultural prescription to "move on" and "withdraw energy from the one who has died to invest it elsewhere," such an approach endorses the normative goal of reconstructing the bond to the deceased rather than relinquishing it (Neimeyer 2001). When mourners seek to access the "back story" of their relationship with the loved one, they grapple with implicit questions like: *How can I recover or reconstruct a sustaining connection with my loved one that survives his or her death? What memories of the relationship bring pain, guilt or sadness, and require some form of redress or reprieve now? How might this forgiveness be sought or given? What memories of the relationship bring joy, security or pride, and invite celebration and commemoration? What lessons about living or loving have I learned during the course of our shared lives? What would my loved one see in me that would give him or her confidence in my ability to weather this hard transition?* (Neimeyer and Thompson 2014). Two additional theories that subscribe to a similar view of the continuing bond as a potentially adaptive resource (Klass et al. 1996) are narrative therapy (Hedtke and Winslade 2004) and the Two-Track Model of Bereavement (TTMB) (Rubin 1999).

According to a narrative therapy perspective anchored in the work of Michael White and David Epston, the dominant cultural narrative that views death only through a lens of loss and presses for "closure" and "letting go" does violence to the relational web that sustains love and community, even beyond the physical presence of the other. Thus, rather than advocating "saying goodbye" as the dominant metaphor for grief work, the goal of bereavement support becomes to "say hello again," in a sense restoring (and re-storying) a "conversation" with and about the loved one that was interrupted by death (Hedtke and Winslade 2004). Support groups conducted along these lines therefore concentrate not solely on expressing and coping with painful grief-related affect associated with those who were lost, but instead on fostering *remembering conversations* that celebrate the continued relevance of the relationship to the deceased in the lives of survivors (Hedtke 2012a). From this vantage point group facilitators might well prompt members with invitations to "introduce their loved ones" to the group (Hedtke 2012b), using questions such as *Who was ____ to you? What did knowing ____ mean to you? Do particular stories come to mind that ____ would want others to know about his life? What did ____ teach you about life, and perhaps about managing the circumstances you face currently? What difference might it make to keep her memory close to you?* From this perspective the mourner is encouraged to retain a vital connection to the loved one, carrying forward his or her symbolic and social presence in the mourner's own life story.

The Two-Track Model of Bereavement (TTMB) adopts a similar ethic, but stretches it in more clinical directions. In the work of Rubin and his colleagues (Rubin et al. 2009), adaptation to bereavement proceeds along two tracks simultaneously, with challenges and impediments arising on either or both. The first and more visible is the track of *biopsychosocial functioning*, which comprises much of the manifest symptomatology of grieving—depression, anxiety, changed relationships with others, a diminished sense of self, somatic concerns and impaired functioning in work and other social roles. It is problems that occur at this level that frequently draw the attention of concerned friends and family, and that constitute the most obvious targets of intervention for professionals. But it is the second track, concerned with the ongoing *relationship with the deceased*, which represents the distinctive contribution of the TTMB. Here, the focus is not merely on the historical character of the relationship with the loved one, but also on how it continues to find expression in significant affect evoked when memories are revisited or triggered, in spontaneous storytelling or ritual connection to the deceased, and on relevant strengths and conflicts in the relationship that invite attention in the course of therapy. By directing assessment and intervention to both tracks of the model, the TTMB extends the predominant concern with symptom management in grief therapy, offering a variety of practices for relational work between the mourner and the deceased (Rubin et al. 2011). Two such procedures derived from humanistic and expressive therapies illustrate this focus.

Imaginal Dialogues

As a performative intervention, fostering imaginal dialogues with the bereaved goes beyond talking *about* the deceased, and conjures the prospect of talking *to* the deceased in an experientially intense, emotionally "real" way. "Invoking an alliance with the deceased" in a triadic, rather than merely dyadic, relationship between therapist and client (Rynearson 2012) can take many forms, including "corresponding" with the dead about the mourner's present state, unanswered questions, and relational needs (e.g., for forgiveness or the affirmation of love) (Neimeyer 2012b) and guided imagery to conjure the loved one's presence (Jordan 2012). One particularly potent intervention along these lines draws on *chair work* procedures developed within emotion-focused therapy (Greenberg 2010), in which the client is encouraged to place the deceased symbolically in an empty chair facing the client's own, and address concerns in the relationship in a first- and second-person, present tense voice (e.g., "*I feel so lost since your death.... You were the only one who really understood and cared.*"). In most cases the client is then encouraged to switch chairs, loan the loved one his or her own voice, and respond as the deceased might to the client's statements. The therapist choreographs the continuing exchange, prompting the client toward emotional immediacy, honesty and depth in each chair, and directing a change of positions at poignant moments in the dialogue. Just as a theatrical drama performs a (usually scripted) story for an audience, so too imaginal dialogues invite performance of the implicit story of the client's relation to the deceased, but typically with the therapist and clients as the only audience. Detailed procedures for the introduction, performance and processing of chair work in the specific context of grief therapy are now available (Neimeyer 2012a).

Research on empty chair monologues by bereaved spouses documents the intimate link between themes of self- and other-blame in the chairing and a variety of adverse outcomes (e.g., guilt, depression, anger) (Field and Bonanno 2001). Moreover, Complicated Grief Therapy, which uses imaginal dialogues with the deceased as a mainstay intervention to resolve such issues, has proven more effective in the treatment of prolonged grief disorder than evidence-based therapy for depression in two randomized controlled trials (Shear et al. 2005, 2014).

Returning to the case with which this chapter opened, Carol had been primed to reconnect powerfully with her deceased son Daniel by the evocative retelling of the narrative of his death. There was so much left unsaid in his sudden and horrific dying, so much anger, so much helplessness, so much love. Taking the pillow that represented him from her hands as she offered it to me, I asked Carol if she felt ready to address those unspoken feelings and their associated questions directly to him, as I positioned the pillow in a comfortable leather chair positioned across from her. What followed was a moving, but increasingly coherent conversation between mother and son, as Carol accepted my invitation to both speak from her grieving heart and periodically to take Daniel's chair and offer a response. These responses, affirming his love for his mother, his regret for his addiction, and his hope for family healing did more to promote Carol's self-compassion, forgiveness for her son, and effort to make sense of his life and death than any wise interpretation or psychoeducational skills training I might have provided.

Legacy Work

A wide-angle lens survey of memorial practices across cultures speaks to the near-universal human impulse to recognize and honor the life story of the deceased. In this view anything that serves to preserve or extend that life story tends to alleviate our suffering over the loss, as research on the construction of the deceased person's identity in eulogies and other forms of commemoration suggests (Neimeyer et al. 2014). In the context of grief therapy this impulse can take the form of various photographic, scrapbooking, documentary, dramaturgical and narrative methods (Neimeyer 2012d), as well as a cornucopia of expressive arts techniques (Thompson and Neimeyer 2014). Therapists crafting uniquely relevant *rituals of continuity* or *rituals of affirmation* can draw upon guidelines formulated to help them do so (Doka 2012).

Among the biographical methods that can be helpful in giving meaning to the loved one's life and impact is the *legacy project*, which can serve to consolidate and communicate the story of the deceased (as in memorial blogs or biographies), or to draw upon his or her life or death to undertake some useful form of social action. In the latter case, legacy projects can be as simple as a random act of kindness in honor of the loved one, as by the bereaved mother who, sitting alone in a restaurant, discovered that the large party at the next table was celebrating a baby shower, and leaving in tears, prepaid the party's bill in honor of her child (Cacciatore 2012). Other legacy projects can take the form of sustained social action, as by families of homicide victims taking a stand against violence through pursuing public speaking, promoting safer communities, or offering support to others suffering analogous losses (Armour 2003). For them, such efforts reflected "a fierce commitment to their loved one. Besides being incensed by the needless loss of life, they value what his or her life stands for… [which] propel[s] them in directions that create meaning out of a senseless act" (pp. 531-532). Indeed, countless social justice initiatives have their origins in tragic loss, and the impulse of survivors to create a positive legacy that honors their loved one in its wake.

When their young adult son, Graham, died under ambiguous circumstances, Jennifer and Brian were plunged into a deep grief beyond anything they could have imagined. Grasping to articulate this ineffable desolation, Brian reflected on the "dark irony" "that this thing that so occupies my being, unquestionably the largest, heaviest, and most omnipresent thing I have ever encountered, is… an absence. It is an absence that is more present than the present…. Our lives are divided into many spheres, but by convention, we keep these separate. Yet Graham's absence infiltrates these disparate spheres with a laughing randomness, making a mockery of convention and throwing into great relief how absurd our petty attempts to compartmentalize life are under the glare of such overwhelming loss". Brian's contribution of his poignant reflections to this essay represented a means of honoring his son's life while also acknowledging his death. For her part, Jennifer organized a remarkably comprehensive, artistic, and up-to-date website with informative links to scores of web pages and blogs about grief and the loss of a child, available at http://www.scoop.it/t/grief-and-loss. Unobtrusively but significantly, she saluted her son in a small script at the top of the opening page: Ave, Graham, seed non vale [Hail, Graham, but not goodbye].

Coda

In this brief chapter I have attempted to sketch some of the principles and procedures that can animate the pluralistic practice of grief therapy. Under the umbrella of a meaning reconstruction model of mourning, I have suggested the further relevance of the Dual Process Model and the Two-Track Model of Bereavement, as well as narrative and cognitive behavioral perspectives to understanding some of the core features of processing this event story of the loss and accessing the back story of the changed relationship. Equally, I have tried to convey some of the great variety of clinical procedures, ranging from restorative retelling and directed journaling, to imaginal conversations and legacy work, which can add weight to the toolbox of practicing psychotherapists (Neimeyer 2012d, c). I hope that this framework serves as an open invitation for therapists of many countries and contexts of work to explore the field of grief therapy, as loss may be the one truly universal source of suffering that will touch the lives of every client they serve, usually repeatedly.

But in closing, it may be worth considering whether the pluralistic pursuit of a meaning-oriented grief therapy carries with it any constraints, or whether it implies a free-wheeling eclecticism constrained only by the creativity of the therapist. While this could appropriately be a topic for a chapter in itself, I want to signal my own acknowledgement of both poles of this implied dichotomy. That is, I personally find that the integration of different therapeutic methods feels more coherent when undertaken in a *theoretically progressive* framework, that is, one that considers the candidate theories from which different techniques are being borrowed to be in some sense consistent in their over-arching view of human beings and the enterprise we call psychotherapy (Neimeyer 1993). For example, as illustrated in the case vignettes related above, I can readily enough transition between emotion-focused methods derived from humanistic therapies and narrative procedures stemming from a constructivist or social constructionist epistemology in the course of my work with a given client (even in a single session). This is possible in part because of their coherence with a respectful appreciation of clients as motivated storytellers who are attempting to come to terms with life stories that feel violated or invalidated by loss. Narrative procedures that invite constructive grappling with the significance of the event story of the death and its meaning for their lives, whether written or oral, therefore comfortably find a place in my therapeutic toolbox. Likewise, techniques that foster an engagement with urgent questions about the back story of clients' relationship with the deceased or that embrace and extend its legacy, work together to reaffirm what had value in the loved one's life, and promote its continued relevance for the clients' future. Along with dozens of other specific methods that serve these ends, such techniques offer a plenitude of possibilities for relieving suffering associated with seemingly senseless loss.

On the other hand, even a broad definition of meaning-making in grief therapy does not embrace an "anything goes" eclecticism. Certainly random attempts at pluralism (e.g., drawing out clients anguished narratives of the death in restorative retelling, only to dispute the rationality or evidence base for their statements or conclusions) strike me as incoherent, and frankly aversive. Likewise, highly psychoeducational interventions that merely instruct clients to "stay busy" or modulate their distress through instruction in progressive relaxation strike me as at best incomplete in their focus on mere symptom management. Nor is the simple cathartic expression of grief-related emotion itself sufficient to alleviate suffering associated with bereavement. All of these attempts to simply *minimize* grief-related suffering without engaging its *meaning* fall short of promoting the growth through grief that can be fostered when the goal of bereavement is taken to be *relearning* rather than merely *recovery*.

Ultimately, however, my practice of grief therapy is informed by a large dose of pragmatism, leavened by my own sense of integrity, and a still deeper respect for the integrity of the client. By developing a strong sense of presence to our relationship, and attending to what a given client *needs* and *is ready for* at a given moment of therapy, I feel in the best position to select or co-construct with the client a way forward in language, experience and action that works for us both, as we seek to address the nuances of the loss, and configure a meaningful life beyond it. I trust that the reader will draw on a similar awareness of self and others to orient to the pluralistic practice of grief therapy.

References

Armour, M. (2003). Meaning making in the aftermath of homicide. *Death Studies, 27*, 519–540.

Boelen, P. A., van den Hout, M., & van den Bout, J. (2006). A cognitive-behavioral conceptualization of complicated grief. *Clinical Psychology: Science and Practice, 13*, 109–128.

Boelen, P. A., de Keijser, J., van den Hout, M., & van den Bout, J. (2007). Treatment of complicated grief: A comparison between cognitive-behavioral therapy and supportive counseling. *Journal of Clinical and Consulting Psychology, 75*, 277–284.

Bryant, R., Kenny, L., Joscelyne, A., Rawson, N., Maccallum, F., Cahill, C., Hopwood S, Aderka I, Nickerson, A. (2014). Treating prolonged gried disorder: A randomized clinical trial. *Journal of the American Medical Association Psychiatry*. doi:10.1001/jamapsychiatry.2014.1600.

Burke, L. A., Neimeyer, R. A., Smigelsky, M. A., Gibson, B. W., Ali, K. S., & Clark, K. A. (2015). Risk factors for anticipatory grief in family members of terminally ill veterans receiving palliative care services. *Journal of Social Work in End-of-Life & Palliative Care, 11*, 244–266. doi:10.1080/15524256.2015.1110071.

Cacciatore, J. (2012). The kindness project. In R. A. Neimeyer (Ed.), *Techniques of giref therapy: Creative practices for counseling the breaved* (pp. 329–331). New York: Routledge.

Coleman, R. A., & Neimeyer, R. A. (2010). Measuring meaning: Searching for and making sense of spousal loss in later life. *Death Studies, 34*, 804–834.

Currier, J. M., Holland, J. M., & Neimeyer, R. A. (2006). Sense making, grief and the experience of violent loss: Toward a mediational model. *Death Studies, 30*, 403–428.

Doka, K. (2012). Therapeutic ritual. In R. A. Neimeyer (Ed.), *Techniques of grief therapy: Creative practices for counseling the bereaved* (pp. 341–343). New York: Routledge.

Field, N. P., & Bonanno, G. A. (2001). The impact of self-blame and blame toward the deceased on adaptation to conjugal bereavement: A five-year follow-up. *American Behavioral Scientist, 44*, 764–781.

Greenberg, L. S. (2010). *Emotion focused psychotherapy*. Washington, DC: American Psychological Association.

Hedtke, L. (2012a). *Bereavement support groups: Breathing life into stories of the dead*. Chagrin Falls: Taos Institute Publications.

Hedtke, L. (2012b). Introducing the deceased. In R. A. Neimeyer (Ed.), *Techniques of grief therapy: Creative practices for counseling the bereaved* (pp. 253–255). New York: Routledge.

Hedtke, L., & Winslade, J. (2004). *Remembering lives*. Amityville: Baywood.

Holland, J. M., Currier, J. M., & Neimeyer, R. A. (2006). Meaning reconstruction in the first two years of bereavement: The role of sense-making and benefit-finding. *Omega, 53*, 173–191.

Holland, J. M., Currier, J. M., Coleman, R. A., & Neimeyer, R. A. (2010). The Integration of Stressful Life Experiences Scale (ISLES): Development and initial validation of a new measure. *International Journal of Stress Management, 17*, 325–352.

Holland, J. M., Currier, J. M., & Neimeyer, R. A. (2014). Validation of the integration of stressful life experiences scale – Short form in a bereaved sample. *Death Studies, 38*, 234–238. doi:10.1080/07481187.2013.829369.

Janoff-Bulman, R., & Berger, A. R. (2000). The other side of trauma. In J. H. Harvey & E. D. Miller (Eds.), *Loss and trauma*. Philadelphia: Brunner Mazel.

Jordan, J. R. (2012). Guided imaginal conversations with the deceased. In R. A. Neimeyer (Ed.), *Techniques of grief therapy* (pp. 262–265). New York: Routledge.

Keesee, N. J., Currier, J. M., & Neimeyer, R. A. (2008). Predictors of grief following the death of one's child: The contribution of finding meaning. *Journal of Clinical Psychology, 64*, 1145–1163.

Kelly, G. A. (1955). *The psychology of personal constructs*. New York: Norton.

Klass, D., Silverman, P. R., & Nickman, S. (1996). *Continuing bonds: New understandings of grief*. Washington: Taylor & Francis.

Lichtenthal, W. G., & Cruess, D. G. (2010). Effects of directed written disclosure on grief and distress symptoms among bereaved individuals. *Death Studies, 34*, 475–499.

Lichtenthal, W. G., & Neimeyer, R. A. (2012). Directed journaling to facilitate meaning making. In R. A. Neimeyer (Ed.), *Techniques of grief therapy* (pp. 161–164). New York: Routledge.

Neimeyer, R. A. (1993). Constructivism and the problem of psychotherapy integration. *Journal of Psychotherapy Integration, 3*, 133–157.

Neimeyer, R. A. (Ed.). (2001). *Meaning reconstruction and the experience of loss*. Washington, DC: American Psychological Association.

Neimeyer, R. A. (2002). *Lessons of loss: A guide to coping*. Memphis: Center for the Study of Loss and Transition.

Neimeyer, R. A. (2006). Narrating the dialogical self: Toward an expanded toolbox for the counselling psychologist. *Counselling Psychology Quarterly, 19*, 105–120.

Neimeyer, R. A. (2009). *Constructivist psychotherapy*. London/New York: Routledge.

Neimeyer, R. A. (2012a). Chair work. In R. A. Neimeyer (Ed.), *Techniques of grief therapy* (pp. 266–273). New York: Routledge.

Neimeyer, R. A. (2012b). Correspondence with the deceased. In R. A. Neimeyer (Ed.), *Techniques of grief therapy* (pp. 259–261). New York: Routledge.

Neimeyer, R. A. (2012c). Retelling the narrative of the death. In R. A. Neimeyer (Ed.), *Techniques of grief therapy* (pp. 86–90). New York: Routledge.

Neimeyer, R. A. (Ed.). (2012d). *Techniques of grief therapy: Creative practices for counseling the bereaved*. New York: Routledge.

Neimeyer, R. A. (2015). Meaning in bereavement. In R. E. Anderson (Ed.), *World suffering and quality of life*. New York: Springer.
Neimeyer, R. A. (2016a). Complicated grief: Assessment and intervention. In J. Cook, S. Gold, & C. Dalenberg (Eds.), *APA handbook of trauma psychology*. Washington, DC: American Psychological Association.
Neimeyer, R. A. (2016b). Meaning reconstruction in the wake of loss: Evolution of a research program. *Behaviour Change*. doi:10.1017/bec.2016.4.
Neimeyer, R. A. (Ed.). (2016c). *Techniques of grief therapy: Assessment and intervention*. New York: Routledge.
Neimeyer, R. A., & Thompson, B. E. (2014). Meaning making and the art of grief therapy. In B. E. Thompson & R. A. Neimeyer (Eds.), *Grief and the expressive arts: Practices for creating meaning* (pp. 3–13). New York: Routledge.
Neimeyer, R. A., & Young-Eisendrath, P. (2015). Assessing a Buddhist treatment for bereavement and loss: The Mustard seed project. *Death Studies, 39*, 263–273.
Neimeyer, R. A., Klass, D., & Dennis, M. R. (2014). Mourning, meaning and memory: Individual, communal and cultural narration of grief. In A. Batthyany & P. Russo-Netzer (Eds.), *Meaning in existential and positive psychology* (pp. 325–346). New York: Springer.
Prigerson, H. G., Horowitz, M. J., Jacobs, S. C., Parkes, C. M., Aslan, M., Goodkin, K., Raphael, B., Marwit, S. J., Wortman, C., Neimeyer, R. A., Bonanno, G. A., Block, S. D., Kissane, D., Boelen, P., Maercker, A., Litz, B. T., Johnson, J. G., First, M. B., …, Maciejewski, P. K. (2009). Prolonged grief disorder: Psychometric validation of criteria proposed for DSM-V and ICD-11. *PLoS Medicine, 6*(8), 1–12.
Rubin, S. S. (1999). The Two-Track Model of Bereavement: Overview, retrospect and prospect. *Death Studies, 23*, 681–714.
Rubin, S. S., Bar Nadav, O., Malkinson, R., Koren, D., & Michaeli, E. (2009). The Two-Track Model of Bereavement Questionnaire (TTBQ): Development and validation of a relational measure. *Death Studies, 33*, 305–333.
Rubin, S. S., Malkinson, R., & Witztum, E. (2011). *Working with the bereaved*. New York: Routledge.
Rynearson, E. K. (Ed.). (2006). *Violent death*. New York: Routledge.
Rynearson, E. K. (2012). Invoking an alliance with the deceased after violent death. In R. A. Neimeyer (Ed.), *Techniques of grief therapy* (pp. 91–94). New York: Routledge.
Rynearson, E. K., & Salloum, A. (2011). Restorative retelling: Revisiting the narrative of violent death. In R. A. Neimeyer, D. Harris, H. Winokuer, & G. Thornton (Eds.), *Grief and bereavement in contemporary society: Bridging research and practice* (pp. 177–188). New York: Routledge.
Saindon, C., Rheingold, A., Baddeley, J., Wallace, M., Brown, C., & Rynearson, E. K. (2014). Restorative retelling for violent loss: An open clinical trial. *Death Studies, 38*, 251–258.
Shear, M. K., Frank, E., Houch, P. R., & Reynolds, C. F. (2005). Treatment of complicated grief: A randomized controlled trial. *Journal of the American Medical Association, 293*, 2601–2608.
Shear, M. K., Boelen, P. A., & Neimeyer, R. A. (2011). Treating complicated grief: Converging approaches. In R. A. Neimeyer, D. Harris, H. Winokuer, & G. Thornton (Eds.), *Grief and bereavement in contemporary society: Bridging research and practice* (pp. 139–162). New York: Routledge.
Shear, M. K., Wang, Y., Skriskaya, N., Duan, N., Mauro, C., & Ghesquiere, A. (2014). Treatment of complicated grief in elderly persons: A randomized clinical trial. *Journal of the American Medical Association Psychiatry*. doi:10.1001/jamapsychiatry.2014.1242.
Stroebe, M., & Schut, H. (1999). The dual process model of coping with bereavement: Rationale and description. *Death Studies, 23*, 197–224.
Stroebe, M., & Schut, H. (2010). The dual process model of coping with bereavement: A decade on. *Omega, 61*, 273–289.
Thompson, B. E., & Neimeyer, R. A. (Eds.). (2014). *Grief and the expressive arts: Practices for creating meaning*. New York: Routledge.

Chapter 11
Why People Might Be Reluctant to Alleviate the Suffering of Others

Paul C. Rosenblatt

Introduction

I am haunted by a telephone survey carried out in the United States, Canada, and Mexico in May, 1995, by The Families and Work Institute, asking people, "How concerned are you about people not caring about others in [your country]?" The majority of respondents in each of the three countries said that they were concerned a great deal that many people in their country did not care about others in their country. If many people are not concerned about others in their own country, how likely are they to do anything about suffering in their country, let alone in other countries? If many people do not care whether others suffer and do not act to alleviate the suffering of others, it is likely that many people who suffer would be doing much better if more people cared.

This chapter explores answers to the question: Why might people be unwilling to act to alleviate the suffering of others? With answers to this question perhaps there would be ways to engage at least some of those who do not act to alleviate suffering. This chapter then explores ideas about sources of resistances to acting to alleviate suffering. The ideas fall into seven categories that have received substantial attention in the social psychological and sociological literature. The categories indicate areas that seem relevant to policy making and productive self-examination. I have ordered the seven categories on a continuum of resistance to helping others from resistance that might be easiest to overcome to resistance that might be most difficult to overcome. Of course, what lies underneath a resistance might make something that looks easy to overcome very difficult to overcome and something that looks virtually impossible to overcome actually not so difficult to overcome. But still the order offers a preliminary sense of which resistances might be less difficult and which might be more difficult to overcome. The seven categories are (1) not

P.C. Rosenblatt (✉)
Department of Family Social Science, University of Minnesota, Saint Paul, MN, USA
e-mail: prosenbl@umn.edu

R.E. Anderson (ed.), *Alleviating World Suffering*, Social Indicators Research Series 67, DOI 10.1007/978-3-319-51391-1_11

knowing what to do, (2) fear of being inadequate or making mistakes, (3) diffusion of responsibility for helping others in need, (4) obliviousness to the suffering of others, (5) defensive reactions to the suffering of others, (6) reluctance to pay the cost (in money, effort, time, or reputational risk) that could be involved in helping others, and (7) not caring.

Perhaps any person's reluctance to alleviate the suffering of others may be driven by a combination of the seven factors, but discussing the factors one at a time makes it easier to explore the issues and, in many instances, reflects accurately the approach taken in the cited academic literature. Another thing to say here is that this analysis focuses primarily on the alleviation of suffering, because that is largely the focus of the research literature this chapter draws on, though as is made clear in the discussion at the end of the chapter, ethical analyses often give as much attention to prevention as to alleviation of suffering.

The analysis in this chapter reveals how contemporary Western culture and human psychology work together to block many people from doing much, if anything, to help those who are suffering, to care about them, or even to know anything about them. That can be taken to mean that at least some people who currently do little or nothing to help those who are suffering or even to be aware of them and their suffering can overcome their psychological, cultural, social, and sociological barriers to acting to ameliorate suffering. Some people, for example, can be educated about obliviousness, defensive reactions to the suffering of others, not knowing what to do, ways to help that fit within money and time budgets, fear of beginner inadequacy or error in trying to help others, and diffusion of responsibility. And that education, and public policies that support that education, may help to overcome those barriers to helping others. In addition, it is possible that people who do not care about the suffering of others can begin to care if the others become human, real, and of worth for them through education, personal contact, and policy changes that alter or create public discourse about those who are suffering.

Not Knowing What to Do

People might be unwilling to help someone who is suffering because they do not know what to do. It might not be clear what would help, or one might not have a route to providing help. Also, one might not know what to do because one does not trust the information one has about the suffering and its context. Furthermore, it is hard to know what, if anything, to do if one is embedded in a social system that makes it seem inappropriate to provide help to those who are suffering. For example, one might not know anyone else who is providing help. And there might be organizations, for example, Doctors Without Borders, that seem to be dealing effectively with the suffering one is focused on. If others seem to be competently dealing with the suffering, people might not help because they do not think there is anything they can do that is not already being done.

People who hold back from helping because they do not know what to do might not realize that sometimes there is something easy to provide that could be of real help. And, related to this, the governmental and nongovernmental organizations that provide help to many people do not necessarily provide anything close to what people need. Some people who are suffering might need extremely expensive medical treatment or some other costly help, but sometimes things that are well within one's power and ability to provide make a big difference. For example, in a study of women who had experienced perinatal loss (Rosenblatt and Burns 1986), some women said that sometimes what helped them with their grief, sorrow, and suffering was a brief conversation with someone else who had had a similar loss. Someone saying something like, "I've been there, and I understand," made a real difference for some women. What follows are additional things that many could provide that might make a big difference for people who are suffering.

Being There Bereaved people often express appreciation for others who were there for them (e.g., Rosenblatt 2000, pp. 163–171, writing about grieving parents). Someone who shows up at the funeral, pays visits to grieving parents, calls periodically, and possibly comes by to help with household chores like the laundry or cleaning the kitchen may be deeply appreciated. With many people dropping away from and even avoiding people who are suffering (Rosenblatt 2000, pp. 168–170) a person who shows up now and then can be deeply appreciated. Similarly, adolescents suffering with cancer put great value on the "being there" of those family members and friends who kept on visiting them (Woodgate 2006).

Witnessing A "witness" to the suffering of another is a person who attends to the suffering and acknowledges it. Often witnesses to the suffering of another communicate their witnessing with the people who are suffering. And that communication may be experienced by those who are suffering as caring about and respecting them (e.g., Kennedy 2008). Witnessing is at the very least a form of support for those who are suffering. It can also be an act that starts a process of preventing future suffering, for example, when people publicly witnessing injustice motivate changes that end the injustice.

Listening "Being there" and "witnessing" can have great value, but they can go on without much or any listening to people who are suffering. But one thing that can be done that might be appreciated by some who are suffering is to listen to them. Some people who are suffering may not want to talk about things. But among those who do, some have never talked about their suffering with anyone, perhaps because they thought nobody wanted to hear, was interested, or knew about their suffering. So having someone who listens can be greatly appreciated, because finally someone knows, because being able to tell the story of one's suffering can help make sense of what one has experienced, and because the sharing may help one to feel less lonely. In my interview research on bereaved parents (Rosenblatt 2000), a number of interviewees said that the interview with me, often many years after their loss, was the first time someone listened well and heard the whole story of the child who died, the death, and its aftermath, and they greatly appreciated my listening.

Help with Basic Material Needs Some suffering people have desperate material needs—food, water, shelter, basic medical care, clothing, blankets. Part of the suffering of many people—those fleeing war zones, for example—is that their basic physical needs are not being met. So sometimes what a person who wants to help can do is to help with basic physical needs.

Giving People What They Say They Want Sometimes would-be helpers of those who are suffering assume they know what those who are suffering need. But it is far better to ask people who are suffering what they want and to attempt to meet those wants than to guess what is wanted. Don't assume, for example, that a newly arrived refugee needs blankets; best to ask her what she wants, and if she says she wants to telephone relatives, take a shower, and get laces for her shoes, it seems best to help with that. That does not mean things are simple. One might not be in a position to ask people what they want, to understand what they say, or to give them what they say they want. People who are suffering may not know what they want, may not trust others enough to tell them what they want, or may not be in a position to lay out what could be a very long or very personal list of wants. Furthermore, some people who are suffering may not want to worry others, perhaps particularly close family members, by telling them what they want (e.g., Rober and Rosenblatt in press, writing about a prisoner of war telling his family things are okay when that was not true). And even if people say what they want, that does not mean they can speak for others who are suffering in the same situation. Still, one reasonable and responsible route toward helping those who are suffering is to ask them what they want. And from a related ethical perspective, Mayeroff (1971) argued that one cannot help another by assuming one knows what the other needs; one must understand what the other needs, and that often means, as Mayeroff saw it, a commitment to continuous learning about the other.

Fear of Beginner Inadequacy or Error

Possibly some people do not help because they fear that whatever they might do to try to alleviate suffering would be inadequate or even harmful, and this may be especially so if people are beginners at trying to alleviate suffering. In fact, as society has become more differentiated into professionals with a diversity of specializations a society-wide ideology has developed that one needs to be an experienced professional to provide effective help. And part of that ideology is that an untrained and inexperienced beginner is likely to do great harm if trying to help someone who is suffering. I have no doubt that some who suffer only can be helped by the right kind of professional. I also have no doubt that some amateurs and beginners who try to help people who are suffering do great harm. However, I also think beginners are often of great help, that in offering, for example, food and shelter, human decency, basic human contact, safety, or listening, they provide great help to someone who is suffering.

Also some professionals are disappointingly unhelpful to some who suffer (see, for example, Coulehan 2012). This is so because professional education and formal programs for helping the suffering can get in the way of being an empathic, caring, helpful human. Some professional approaches to helping can lead to a bureaucratization of help such that the highest priority in the "care" situation is not the amelioration of suffering but record keeping and conformity to rules, and in the process of bureaucratization people who are suffering will not only not be helped much to deal with their suffering but may also come to feel that they do not matter as individuals in the care setting. Professional education and formal programs for helping can also lead to diagnostic categorizing of someone who is suffering being the primary form of "help," and the focus on diagnostic categorization can lead a professional to have minimal capacity to care, listen, understand, or meet the needs of a person who is suffering (e.g., Sweet and Wilson 2011). With many professionals so wrapped up in activities that do little or nothing to address suffering, in some situations amateur helpers may do more to alleviate suffering—for example, in hospice facilities the volunteer who visits patients, the patient in the next bed, or the cleaning person. Their freedom from the constraints and demands that burden professionals may allow their basic humanity and caring to be expressed in ways that are helpful to the person who is suffering.

Care of the dying is a particularly poignant area in which fear of inadequacy or error might lead to great suffering. People who are at the end of life and are in extreme pain may be much more comfortable in their last days if treated with pain-killing medication. But some family members and physicians prefer that a dying person in their care not receive such palliative care. They may fear that the palliation may accelerate the death. They may be unwilling to allow their loved one to be sedated because of concerns about addiction, not that someone with days to live could be addicted for very long. They may feel that it would be a mistake to put the sick person on any medication that might make the person's thinking less clear and thus make it harder for the person to communicate, though great pain also clouds thinking and makes communication difficult. In a sense the palliative care movement, which has led to important developments in hospice care and palliative medicine, was created in reaction to the power of those who fear beginner inadequacy or error in palliation and because of that favor doing nothing to ameliorate end of life suffering. The palliative care movement has had great success, but many family members and physicians still oppose palliation.

Diffusion of Responsibility for Helping Others in Need

Some people who do nothing to alleviate suffering may think that others are acting to alleviate the suffering. That resonates with a line of research showing that when someone seems in need, for example, when a woman outside on a dark night is screaming for help, many people are unlikely to help because they think that others know better what is going on and would act if something was needed (Latane and

Darley 1970; Staub 2001). From that perspective, the greater the number of people who seem aware and potentially could do something, the less inclined any given person is to do something. But then additional research in that area shows that it is not just diffusion of responsibility but also not being sure what is going on, thinking what is going on may be legitimate, fearing being a spoil-sport, a tattletale, or inappropriately deviant in speaking out (Arluke 2012), and fearing the disapproval of others (Staub 2001). From another perspective, diffusion of responsibility can be linked to obliviousness (which is discussed in the next section of this chapter) in that bystanders may work at not knowing what is going on, even about mass killings (e.g., Staub 2011, p. 195).

From a different but related perspective, the extreme complexity of modern society and the existence of a vast array of specialists sets up the possibility of diffusion of responsibility in many situations of suffering. A person might ask, "Why should I help someone who is suffering when there are clinical psychologists, palliative care doctors, pain clinics, a wide array of organizations that help people in need, government agencies responsible for helping people with this or that kind of need, and so on?" That suggests that to some extent to overcome diffusion of responsibility people who could do something to alleviate the suffering of others may have to be persuaded, when it is true, that professionals, help organizations, and government agencies are not doing the job well enough or not serving all the people who are suffering and need help.

Obliviousness to the Suffering of Others

People are oblivious to almost everything that goes on in the world, including much that goes on around them (Rosenblatt 2009), so it is not surprising that many people are oblivious to the suffering of others. There are many reasons for obliviousness. There is far more going on than any human can attend to. Then, too, typically the news media report little of the suffering associated with warfare, political and economic oppression, human rights violations, epidemics, famine, or natural disasters. For example, in relationship to the Iraq war the emphasis in the mass media in the United States and Scotland has from the start been on what the national government wants to communicate to the public (Altheide and Grimes 2005; Robertson 2004), and that does not include specifics on the horrible loss of life, gruesome injuries, lives disrupted, families torn apart, psychological difficulties, forced migration, and what Iraqis victimized by the war have to say (Altheide and Grimes 2005; Robertson 2004). Thus, many people may be oblivious to the suffering of others because they have too much to attend to and because the news media makes it easy to be oblivious to the suffering of others.

Even with regard to those who are nearby, one may not know of or notice their suffering—for example, the suffering of the sexually abused neighbor, the colleague who is a victim of racism, the friend with a painful illness, or the relative who is grieving (Fidyk 2011). This obliviousness is typically reinforced by the priorities for what to pay attention to set by the family system in which a person lives (Rosenblatt 2009). A person's obliviousness in difficult situations can also be about a cultural value of something like minding one's own business (King and Sakamoto 2015).

Then, too, there is considerable evidence that some people tune out, are oblivious to, or trivialize the suffering of those in social categories of which they think poorly (e.g., Cargile 2015; Fourie et al. 2013). So, for example, a white person who thinks poorly of black people might not attend to the suffering of black people. The tuning out may involve obliviousness to feelings, and hence a failure to empathize, or it might involve inattention to events affecting people who are not thought well of. From that perspective, in order to care enough about others in social categories one thinks poorly of to pay attention to their suffering and to empathize with them, there might have to be something like a rehumanization of those others (Fourie et al. 2013). A step toward doing that is to make the others in important ways count as individuals who matter. Another possibility is to consider all humans to be valuable and worth helping, and that can make an empathic and helping response not calculative but just something one should do (Monroe 2015).

Obliviousness can blend into willful ignorance. Willful ignorance no doubt has many sources. Among them is the willful ignorance of those who work hard to limit the information they receive that could tell them that they are responsible for suffering (McGoey 2012).

Defensive Reactions to the Suffering of Others

Many people feel uncomfortable with the suffering of others or are threatened by it, and that may lead them to defensive distancing, tuning out, or denying the suffering (Cohen 2001; Fidyk 2011). For example, many bereaved parents report how, after their child's funeral, many acquaintances, friends, and relatives drift away and even actively avoid them (Rosenblatt 2000, pp. 93–96). The bereaved parents go from a funeral at which many people show caring and support to often being isolated and with almost no support. And some people who give reasons for not providing support to bereaved parents say things that could be understood as defensive. For example, some parents of living children say it is too threatening and uncomfortable to interact with parents who have had a child die, because the bereaved parents are powerful reminders of the vulnerability of all children (Rosenblatt 2000, p. 94).

Similarly, the farming neighbors of a farm family in such grave economic trouble that they seem likely to lose their farm may avoid them in part because it is too threatening to confront their own economic vulnerability (Wright and Rosenblatt 1987). Related to this, some people blame victims of natural disasters for what has happened to them in a way that seems to be in part defensiveness about their own vulnerability to natural disasters. For example, some people blamed victims of Hurricane Katrina for their suffering in ways that could be taken as defensive denial of government failures to protect the public against natural disasters through maintenance of Gulf Coast wetlands, dikes, and the like (e.g., Napier et al. 2006).

Defensive distancing can also be linked to the possibility of feeling guilty for not suffering. People experiencing privilege and good fortune may feel guilty about not suffering when others are suffering. One way out of feeling such guilt is to blame those who suffer for causing their own suffering, thus absolving oneself of guilt, suppressing it, and possibly eliminating feelings of obligation to help (Xu et al. 2011). But then, the issue is not simple, because it also seems that people who do not have relevant experiences of suffering tend to underestimate the pain that people who are suffering feel (Nordgren, Banas, and MacDonald 2011). Also, some people who might help alleviate suffering can be turned off by campaigns to raise money to help alleviate suffering if the campaigns are designed to make people feel guilty if they do not help (Cohen 2001 p. 215).

People who feel responsible for the suffering of others may be motivated (by strong guilt feelings or empathy) to provide help for those whose suffering they feel they caused. But feelings of guilt may motivate other actions (O'Connor et al. 2012), among them blaming the suffering of the other on the other (e.g., van den Bos and Maas 2009). Related to this, there is evidence that perpetrators often deny the suffering of their victims, see the suffering as deserved, or see the suffering as much less than what the victims experience (e.g., Eckhardt et al. 2013). And in the United States, which through government, military, and economic action causes great suffering to tens of millions of people around the world, there are questions about whether ordinary citizens typically feel at all responsible for the suffering their government causes. In fact, many in the United States may act as though there is a division of labor such that the federal government will pay attention to the deaths and destruction it causes and ordinary citizens will pay attention to their own lives (Rosenblatt 2009, p. 45). And at the level of political ideology, there are strains of thought, for example, "neoliberalism," that can be understood as seeing victims of almost anything as responsible for what has happened to them, which absolves the social and political collective for responsibility about who is impoverished, undereducated, discriminated against, or targeted by violence (Stringer 2014).

Perhaps defensive denial of personal responsibility is reflected in people not perceiving that their government has caused suffering and that they have some responsibility for that suffering (because it's their government that caused the suffering). Thus, it is possible that many in the United States who have no interest in helping suffering Latin Americans who are trying to flee to the United States are in denial about how the suffering of Latin Americans has been and is being caused by U.S. economic and trade policies, U.S. policies of supporting right wing oligarchs and military oppression in Central America, and U.S. drug policies. Similarly, one can see those in the United States who want to stop refugees from Syria, Iraq, Afghanistan, Libya, and Yemen from coming to the United States as possibly being in defensive denial about how the suffering of these refugees is largely due to U.S. military, intelligence agency, and military contractor activities in the countries these refugees are fleeing.

At another level, defensive denial could be operating in people who espouse a religious ideology that advocates helping the needy, the poor, the hungry, and others who are suffering and yet who strongly oppose helping those who are suffering. Some such people even advocate strongly for actions that will increase the suffering of many. In these instances the defensive denial might be that the religious doctrine is relevant to the suffering of many who are somehow different from oneself. One might call this "footnote denial." By that I mean that people understand the meaning of their religious doctrine about helping those who are in need to be footnoted so that it is only about certain other people. Footnotes will differ from believer to believer, but it may be common to understand the doctrine not to apply to the suffering of people of other religions, races, or nationalities.

Finally, in considering defensive reactions to the suffering of others, some people may feel so overwhelmed by how much suffering there is in the world that they feel paralyzed and incapable of acting constructively. Consider, for example, at any one time there are dozens of bloody armed conflicts going on in the world and innumerable instances of human rights violations (including torture, sexual slavery, assassination of political dissenters, child labor, child sexual abuse, and children forced to be soldiers in warfare) (Rosenblatt 1995). With so much suffering in the world one can feel overwhelmed emotionally; there can be too much flooding in on one. And that can lead to ego-defensive closing down and denial.

Unwillingness to Pay the Cost in Money, Effort, Time, or Personal Discomfort

Some people may hold back and choose not to help those who suffer because they cannot or will not pay the cost in money, effort, time, or personal discomfort. In principle they could do something, but in their estimation the potential cost to them is steep enough to deter them from acting. That may suggest that people who have less money are less likely to help others, but actually the opposite seems to be true. People who are not well off economically may be *more* likely to provide help for others (Miller et al. 2015; Piff et al. 2010). One can take this to mean that sharing of meager resources is more common among those with less, whereas for those with substantial resources there may be more inclination not to share. Perhaps it also suggests that those with fewer resources are less calculative, less into assessing what they gain and lose from doing something, than those with more resources.

Perhaps one possibility for motivating people who are unwilling to give up any of their money, effort, time, or comfort would be to make the perceived benefit of helping seem quite high relative to the cost. Then they get a bargain, as it were. For example, being able to show that what is for them a small fraction of their assets, effort, or time can feed a starving family for a year, restore a thirsty village's water supply, or cure a child of a disease that was about to kill her might motivate them to help.

People who are unwilling over a long period of time to provide more than an infinitesimal amount of their resources to those who are suffering, for example, well-off people who do nothing for people who are suffering other than donate $5 a year to each of three causes, may feel good about the little that they do. Perhaps many token donors are not qualitatively different from those who do nothing for others who are suffering. But their existence raises questions about how much is more than a token, how much is a fair share, and how much is enough. From the perspective of those who are suffering one can imagine that it can seem extremely selfish and insensitive for someone living well materially not to provide the resources he or she could well afford that would spare perhaps many from considerable suffering. From the perspective of the person who donates only a small amount there may be possibly valid concerns about the efficacy and trustworthiness of the process of getting a charitable donation to those who have real need. Even direct giving to those who seem needy may be complicated by possibly valid concerns about the uses to which the donation will be put. Related to this, some who give little or nothing may be engaged in a cost/benefit analysis in which anything they provide has a cost to them and they may not have much reason to think that what they give will benefit them, even indirectly through knowing that someone else was grateful for what they gave or that someone's suffering was reduced (Zagefka and James 2015). One could take that line of thinking as a failure of empathy, but it also may be about the stingy donor not having evidence that charitable action will make a difference.

Not Caring

The fact that some people do not care that others are suffering seems a qualitatively different matter to deal with than the six sources of resistance to helping others discussed so far. With each of the previous six, there seems to be potential to want to do something if a crucial source of resistance to helping others is overcome. With "not caring" this issue is that to some people it does not matter that others suffer. People are less likely to do something to alleviate the suffering of others if they have no concern for the welfare of the others and feel no personal responsibility for their well-being (Staub 2001). But perhaps "not caring" can be overcome. One possibility for change is for those who are thought so little of to be humanized (Staub 2011 p. 327), for example, through positive contact and through vivid and touching stories and pictures in the media. However, positive contact is difficult to achieve in a world where those who dehumanize others are often geographically and culturally distant from the others who suffer, and it is not a simple matter to communicate across language, culture, and experiential differences. And television (along with other media) arguably does more to make those who are suffering, particularly, perhaps, in great disasters, subjects of passive spectatorship by those who learn of their suffering through the media (Chouliaraki 2006). And the position of passive spectatorship is a position that is unlikely to engage empathic and caring understanding or desire to help.

People also may not care about the suffering of others when they are given information about the suffering that is too abstract to engage their capacity for empathy and caring (Slovic et al. 2013). Statistics and abstract news reports about suffering may not make a difference to them. But more concrete information, such as the photo of a child lying dead in the surf or the emotional testimony of a torture victim, may motivate people who are unmoved by statistics and abstract news reports. But from another perspective, the key to developing empathy might be, for many people, rooted in their own suffering (Erikkson 1992). Having an experience of suffering that one can remember, acknowledge, and allow oneself to have feelings about might be a powerful foundation for empathizing with the suffering of others.

Discussion

The telephone survey data described at the beginning of this chapter, reporting that many people in the United States, Canada, and Mexico said they were concerned a great deal that people in their country did not care about others in their country, makes sense in terms of the literature and ideas discussed in this chapter. There are many factors that could lead people to do nothing to help others who are suffering and, in many instances, to seem not to care. But still, the reasons laid out in this chapter for some people not ever to try to alleviate the suffering of others points to ways that resistance to trying to help those who are suffering might be overcome. No doubt some people can be educated about obliviousness, defensive reactions to the suffering of others, not knowing what to do, ways to help that fit within money and time budgets, fear of beginner inadequacy or error in trying to help others, and diffusion of responsibility. And that education may help overcome those barriers to helping others. In addition, it is possible that people who do not care about the suffering of others can begin to care if the others are humanized in some way. In general, there is hope that some of those who do nothing to alleviate the suffering of others may come to change their ways.

Contrarian Views

This chapter takes the position that we have a responsibility and obligation to help those who are suffering and to act in ways that will prevent suffering. It is rooted in a universalistic position that many who write about ethics and morality lean toward (e.g., Peter Singer 1993), a position that advocates treating all humans with the same care and respect one would want for oneself. Thus, the ethical thing to do is to value the interests of others as much as one values one's own interests. However, there is a contrarian view from which one could argue that human systems need a division of labor such that only some people try to alleviate the suffering of others. For example, it may be best if the only people who offer help to the suffering are those who are good at empathizing with others, care strongly, and have sufficient knowledge and experience.

Another contrarian view is that the focus in this chapter is too much on direct action to alleviate suffering and not enough on attending to causes of suffering and trying to block those causes from operating to cause suffering. From that perspective one might argue that too much effort is put into helping suffering people and not enough is put into neutralizing causes of suffering. Of course, immediate needs are very important. A person who is starving or needs immediate medical attention has needs that, from the view that we must all act to ameliorate suffering, must be met now. But sometimes a big-picture view of suffering suggests that a great deal of suffering, the suffering of even billions of people, might be prevented if we could work effectively to reduce what causes such suffering. People in the United States may feel enormous social pressure (including, perhaps, genuinely well-justified fear of retaliation) not to be activists working to change policies of the U.S. government and major corporations by demanding, for example, an end to U.S. military aggression (and the aggression of U.S. military allies) around the world. But effective activism directed at U.S. military and corporate actions that cause suffering may reduce or prevent the suffering of billions of people.

The Context for Not Caring

It is common for government and corporate leaders who cause great suffering (and even mass murder) to deny their responsibility (Cohen 2001). In denying the great suffering they have caused, leaders use a wide range of well-developed discourse strategies to divert the public from understanding the suffering that has been caused and/or the crucial role of these officials in causing that suffering (Hansson 2015). In rare instances some lower-level government and corporate harm-doers may be tried for their crimes (Boyanowsky 2015, writing about disasters involving defective dams in Italy), but higher level leaders seem always to escape legal consequences (Boyanowsky 2015; Voigt and Thornton 2015, writing about Hurricane Katrina and its aftermath in New Orleans). Thus one part of the context for members of the general public not caring about suffering is the denial of suffering by government and corporate officials who have key roles in causing suffering and who use a host of rhetorical devices to bolster their denial. These rhetorical devices include not only claims that whatever happened is not their responsibility but also victim-blaming, distracting and frightening the public (there are terrorists everywhere and they are a great danger to you), and focusing on the importance of being patriotic (don't you dare think that the U.S. government and U.S. corporations that promote war are doing terrible things).

Next Steps

This essay has addressed key reasons why people might not help others who are suffering. Situations are complex and variable and the reluctance of many to alleviate the suffering of others may represent combinations of two or more of the seven factors explored in this chapter, which could mean that simple approaches to motivating more assistance to those who are suffering may not work. But still we hopefully can move forward with engaging more people to act to alleviate the suffering of others. If the vast amount of suffering worldwide is to be alleviated, ideally as many people as possible must step up and act. But in the absence of that, perhaps those who are able and willing to act might ideally be given as much support for their efforts as possible and as much help at being as good as they can be in what they do. This is not to say that there is always agreement about what is appropriate amelioration of suffering. For example, family members might disagree about what is the best way to ameliorate the suffering of a woman who just learned of her husband's death (Rober and Rosenblatt 2013). Nor is it to say that there is necessarily agreement about what suffering should be ameliorated. For example, whereas some might be rather quick to ameliorate the suffering of grief with medications and psychotherapy, others might be much more inclined to respect grieving as necessary and appropriate and to assume it would be best to allow it in most instances to run its course (Rosenblatt 2012). Nevertheless, the vast amount of suffering around the world calls out for amelioration.

References

Altheide, D. L., & Grimes, J. N. (2005). War programming: The propaganda project and the Iraq war. *The Sociological Quarterly, 46*, 617–643.

Arluke, A. (2012). Bystander apathy in animal abuse cases: Exploring barriers to child and adolescent intervention. *Anthrozoos, 25*(1), 5–23.

Boyanowsky, E. (2015). A recipe for a toxic culture. *Ecopsychology, 7*(2), 84–86.

Cargile, A. C. (2015). Prejudice and openness to the other: Investigating responses to testimonies of race-based suffering. *Race and Social Problems, 7*, 198–212.

Chouliaraki, L. (2006). *The spectatorship of suffering*. London: Sage.

Cohen, S. (2001). *States of denial: Knowing about atrocities and suffering*. Cambridge: Polity Press.

Coulehan, J. (2012). Suffering, hope, and healing. In R. J. Moore (Ed.), *Handbook of pain and palliative care: Biobehavioral approaches for the life course* (pp. 717–731). New York: Springer.

Eckhardt, C. I., Sprunger, J. G., & Hamel, J. (2013). Intimate partner violence perpetrators. In L. Grossman & S. Walfish (Eds.), *Translating psychological research into practice* (pp. 443–451). New York: Springer.

Erikkson, K. (1992). The alleviation of suffering: The idea of caring. *Scandinavian Journal of Caring Sciences, 6*, 119–123.

Fidyk, A. (2011). Suffering with: Seven moments of ignorance. In E. Malewski & N. Jaramillo (Eds.), *Epistemologies of ignorance in education* (pp. 129–165). Charlotte: IAP Information Age.

Fourie, M. M., Gobodo-Madikizela, P., & Stein, D. J. (2013). Empathy, forgiveness, and reconciliation: The Truth and Reconciliation Commission in South Africa. In M. Linden & K. Rutkowski (Eds.), *Hurting memories and beneficial forgetting: Posttraumatic stress disorders, biographical developments and social conflicts* (pp. 227–240). Amsterdam: Elsevier.

Hansson, S. (2015). Discursive strategies of blame avoidance in government: A framework for analysis. *Discourse & Society, 26*, 297–322.

Kennedy, R. (2008). Subversive witnessing: Mediating indigenous testimony In Australian cultural and legal institutions. *Women's Studies Quarterly, 36*(1–2), 58–75.

King, R. U., & Sakamoto, I. (2015). Disengaging from genocide harm-doing and healing together between perpetrators, bystanders, and victims in Rwanda. *Peace and Conflict: Journal of Peace Psychology, 3*, 378–394.

Latane, B., & Darley, J. M. (1970). *The unresponsive bystander: Why doesn't he help?* New York: Appleton-Century Crofts.

Mayeroff, M. (1971). *On caring*. New York: Harper Perennial.

McGoey, L. (2012). The logic of strategic ignorance. *British Journal of Sociology, 63*, 553–576.

Miller, J. G., Kahle, S., & Hastings, P. D. (2015). Roots and benefits of costly giving: Children who are more altruistic have greater autonomic flexibility and less family wealth. *Psychological Science, 26*, 1038–1045.

Monroe, K. R. (2015). Empathy and our relations to others. In A. Laitinen & A. B. Pessi (Eds.), *Solidarity: Theory and practice* (pp. 88–104). Lanham: Lexington Books.

Napier, J. L., Mandisodza, A. N., Andersen, S. M., & Jost, J. T. (2006). System justification in responding to the poor and displaced in the aftermath of Hurricane Katrina. *Analyses of Social Issues and Public Policy (ASAP), 6*(1), 57–73.

Nordgren, L. F., Banas, K., & MacDonald, G. (2011). Empathy gaps for social pain: Why people underestimate the pain of social suffering. *Journal of Personality and Social Psychology, 100*, 120–128.

O'Connor, L. E., Berry, J. W., Lewis, T. B., & Stiver, D. J. (2012). Empathy-based pathogenic guilt, pathological altruism, and psychopathology. In B. Oakley, A. Knafo, G. Madhavan, & D. S. Wilson (Eds.), *Pathological altruism* (pp. 10–30). New York: Oxford University Press.

Piff, P. K., Kraus, M. W., Cote, S., Cheng, B. H., & Keltner, D. (2010). Having less, giving more: The influence of social class on prosocial behavior. *Journal of Personality and Social Psychology, 99*, 771–784.

Rober, P., & Rosenblatt, P. C. (2013). Selective disclosure in a first conversation about a family death in James Agee's novel A Death in the Family. *Death Studies, 37*, 172–194.

Rober, P., & Rosenblatt, P. C. (in press). Silence and memories of war: An autoethnographic exploration of family secrecy. *Family Process*

Robertson, J. W. (2004). People's watchdogs or government poodles? Scotland's national broadsheets and the second Iraq war. *European Journal of Communication, 19*, 457–482.

Rosenblatt, P. C. (1995). Human rights violations. In C. R. Ember & M. Ember (Eds.), *Research frontiers in anthropology* (Vol. 4, pp. 183–202). Englewood Cliffs: Prentice-Hall.

Rosenblatt, P. C. (2000). *Parent grief: Narratives of loss and relationship*. Philadelphia: Brunner/Mazel.

Rosenblatt, P. C. (2009). *Shared obliviousness in family systems*. Albany: State University of New York Press.

Rosenblatt, P. C. (2012). The concept of complicated grief: Lessons from other cultures. In M. Stroebe, H. Schut, & J. van den Bout (Eds.), *Complicated grief: Scientific foundations for health professionals* (pp. 27–39). New York: Routledge.

Rosenblatt, P. C., & Burns, L. H. (1986). Long term effects of perinatal loss. *Journal of Family Issues, 7*, 237–253.

Singer, P. (1993). *Practical ethics* (2nd ed.). New York: Cambridge University Press.

Slovic, P., Zionts, D., Woods, A. K., Goodman, R., & Jinks, D. (2013). Psychic numbing and mass atrocity. In E. Shafir (Ed.), *The behavioral foundations of public policy* (pp. 126–142). Princeton: Princeton University Press.

Staub, E. (2001). Emergency helping, genocidal violence, and the evolution of responsibility and altruism in children. In R. J. Davidson & A. Harrington (Eds.), *Visions of compassion: Western scientists and Tibetan Buddhists examine human nature* (pp. 165–181). New York: Oxford University Press.

Staub, E. (2011). *Overcoming evil: Genocide, violence conflict, and terrorism*. New York: Oxford University Press.

Stringer, R. (2014). *Knowing victims: Feminism, agency and victim politics in neoliberal times*. New York: Routledge/Taylor & Francis.

Sweet, G. S., & Wilson, H. J. (2011). A patient's experience of ward rounds. *Patient Education and Counseling, 84*(2), 150–151.

van den Bos, K., & Maas, M. (2009). On the psychology of the belief in a just world: Exploring experiential and rationalistic paths to victim blaming. *Personality and Social Psychology Bulletin, 35*, 1567–1578.

Voigt, L., & Thornton, W. E. (2015). Disaster-related human rights violations and corruption: A 10-year review of post-Hurricane Katrina New Orleans. *American Behavioral Scientist, 59*, 1292–1313.

Woodgate, R. L. (2006). The importance of being there: Perspectives of social support by adolescents with cancer. *Journal of Pediatric Oncology Nursing, 23*(3), 122–134.

Wright, S. E., & Rosenblatt, P. C. (1987). Isolation and farm loss: Why neighbors may not be supportive. *Family Relations, 36*, 391–395.

Xu, H., Begue, L., & Shankland, R. (2011). Guilt and guiltlessness: An integrative review. *Social and Personality Psychology Compass, 5*, 440–457.

Zagefka, H., & James, T. (2015). The psychology of charitable donations to disaster victims and beyond. *Social Issues and Policy Review, 9*(1), 155–192.

Part III
Improving Global Development, Healthcare and Poverty Reduction

Chapter 12
Addressing the Structural Causes of World Suffering

Jason Hickel

Introduction

It is difficult to imagine a more vital measure of a civilization than the extent to which its citizens suffer. We inherit this view from a long tradition of Western philosophy. Thinkers like Thomas Hobbes and John Locke sought to justify civilization on the basis that it reduced the suffering that characterized life in the so-called state of nature, which was supposedly nasty, brutish, and short. How does our global civilization fare when assessed on these terms? As globalization consolidates our world into a single transnational system, are people's lives getting better or worse? Is human suffering increasing or decreasing, in aggregate? One common way to answer this question is to look at the statistics on global poverty and hunger. Recently the main institutions of the international development industry – the World Bank, UN agencies, international NGOs like Oxfam and World Vision, and government departments like the United States Agency for International Development (USAID) and Britain's Department for International Development (DfID) – have united around a powerful narrative claiming that global poverty and hunger have been declining dramatically over the past decades, thanks to foreign aid and the Millennium Development Goals. This essay provides evidence that such a narrative is misleading at best, and intentionally inaccurate at worst. In reality, global poverty and hunger have been worsening significantly over the past few decades, since accurate records began in 1981. According to these measures, then, the development industry has failed to alleviate human suffering, despite delivering more than $3.3 trillion dollars in aid over this period. The reason that the development industry is failing is because it refuses to address the root causes of poverty. It tends to see poverty as a purely endogenous problem, and ignores the external political and

J. Hickel (✉)
Faculty of Anthropology, London School of Economics and Political Science,
London WC2A 2AE, UK
e-mail: j.e.hickel@lse.ac.uk

R.E. Anderson (ed.), *Alleviating World Suffering*, Social Indicators Research
Series 67, DOI 10.1007/978-3-319-51391-1_12

economic forces that are much more causally significant. In order to be effective, our solutions to poverty and other dimensions of world suffering need to address the power imbalances and financial biases in the global economy. The final section of this chapter offers some ideas toward this end.

How Bad Is World Suffering, Really?

This question quickly draws us into contested terrain, and the stakes are very high. The dominant narrative draws on the UN's Millennium Development Goals (MDGs). In 2015, the United Nations published the final report of the MDGs. The report led with a glowing, good-news narrative about how the world is getting better. It claimed that the MDGs succeeded in cutting absolute poverty rates in half, and hunger rates nearly in half. On poverty, the report states: "The poverty rate in the developing regions has plummeted, from 47% in 1990 to 14% in 2015." On hunger, the report states: "Projections indicate a drop of almost half in the proportion of undernourished people in the developing regions, from 23.3% in 1990–1992 to 12.9% in 2014–2016. This is very close to the MDG hunger target" (United Nations 2015).

These claims have been repeated by the development sector and the media, with little to no critical scrutiny. It is a powerful story. For those who have an interest in defending the status quo of the global economic system, the good-news narrative about poverty and hunger serves as a potent political tool. It lends a kind of moral justification to the present order and its logic of growth, liberalization, privatization, and increasing corporate power. It tells us that whatever we're doing is working, so we need to do more of it. Sometimes this argument is quite explicit. *The Spectator* recently published an article titled "What Oxfam doesn't want you to know: global capitalism means less poverty than ever." Leading with the MDG statistics on poverty and hunger, the author (Nelson 2015) argued that all the attention focused on social inequality and wealth accumulation among the 1% is misplaced. The 1% may now have more wealth than the rest of the world's population combined, but this skewed distribution is justified because the very system that has made them so rich has also reduced poverty in developing countries.

But a number of scholars, including myself, have been pointing out that this good-news narrative is not accurate. The UN has effectively manipulated the data to make it appear as though poverty and hunger are being reduced when in fact they are not. Here I will offer only a cursory overview of this argument, which I have developed more fully elsewhere (Hickel 2016).

So what is wrong with the official poverty and hunger statistics? The first step is to understand that the main precedent for MDG-1, which is the goal on poverty and hunger, was the agreement made at the World Food Summit that was held in 1996 in Rome. The world's governments pledged for the first time to reduce the absolute number of undernourished people to half their present level by no later than 2015. In the Rome Declaration, the focus was very clearly on absolute numbers. But when the Millennium Declaration was signed in 2000, the goalposts were changed quite dramatically. They shifted from halving the *absolute number* of poor and hungry people to halving the *proportion* of poor and hungry people as a percentage of the world's population. This made the goal much easier to achieve, simply because it could take advantage of population growth. Later, when MDG-1 was formulated, the goal was diluted yet again. First, it was changed from halving the proportion of poor and hungry people in the whole world to halving the proportion in *only developing countries*. This change – which was not publicized, and which journalists failed to notice – allowed them to take advantage of a much faster-growing denominator. There was also a second major change: the baseline was moved from 2000 back to 1990. This translated to a higher baseline proportion of poor and hungry, gave the UN much more time to accomplish the goal, and allowed them to retroactively claim the big gains against poverty and hunger achieved by China in the 1990s, which of course had nothing at all to do with the MDGs, and took place before the MDGs were even conceived. By redefining the goals in this way, the UN has created the powerful impression that poverty and hunger have been reduced when in fact the reality of it is not so rosy (Pogge 2004, 2009, 2010).

Another key issue is that the poverty and hunger lines themselves have been massaged in ways that support the good-news narrative (Reddy and Pogge 2005). The very first international poverty line (IPL) was set by the World Bank at $1.02 per day. Using this line, it was clear that global poverty was rising steeply. In its 2000 annual report the World Bank announced that "the absolute number of those living on $1 per day or less *continues to increase*. The worldwide total rose from 1.2 billion in 1987 to 1.5 billion today and, if recent trends persist, will reach 1.9 billion by 2015" (emphasis mine). These figures projected a troubling trend. Then, 3 years later, the World Bank announced the exact opposite story: poverty was not increasing but rather decreasing, by 400 million people between 1981 and 2001 (Chen and Ravallion 2004). How did this happen? Because the World Bank changed the IPL, rebasing it to new Purchasing Power Parity (PPP) figures – from $1.02 per day (at 1985 PPP) to $1.08 per day (at 1993 PPP). While this new IPL appeared to be higher, it was in fact *lower* in real terms, and therefore made it seems as though there were fewer people in poverty than there were before. The new IPL went live in 2000, just in time for the MDGs to use it as their official measure. In 2008, there was a second change to the IPL. It was shifted to $1.08 per day (at 2005 PPP). Once again, this made the poverty reduction trend look better, creating the illusion that an additional 121 million people had been lifted from poverty overnight, even though nothing had changed in the real world. This has to do with the fact that PPP figures tend to discriminate against poor people. PPP assesses the prices of a broad basket of goods, but poor people spend the majority of their income on a single good – food – the price of which tends to rise faster than that of other goods. As a consequence, PPP figures overstate the purchasing power of poor people by about 50% (Cimadamore et al. 2016: 6).

The upshot of this is that much of the gains that the MDGs have reported against poverty have been due to changes in the poverty line, rather than to actual changes in the real world. The same story applies to the hunger goal. For most of the MDG period, the UN's Food and Agricultural Organization (FAO) was reporting that global hunger numbers were *rising*, not falling. In 2009, the FAO reported that the food price crisis had pushed 150 million additional people into hunger, bringing the global total up to 1023 million – a 21% increase from 1990 (FAO 2009). The MDGs' hunger goal was set to be a catastrophic failure. But then, with only 3 years to go before the expiry of the MDGs, the FAO began telling the exact opposite story. The UN's 2013 report announced: "Progress in reducing hunger has been more pronounced than previously believed, and the target of halving the percentage of people suffering from hunger by 2015 is within reach" (United Nations 2013). How did this happen? Because at the eleventh hour the FAO introduced a new "improved" methodology, which transformed a steadily rising trend into a steadily falling one. The new methodology made two key changes: first, it excluded the impact of the food price crisis, and second it pushed the hunger threshold lower, making it seem as though fewer people were hungry than before. Independent scholars have been highly critical of this move (Caparros 2014; Moore- Lappé et al. 2013a, b).

A More Accurate View of Poverty

Beyond critiquing the questionable methodological changes that lie behind the official poverty and hunger statistics, we also need to question the way that poverty and hunger are measured in the first place. The international poverty line (IPL) is based on the national poverty lines of the 15 poorest countries. But we don't really know how accurate these lines are – some of them have been set using very poor data. Plus, they tell us little about what poverty is like in even slightly better-off countries. The IPL generally underestimates poverty when compared to national lines. In India, for example, national data shows that absolute poverty is twice as high as the IPL suggests (NDTV 2014; Prashad 2014). In Mexico and Sri Lanka, the figure is about ten times as high (Cimadamore et al. 2016; World Bank 2000: 237). Recent research shows that in most countries the IPL is actually not sufficient for basic human survival. In India a child living just above the IPL has a 60% risk of being underweight. In Niger, babies born just above the IPL face an infant mortality risk of nearly 20% – which is three times the world average (Wagstaff 2003).

If $1.25 is not sufficient to guarantee basic nutrition or infant survival, then we cannot claim that lifting people above this line means bringing them out of poverty. Research by economist Peter Edward (2006) shows that in order to achieve normal human life expectancy of just over 70 years, people need 3.9 times *more* than the IPL, or about $5 per day (in 2005 PPP). This is what Edward calls the "ethical poverty line," and it is probably the best global line currently available. The ethical poverty line has confirmation from a number of sources. Rahul Lahoti and Sanjay Reddy (2015) argue that people need about $4.50 per day to achieve minimum basic nutrition. The New Economics Foundation (2010) shows that people need about $5.87 per day to significantly reduce infant mortality.

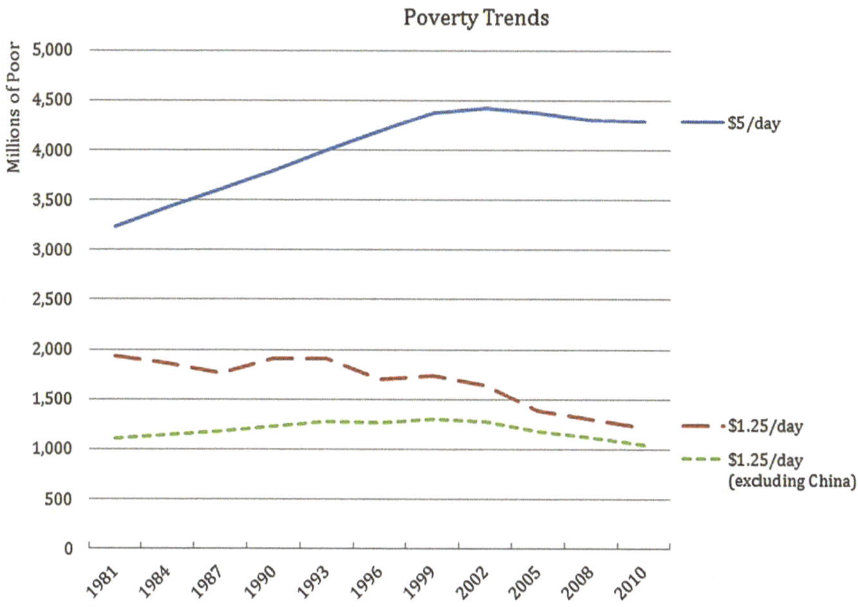

Fig. 12.1 Global poverty trends (Based on data from PovcalNet at 2005 PPP)

So what happens if we measure poverty at this more accurate level – at $5/day? We see that the global poverty headcount is closer to 4.3 billion people, even according to the World Bank's own calculations (see Fig. 12.1). That is 4 times more than the UN would have us believe. And, what is more, the number has risen steadily since 1981, with only a slight drop off after 2000 when the MDGs signaled that poor countries could prioritize social spending – an option denied to them under the structural adjustment programs imposed during the 1980s and 1990s (which I will describe below). According to this measurement, the number of poor people in the world today is one billion higher than it was in 1981.

During the course of the MDGs, many scholars called for the World Bank to upgrade its poverty line to reflect this more accurate view of the problem, but the World Bank consistently refused. They insisted on using the discredited dollar-a-day figure, for it is the only way to show any meaningful progress against poverty. In 2015, after the conclusion of the MDGs, the World Bank did announce a new poverty line of $1.90 per day. At first glance, it seemed to many that the Bank had finally admitted that the old line was too low, and raised it to a more meaningful level. But in reality the Bank didn't raise the line at all – it simply rebased it to the latest PPP standards (from 2011). Once again, the new line is effectively lower than the old one, in real terms, and therefore makes it seem as though there are fewer poor people than before. After rolling out the new poverty line, just in time for the new Sustainable Development Goals (SDGs), the Bank suddenly announced that the global poverty headcount had decreased by 100 million people overnight, and that the poverty reduction trend has been declining more rapidly than we used to

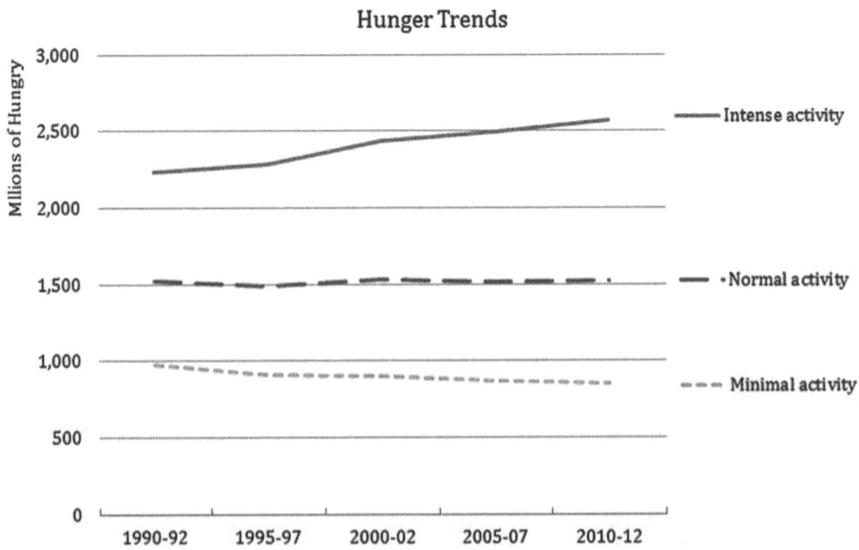

Fig. 12.2 Global hunger trends (Based on data from FAO 2009)

believe. It is important to note that this new poverty line brings us no closer to the ethical poverty line. If we rebase the ethical poverty line to the same PPP standard, it comes out as $7.40 per day (Hickel 2015).

A More Accurate View of Hunger

What about hunger? Even if we choose to accept the FAO's questionable new methodology, there are serious questions to be asked about the core definition of hunger that lies behind the dominant narrative. The FAO counts people as hungry only when their caloric intake becomes "inadequate to cover minimum needs for a sedentary lifestyle" for "over a year" (FAO 2012). So if a person is hungry for 11 months in a row, the FAO does not count them as hungry. And of course most poor people do not live sedentary lifestyles; rather, they are usually engaged in demanding physical labor, so in reality they need much more than the FAO's minimum caloric threshold. Even the FAO admits that this is true, acknowledging that "many poor and hungry people are likely to have livelihoods involved in arduous manual labor" and thus require caloric intake adequate for what it terms "normal" or "intense" activity (FAO 2012: 12). So what does global hunger look like at these more accurate levels? According to the "normal activity" threshold, the hunger headcount is about 1.5 billion, and according to the "intense activity" threshold it is more than 2.5 billion (see Fig. 12.2). And the numbers are rising, not falling. But even these figures are probably conservative. The FAO's definition of hunger counts only calories, so people who suffer from nutrient deficiencies fall through the cracks – a condition that affects about 2.1 billion people worldwide, even according to the FAO's own estimates (FAO 2012: 23). In fact, the FAO admits that its definition of hunger is "narrow", "very conservative," and thus "clearly insufficient" to inform policy.

The implications of this reality are profound. The fact that poverty and hunger trends have been worsening means the business-as-usual model of development is not working, and calls the legitimacy of our global economic system into question, for it is evidently failing the majority of humanity. The development industry has been active for many decades, and yet the number of poor and hungry people in the world has been generally growing, not shrinking.

Why Is Economic Development Failing?

The development industry is failing because it fails to address the real causes of poverty. It assumes that poverty is primarily an endogenous phenomenon, having to do with the domestic conditions of poor countries, as if poor countries are islands disconnected from the rest of the world. All they need is a bit of technical assistance and the right policies, and they should be on their way to full industrialization. It is the classic view of individual responsibility mapped onto the nation state. This view has some merit, of course, but its main problem is that it ignores the past 500 years of global political economy, during which the world system – to use Immanuel Wallerstein's phrase – was constructed in the interests of a relatively small number of rich countries. Colonialism played a significant role in this process. European powers protected their own markets with high trade tariffs, but forced their colonies to adopt low tariffs. These "unequal treaties" effectively prevented industrialization in most of the global South, while enabling it in the global North. Denied the opportunity for industrial development, global South countries were made to serve as suppliers of cheap raw materials and consumers of European manufactures (see Pomeranz 2001; Davis 2002). We cannot understand the condition of global suffering today without acknowledging this history.

But it is the post-colonial era that I wish to focus on here. After the end of colonialism in the 1950s, many newly independent global South countries followed the Keynesian model of development that had been working so well in the West. They made strategic use of land reforms to help peasant farmers, labor laws to boost workers' wages, tariffs and import substitution to protect and grow local businesses, and resource nationalization to help fund public housing, healthcare, and education. This was the heyday of what scholars call "developmentalism." Developmentalist policies sustained high per capita income growth rates across the global South of 3.2% on average during the 1960s and 1970s. It was a kind of development miracle, and many global South countries were making rapid progress against poverty and hunger. One might assume that Western governments would celebrate this good news; after all, they had long claimed to be in favor of development in the global

South. But they were not amused. Developmentalism meant that Western states were losing their access to the cheap raw materials they had enjoyed during colonialism, and were losing access to global South markets because they had to compete with high tariffs and import substitution.

Structural Drivers of Poverty

Western states were eager for a solution to this problem, and eventually they got it. When a debt crisis hit the global South in the early 1980s, due in large part to a sudden hike in interest rates by the US Federal Reserve (known as the Volcker Shock), developing countries came to the brink of defaulting on their external debt. The United States refused to permit default, however, because it would put overexposed Wall Street banks at risk of collapse. Instead, they used the IMF to roll over the debts of developing countries and impose "structural adjustment programs," which included a cocktail of austerity, market liberalization, and privatization – the exact opposite policies to developmentalism. We can think of this as a massive bank bailout. It was a way of guaranteeing debt repayment by funneling all existing resources in global South countries back to the creditors (in this sense, structural adjustment programs were very similar to the debt restructuring deals imposed on Greece after 2009). The World Bank followed suit, and made all of its new development loans conditional on the adoption of structural adjustment programs.

The World Bank and IMF assured us that structural adjustment would help stimulate the economies of poor countries. But exactly the opposite happened. Instead of helping poor countries, structural adjustment ruined them. Per capita income growth in developing world collapsed, from the 3.2% it enjoyed during the 1960s and 1970s down to 0.7% during the 1980s and 1990s. In total, Global south countries lost an average of $480 billion per year in potential GDP during the structural adjustment period (Pollin 2005: 133). Structural adjustment was particularly destructive in Sub-Saharan Africa. The GNP of the average country in the region *shrank* by around 10%, and the number of people in absolute poverty doubled. Globally, around 1.2 billion people were added to the ranks of the poor between 1980 and 2000, as we can see Fig. 12.1 at the $5/day line. It would be hard to overstate the extent of human suffering that these numbers represent. Structural adjustment was the greatest single cause of poverty in the twentieth century, after colonialism. And, ironically, it was conducted under the banner of "development".

Why were structural adjustment policies reproduced for so long, despite the fact that they were so obviously destructive? One of the main reasons has to do with skewed voting power in the World Bank and IMF. The global South, which has more than 80% of the world's population, has less than 50% of the vote. The remainder is controlled predominantly by a small handful of rich countries, and the US enjoys veto power over all major decisions. Another key issue is that the World Bank and IMF enjoy sovereign immunity, which means it is impossible to sue them when their policies cause economic crisis or human devastation. Their sovereign immunity produces a kind of moral hazard: because they bear no accountability for their actions, they have been able to continue these destructive practices with impunity. By the end of the 1990s, when it became clear that structural adjustment was causing such harm, the IMF and World Bank were forced to back down from it. They officially scrapped structural adjustment programs and replaced them with Poverty Reduction Strategy Papers (PRSPs); but behind the more palatable name, PRSPs operate on exactly the same principles, albeit with slightly less coercion.

For the most part, the development industry ignores these major structural drivers of poverty. And there are many others worth noting. In the World Trade Organization (WTO), bargaining power is determined by market size, so Western powers hold most of the cards. This explains why the WTO has forced the global South to abolish subsidies for its agricultural sector (the one sector in which it actually has comparative advantage) while allowing the US and EU to pay enormous subsidies to their own farmers, who then flood global markets with cheap grain and undercut producers in the South. Due to tariff imbalances like these, enshrined in the Uruguay Round of the WTO, global South countries are deprived of more than $700 billion each year in export revenues (Sogge 2002: 35). Imbalances in WTO governance also explain why the WTO prevented the global South from manufacturing generic antiretroviral medicines during the HIV/AIDS epidemic, leading to millions of preventable deaths.

There is another dimension of this story worth discussing. The trade liberalization that has been imposed on poor countries by the IMF, World Bank, and WTO allows multinational corporations to scour the planet in search of the cheapest labor. As a result of this hyper-mobility, countries have to compete for foreign investment by driving wages down. On top of this, "free trade" agreements often restrict union activity, and empower corporations to sue governments (in investor-state dispute settlement tribunals) if they improve labor standards. The result of this carefully constructed system is that workers in the global South earn only a fraction of the wages that workers in rich countries receive for the same productivity. In 1966, at the end of colonialism, economist Samir Amin calculated that developing countries were losing $161 billion (in 2015 dollars) each year through undervalued labor (Amin 1976: 144). Economist Gernot Kohler (1998) updated this figure for 1996, at the height of the globalization era, and found that annual losses had risen to $2.66 trillion.

Aid in Reverse

The point here is that it makes very little sense to focus on improving endogenous conditions for poverty eradication when by far the most significant drivers of poverty have to do with the structure of the global political economy. This seems a simple point, but the development industry does an effective job at avoiding it. Instead of looking at root causes, the industry distracts our attention with a narrative about aid. According to this narrative, rich countries bear no responsibility for the poverty of poor countries; quite the contrary, they reach out across the chasm and give generously of their surplus. How this surplus has been acquired is never questioned. And the claim made by figures like Jeffrey Sachs is that if rich countries just give enough aid, they will be able to help boost poor countries onto the development ladder. Of course in most cases it's not that poor countries aren't able to climb the ladder of their own accord – it's that they have been actively prevented from doing so. But the discourse of aid obscures this crucial fact.

Rich countries give around $140 billion per year in aid to poor countries. With disbursements like this, it is difficult to argue that rich countries don't have the best interests of poor countries in mind. But if we look more closely, we see that these aid disbursements from rich countries to poor countries are vastly outstripped by the wealth that flows in the opposite direction.

Consider tax evasion, for instance – one of the biggest media stories of the past few years. Western citizens have recently become concerned about the fact that giant corporations like Google and Starbucks are not paying their fair share of taxes in their countries; like many other major multinational corporations, they are stashing their wealth away in secretive offshore tax havens. Yet the real victims of the tax evasion system are not rich countries but poor countries. Global Financial Integrity calculates that up to $1.1 trillion flows illegally out of poor countries into Western accounts and tax havens each year, mostly through trade misinvoicing (Kar and Spanjers 2015). And then there is abusive transfer pricing, which probably costs the poor countries another $879 billion annually.[1] Together, these two figures add up to about 14 times the size of the aid budget. These outflows deprive poor countries of a vital source of tax revenue and capital investment – money that is essential for funding development.

And then there is debt service. Since the official aid budget includes loans and debt cancellation, it only makes sense that we should include debt service payments as part of the equation as well. Today, poor countries pay about $732 billion in total external debt service each year (according to the World Development Indicators), much of it on the compound interest of loans already paid off many times over, and some of it on loans accumulated in the past by illegitimate dictators, often backed by Western powers. Debt service alone amounts to more than 5 times the size of the aid budget.

We can see these figures as direct cash transfers from poor countries to rich countries. But there are many other flows of wealth and income that are being siphoned from the global South that we need to take into account. For example, Action Aid reports that multinational corporations extract about $138 billion from developing countries each year in tax holidays, which are different from tax evasion and avoidance (Balleny 2013). This figure alone nearly cancels out the global aid budget. For another example, we can look at the WTO's agreement on intellectual property rights (TRIPS), which forces developing countries to pay $60 billion annually –

[1] Raymond Baker (2005) estimates that the extent of transfer pricing is probably roughly the same as that of trade misinvoicing. According to Kar and Spanjers (2015), illicit flows due to trade misinvoicing amounted to $879 billion.

nearly half the aid budget – in extra patent licensing fees for the use of technologies and pharmaceuticals that are often essential to development and public health (Raman 2015). And this is to say nothing of other structural costs the global South suffers, such as those due to climate change, which is primarily the result of historical emissions from Europe and the United States. The costs of climate change in the global South are currently estimated at $571 billion per year; nearly six times the aid budget, according to the 2010 report of the Climate Vulnerability Monitor. Then there are forms of extraction that are more difficult to quantify, such as the 133 million acres of land (more than four times the size of England) that has been grabbed in developing countries over the past decade, according to the Land Matrix database.

These are just a few of the costs and outflows that we might tabulate. What emerges from this exercise is that the discourse of development has it backwards. Rich countries aren't developing poor countries; poor countries are effectively developing rich countries. Aid masks this harsh reality. It makes the takers seem like givers, grants them a kind of moral high ground, and prevents us from recognizing the structural drivers of poverty. This is not to say that aid does no good whatsoever. On the contrary, some of it surely goes a long way toward making people's lives measurably better. The problem is that it doesn't come close to compensating for the damage that the givers of aid themselves inflict. And, more importantly, it distracts us from seeing the broader picture. It hides the patterns of extraction that are actively causing the impoverishment of the global South today, or at least actively impeding meaningful development. If we think about aid in the context of this broader system of flows, it becomes clear that it is little more than political propaganda.

Imagining Solutions

Make the System Fairer

So what might we propose as solutions to these main structural drivers of poverty? Perhaps the most important step is to abolish the debt burdens of developing countries. This move is key to rolling back the power that rich countries exercise over poor countries, and to restoring democratic control over economic policy at the national level. It would also free developing countries to devote their budgets to healthcare, education, and poverty reduction efforts instead of just handing it over in debt service to big banks. Yes, there have been some steps toward debt relief over the past decade or so, but creditors have typically required structural adjustment as a condition for debt relief – so it does little more than perpetuate the problem. To be effective, debt relief needs to be unconditional. Building on this, we might say that all new development aid should be delivered without structural adjustment conditions. Getting rid of structural adjustment will ensure that developing countries have sufficient policy space to use tariffs, subsidies, capital controls, social spending, and other measures they might need for development and poverty reduction. Groups such as the Jubilee Debt Campaign and the Committee for the Abolition of the Third World Debt have been developing proposals on this issue for many years.

Second, we need to democratize the World Bank and the IMF to guarantee fair representation for the world's majority in these key institutions of global economic governance. The veto of the United States should be abolished, and voting power should be allocated according to a more democratic formula. In addition, the sovereign immunity of the World Bank and the IMF needs to be revoked, so we can hold them accountable for their actions. This move is essential to eliminate the moral hazard that presently plagues these institutions, which are free to dish out loans and policy prescriptions without heed for the damage they cause. We also need to democratize the World Trade Organization. All proceedings of the WTO should be made open and transparent with equal participation of all representatives. The exclusive Green Room meetings where rich countries pre-determine many of the WTO's most important decisions need to be discontinued, as do the secretive tribunals that decide the fate of countries accused of breaking WTO trade rules. These basic inequities should be rectified before any further demands for market liberalization are made on developing countries. See Joseph Stiglitz's (2003) work for some compelling initial proposals toward this end.

Third, we need to make the international trade system fairer. We could start by reforming the TRIPS agreement, relaxing patent protections so that poor countries can access the technologies they need for human development – especially generic versions of life-saving medicines. Better yet, we could demand that all life-saving medicines and other essential technologies be available in generic form, effectively decommoditizing them. The inequitable agricultural subsidy system also needs to be reformed, to allow global South countries fair access to Western markets and to protect their domestic markets from being undercut by cheap imports. Stiglitz (2005) has made an interesting proposal for reforming the imbalances of the trade system. He argues that, instead of requiring across-the-board tariff reductions, trade should be conducted with a bias toward poor countries. In his proposal, all WTO members would provide free market access in all goods to all developing countries either smaller or poorer than themselves (in terms of GDP and GDP per capita). This would allow developing countries to benefit from selling to rich-country markets without having to liberalize their own trade rules in return.

Fourth, we need to put a floor on the global "race to the bottom" for cheap labor. If we are going to have a global labor market, it stands to reason that we need a global system of labor standards, something that will guarantee a baseline level of fairness for workers. The single most important component of such a system would be an international minimum wage. The main recommendation out there – put forward by American economist Thomas Palley (2011) – is for the minimum wage to be set at 50% of each country's median wage, so it would be tailored to local economic conditions, costs of living, and purchasing power. As wages increase across the spectrum the floor would move up automatically, so we wouldn't have to constantly pressure politicians to raise the minimum. Under this proposal, all countries would be treated equally, and countries that presently enjoy a comparative advantage through cheap labor would retain that advantage, so there would be minimum disruption. Of course, in some countries median wages are so low that 50% of the median would still leave workers in poverty. So the global minimum would need a second safeguard: wages in each country must be above the national poverty line (Hickel 2013). This system would go a long way toward eliminating poverty, and would help reduce inequality within countries. Raising wages also has positive economic benefits: it stimulates demand and thus facilitates local economic growth, and it does so in a way that doesn't depend on debt (unlike, say, microfinance).

Fifth, we need to put an end to tax evasion. There are a number of ideas toward this end: closing down the tax havens, requiring country-by-country reporting of profits, and introducing penalties for bankers and accountants who facilitate tax evasion. Another popular idea is a global minimum tax on corporations, which would eliminate their incentive to evade national taxes. For a rich exploration of global tax justice solutions, see Pogge and Mehta (2016).

Sixth, ending hunger in particular will require a number of other key interventions. We know that, of all the progress against hunger that the MDGs claim, 50% of it comes from China during the 1990s. We also know that progress against hunger in China during that period was largely the result of land reform, which guaranteed small farmers secure access to land (Moore- Lappé et al. 2013a, b). Land reform is key to food security – but this is the opposite of what the UN is presently doing with the New Alliance for Food Security and Nutrition, which promotes consolidation of agricultural land in corporate hands. The 2014 report of the UN Special Rapporteur on the right to food argues that food security will require protecting small farmers from land grabs and other forms of eviction; ensuring that small farmers have rights to use, save and exchange seeds; regulating financial speculation on food commodities to prevent price spikes; and working towards food sovereignty, which means rolling back corporate control over food systems (De Schutter 2014).

There are many more solutions we might add to this list. By targeting ultimate structural issues, these kinds of interventions would have a monumental impact on poverty across the global South. This approach would not require a single additional dollar of foreign aid. It would, however, require a political struggle, for it would run straight up against the interests of very powerful actors who extract significant material benefit from the present system.

Abandon Preoccupation with GDP Growth

But, in and of itself, this reformist approach does not go far enough. It is easy to assume that if we can just make the economic system *fairer* then poor countries – finally masters of their own economic destinies – will be able to grow their economies, redistribute the gains, and eventually catch up to middle- and high-income countries. This vision sounds nice, and it may have made sense at one time, but as we become increasingly aware of climate change and our planet's resource limits, this promise begins to appear inherently contradictory, and perhaps even illogical. We now know that if everyone in the world lived like the average person in the average high-income country, we would need 3.4 Earths to sustain us, according to the Global Footprint Network. If we all lived like the average American, we would need 4.4 Earths. Clearly global development along the lines of the Western model is not feasible. Even at existing levels of global consumption, we are already overshooting our planet's biocapacity by about 50% each year. In other words, global economic growth is no longer an option – we have already grown too much, in aggregate. Scientists tell us that we are blowing past planetary boundaries at breakneck speed (Steffen et al. 2015).

This overshoot is due almost entirely to excess income and consumption in rich countries. Right now, our planet only has sufficient resources for each of us to consume 1.8 "global hectares" annually – a standardized unit that measures resource use, waste, and emissions. But people in the US and Canada consume about 8 global hectares per person, while Europeans consume 4.7, many times their fair share. If we accept the idea that poor countries will need to grow their economies in order to reduce poverty, we must accept that this will only be feasible if rich countries and rich individuals significantly reduce their over-consumption. In other words, rich countries – and gradually the whole world – need to embark on a path of intentional de-growth and plan a rapid shift to what Herman Daly (2014) has called a "steady-state" economy that maintains material throughput and pollution at ecological equilibrium. Our more optimistic pundits claim that rich countries will be able to maintain GDP growth into the future because technological innovation will gradually decouple growth from material throughput. Sadly there is no evidence that such decoupling is on the horizon. Global material extraction and consumption has doubled over the past 30 years, and accelerated since 2000 (Giljum et al. 2014). Current projections show that by 2040 we will more than double the world's shipping, trucking, and air miles – along with all the stuff those vehicles transport (Scutt 2016).

One key step will be to abandon GDP growth in favor of a saner measure of human progress – one that does not rely on endlessly increasing extraction and consumption (Stiglitz and Sen 2011; Fioramonti 2013). The imperative for GDP growth places human and natural systems under enormous pressure. As long as GDP growth remains the main objective of the global economy, the sensible reformist solutions I have listed above will be impossible. Why? Because the pressure to increase GDP translates into pressure for more loans, more structural adjustment, more "free trade", more land grabs, more deforestation, more extraction, and so on. It is impossible to push against this tide. But there are a number of well-researched alternatives out there. The Genuine Progress Indicator (GPI), for example, starts with GDP and then adds positive factors such as household and volunteer work, subtracts negatives such as pollution, resource depletion, and crime, and adjusts for inequality. A number of US states, like Maryland and Vermont, have already begun to use GPI as a measure of progress, albeit secondary to GDP. Costa Rica is about to become the first country to do so, and Scotland and Sweden may soon follow. Getting rid of the GDP growth imperative would release the pressure that causes so much human suffering, and focusing on GPI would incentivize policies that facilitate good outcomes while diminishing bad ones. It doesn't have to be GPI, of course; it could be any alternative measure. As soon as we are free from the tyranny of GDP, we can have an open discussion about what we really value, and how we want to measure human progress.

Conclusion

When it comes to the question of world suffering, we have allowed ourselves to be lulled into complacency by official reports stating that global poverty and hunger have been decreasing steadily and will soon be eradicated. If we look more closely at the data behind these claims, however, it becomes clear that the problem is not so tractable. In reality, around four billion people remain in poverty today, and around two billion remain in hunger – and the numbers have been generally rising over the past few decades, not falling. This compels us to rethink our approach to alleviating world suffering, as our existing strategy, as embodied by the international development industry, has been failing according to these metrics. Effectively alleviating world suffering requires more than just a bit of aid here and there. It requires targeting root structural causes: the international debt system, structural adjustment, lack of democracy in global governance, unfair trade regimes, poor wages, tax evasion, land grabs, and climate change. Redressing these political imbalances is essential for reducing global poverty and hunger. But in light of our planet's resources limits, we have to go one step further. In addition to making the global economy fairer for the world's majority, the great challenge of the twenty-first century will be to actively shrink our ecological footprint to fit within the planet's boundaries – reducing the material over-consumption of the richer countries while improving human development in the poorer ones.

References

Amin, S. (1976). *Unequal development*. New York: The Harvester Press.

Baker, R. (2005). *Capitalism's Achilles heel: Dirty money and how to renew the free-market system*. Hoboken: Wiley.

Balleny, L. (2013, July 4). Corporate tax breaks cost poor nations $138 billion a year – Report. *Reuters*. http://news.trust.org//item/20130704171338-lvmdw/?source=search. Accessed 1 Aug 2016.

Caparros, M. (2014, September 27). Counting the hungry. *New York Times*. http://www.nytimes.com/2014/09/28/opinion/sunday/counting-the-hungry.html?_r=0. Accessed 1 Aug 2016.

Chen, S. & Ravallion, M. (2004, June). *How have the world's poorest fared since the early 1980s?* World Bank policy research working paper 3341. Washington, DC: World Bank.

Cimadamore, A., Koehler, G., & Pogge, T. (2016). *Poverty and the Millennium Development Goals: A critical look forward*. London: Zed Books.

Daly, H. (2014). *From uneconomic growth to a steady-state economy*. Cheltenham: Edward Eglar.

Davis, M. (2002). *Late Victorian holocausts: El Nino famines and the making of the Third World.* London: Verso.
De Schutter, O. (2014). *Report of the special Rapporteur on the right to food.* New York: United Nations Human Rights Council.
Edward, P. (2006). The ethical poverty line: A moral quantification of absolute poverty. *Third World Quarterly, 37*(2), 377–393.
Fioramonti, L. (2013). *Gross domestic problem: The politics behind the world's most powerful number.* London: Zed Books.
Food and Agricultural Organization. (2009). *State of food insecurity in the world.* Rome: Food and Agricultural Organization.
Food and Agricultural Organization. (2012). *State of food insecurity in the world.* Rome: Food and Agricultural Organization.
Giljum, S., et al. (2014). Global patterns of material flows and their socio-economic and environmental implications. *Resources, 3*, 319–339.
Hickel, J. (2013, June 10). It's time for a global minimum wage. *Al Jazeera English.* http://www.aljazeera.com/indepth/opinion/2013/06/20136910314254268.html. Accessed 1 Aug 2016.
Hickel, J. (2015). Could you live on $1.90 a day? That's the international poverty line. *The Guardian.* https://www.theguardian.com/global-development-professionals-network/2015/nov/01/global-poverty-is-worse-than-you-think-could-you-live-on-190-a-day. Accessed 1 Aug 2016.
Hickel, J. (2016). The true extent of global poverty and hunger: Questioning the good-news narrative of the Millennium Development Goals. *Third World Quarterly, 37*(5), 749–767.
Kar, D., & Spanjers, J. (2015). *Illicit financial flows from developing countries: 2004–2013.* Washington, DC: Global Financial Integrity.
Kohler, G. 1998. *Unequal exchange 1965–1995: World trend and world tables.* http://wsarch.ucr.edu/archive/papers/kohler/kohler3.htm. Accessed 1 Aug 2016.
Lahoti, R. & Reddy, S. (2015). *$1.90 per day: What does it say?* Institute for New Economic Thinking. https://www.ineteconomics.org/ideas-papers/blog/1-90-per-day-what-does-it-say?p=ideas-papers/blog/1-90-per-day-what-does-it-say. Accessed 1 Aug 2016.
Moore-Lappé, F., et al. (2013a). *Framing hunger: A response to the State of food insecurity in the world 2012.* http://www.ase.tufts.edu/gdae/pubs/rp/framinghunger.pdf. Accessed 1 Aug 2016.
Moore-Lappé, F., et al. (2013b). How we count hunger matters. *Ethics & International Affairs, 27*(3), 251–259.
NDTV. (2014, February 20). *Poverty in India 2.5 times the official figure: Study.* http://www.ndtv.com/india-news/poverty-in-india-2-5-times-the-official-figure-study-551445. Accessed 1 Aug 2016.
Nelson, F. (2015, January 19). What Oxfam doesn't want you to know. *The Spectator.* http://blogs.spectator.co.uk/coffeehouse/2015/01/what-oxfam-doesnt-want-you-to-know-global-capitalism-means-theres-less-poverty-than-ever/. Accessed 1 Aug 2016.
New Economics Foundation. (2010). *How poor is poor? Toward a rights-based poverty line.* London: New Economics Foundation.
Palley, T. (2011, July 18). A global minimum wage system. *The Financial Times.* http://blogs.ft.com/economistsforum/2011/07/a-global-minimum-wage-system/. Accessed 1 Aug 2016.
Pogge, T., & Mehta, K. (Eds.). (2016). *Global tax fairness.* Oxford: Oxford University Press.
Pogge, T. (2004). The first United Nations Millennium development goal: A cause for celebration? *Journal of Human Development, 5*(3), 377–397.
Pogge, T. (2009). How world poverty is measured and tracked. In M. Elcke et al. (Eds.), *Absolute poverty and global justice.* Aldershot: Ashgate.
Pogge, T. (2010). Millions killed by clever dilution of our promise. *Crop Poverty Brief.* http://www.crop.org/CROPNewsEvents/Millions-Killed-by-Clever-Dilution-of-Our-Promise.aspx. Accessed 1 Aug 2016.
Pollin, R. (2005). *Contours of descent.* New York: Verso.

Pomeranz, K. (2001). *The great divergence: China, Europe, and the making of the modern world economy*. Princeton: Princeton University Press.
Prashad, V. (2014, November 10). Making poverty history. *Jacobin*. https://www.jacobinmag.com/2014/11/making-poverty-history/. Accessed 1 Aug 2016.
Raman, M. (2015, May 10). WIPO seminar debates intellectual property and development. *Our World is Not For Sale*. http://www.ourworldisnotforsale.org/en/article/wipo-seminar-debates-intellectual-property-and-development. Accessed 1 Aug 2016.
Reddy, S., & Pogge, T. (2005). *How not to count the poor*. New York: Columbia University Academic Commons.
Scutt, D. (2016, April 19). Forecast for worldwide growth of ships, cars, and people – Bernstein Research. *Business Insider*. http://www.businessinsider.com.au/global-crude-oil-demand-emerging-markets-india-china-april-bernstein-2016-4. Accessed 1 Aug 2016.
Sogge, D. (2002). *Give and take: What's the matter with foreign aid?* London: Zed Books.
Steffen, W., et al. (2015). Planetary boundaries: Guiding human development on a changing planet. *Science, 347*(6249), 1259855. doi:10.1126/science.1259855.
Stiglitz, J. (2003). Democratizing the international Monetary Fund and the World Bank: Governance and accountability. *Governance, 16*(1), 111–139.
Stiglitz, J. (2005). *Fair trade for all: How trade can promote development*. Oxford: Oxford University Press.
Stiglitz, J., & Sen, A. (2011). *Mis-measuring our lives*. New York: The New Press.
United Nations. (2013). *Millennium development goals report*. New York: United Nations.
United Nations. (2015). *Millennium development goals report*. New York: United Nations.
Wagstaff, A. (2003). Child health on a dollar a day: Some tentative cross-country comparisons. *Social Science and Medicine, 57*(9), 1529–1538.
World Bank. (2000). *World development report 1999/2000*. Washington, DC: World Bank.

Chapter 13
Refugees and Citizens on the Margins: Sufferings Recognized, Sufferings Denied

Cawo Mohamed Abdi

Introduction

A personal appeal from the United Nations High Commissioner for Refugees opens with the statement "Refugees are among the most vulnerable people in the world." (UNHCR 2011). Dispossession, displacement, and multiple forms of violence anchor our thinking of what and who refugees are. The ultimate outcome of political crisis and violence that pushes millions of people out of the borders of their own nation-states inevitably leads to physical, emotional, economic, and political insecurity that instantaneously transforms lives and futures in ways that were probably unimaginable for most of those affected. The world is witnessing such a disoriented population with the Syrian refugee crisis. This political turmoil is being felt by citizens and nations that are geographically far away (Europe) and by those much closer (bordering countries). New technologies are facilitating this latest refugee crisis to pull our emotional strings in ways that would never have been imagined decades ago when the world was experiencing similar and even worse crises (under Nazism for example), but the suffering of the affected populations could not be witnessed as viscerally as they are today. A globally connected audience watches live as boats dock in Lesbos, Greece, and as the dead bodies of refugees are scattered on the beaches of Turkey, Greece, and Malta.

Suffering and the refugee condition remain intrinsically tied both in the past and in the present. And when we use the words "suffering" or "sufferings" regarding refugees, there is often no expectation to define what we mean by these words. But refugees do not have a monopoly on suffering, nor do they have a monopoly on the urgency to alleviate suffering from our world. Our definition of this concept,

C.M. Abdi (✉)
Associate Professor, Department of Sociology, University of Minnesota, USA
e-mail: cabdi@umn.edu

R.E. Anderson (ed.), *Alleviating World Suffering*, Social Indicators Research Series 67, DOI 10.1007/978-3-319-51391-1_13

therefore, requires us to include myriad other categories in which suffering is also real and just as desperate. As such, this paper engages with the fact that suffering remains the lot of millions of citizens around the globe, most of whose nation-states have not collapsed, but whose daily lives are defined by experiences and conditions that are at times much worse than those experienced by refugees. Highlighting the suffering of "invisible" sufferers is meant to underscore the need for political solutions to alleviate the suffering of refugees, while also drawing attention to competing "victimhoods" and the role legal and legible categories—refugees versus citizens, for example—play in our definitions of suffering.

Linking the injustices and violence experienced by refugees to that which might also prevail for marginalized citizens in the refugee-hosting countries is paramount in order to alleviate all suffering. As we seek solutions to safeguard the rights of refugees, we also need to pressure refugee-hosting governments to safeguard the rights of their own citizens. The paper thus asks: How does our empathy and representation of particular experiences privilege and marginalize some groups while attending to that of others? How and what actions, both local and global, might aid in alleviating the suffering of those most marginalized, regardless of their legal status?

The aim of this chapter is to excavate the denied suffering of South African poor Black citizens, which I argue shapes their relationship with refugees who arrive at their shores in search of safe haven. I showcase how in addition to being a major refugee-hosting nation, a large segment of the Black South African population is mired in much injustice-violence, exclusion, and apathy toward their condition that is comparable to the violence subjected to refugee populations in this country. Again, my goal is not to compare the kinds of suffering, but rather to link the intertwined nature of suffering for both groups and to argue for interventions that are more holistic in the approach to alleviate the suffering of each. I strive to expose the inadequacy that emerges when justice for refugees is sought with little effort to also intervene and change the dehumanizing conditions that the local Black and poor South Africans confront in their daily lives in post-apartheid South Africa. I posit that massive inequality, neglect to attend to the most basic needs of citizens, and the persistent structural violence in South Africa all produce vulnerability and suffering for locals. Alleviating this suffering is crucial to counter the violence and animosity that refugees and migrants confront in this country.

The paper builds on my work with refugees over the past 15 years. I have conducted fieldwork in Kenya, South Africa, Somalia, the United Arab Emirates and the United States. More specifically, the article extends my work in South Africa where refugees and migrants have confronted extreme levels of violence, displacement, and dispossession. Building on previous publications on this topic (Abdi 2015, 2011), I also draw from the secondary data available on South African migrant and native relations and the highly publicized attacks against migrant and refugee businesses and bodies in South African townships and informal settlements.

Suffering as a Concept

In the context of major political upheavals, or political persecution, be it refugee crisis, genocide, apartheid, or ethnic cleansing, what we witness is suffering as a social phenomenon that transcends the individual pain and trauma that the term conjures in our everyday usage. As Kleinman rightly states, it is worthy to study "[S]ocial suffering, its relation to subjectivity, its bodiliness as processes that connect the moral to the medical, the political to the emotional, and the religious to the physiological, and the manner in which it (and with it the human experience of transformation) is being remade in our disordering contemporary world." (Kleinman 1997: 317). Suffering imposed on an individual or a group includes the "insidious assault on dignity" such that institutionalized forms of exclusion and insecurity (physical, psychological, economic, and emotional) cause pain and suffering for millions around the world (Farmer 1996, 2004; Frost and Hoggett 2008). We also know that social suffering in not exclusive to areas of political turmoil but is the lot of subgroups found in the wealthiest nations of the world (Kleinman et al. 1997; Farmer 2004; Koinange 2006; Keaton 2006; Bass 2014). Hurricane Katrina in the United States, or the uprisings of youth in French banlieues expose the third world within the first world, segments of the population that remain off the international media radar until a natural disaster like a hurricane or a riot (New Orleans, Los Angeles, Ferguson, Paris, etc.) reveals to the rest of the world the "other" United States or the "other" France.

In a world where suffering is omnipresent then, alleviating human suffering remains messy and often complex. The most direct humanitarian interventions in refugee crises are more straightforward, as the need to provide basic shelter, medicine, and subsistence to people fleeing or crossing international borders takes precedence over the need for those caught in persistent poverty and violence that might exist in particular neighborhoods in New Orleans or Los Angeles. Even if or when the latter is produced by racism, police brutality, poverty, or centuries-old discrimination, its moral pull remains weak despite the consistent suffering and humiliations that these communities confront in their daily lives. The latter condition is tied to structural violence, a broad term referencing institutionalized forms of exclusion, or as Farmer (2004: 307) puts it "[s]tructural violence is violence exerted systematically—that is, indirectly—by everyone who belongs to a certain social order: hence the discomfort these ideas provoke in a moral economy still geared to pinning praise or blame on individual actors. In short, the concept of structural violence is intended to inform the study of the social machinery of oppression." But what happens when this structural violence is so extreme that it has an impact on the majority of the population and thus leads to crises that massively affect the physical, social, and psychological security of the majority of the population as well as the majority of newcomers?

The above crises is of course distinct from that experienced by refugees who, because of extreme violence, were pushed outside of the borders of their birth places. The 1951 refugee convention continues to define a refugee as "a person who is outside his or her country of nationality or habitual residence; has a well-founded fear of being persecuted because of his or her race, religion, nationality, membership of a particular social group or political opinion; and is unable or unwilling to avail him- or herself of the protection of that country, or to return there, for fear of persecution" (see Article 1A(2)) (UNHCR 2011:5). This category carries the weight given to it as a result of the failure of a given state to provide the protections hypothetically guaranteed for citizens of the modern nation-state system. As such, an anchoring assumption in this definition is that those who are unable or unwilling to cross international borders, even when they experience violence, are not able to access the protection available to those who leave their birth country. Moreover, another premise in this definition is that the receiving country provides social, political, and civic protection to its own citizens and thus is capable of extending this privilege to the non-citizens who now find themselves within its borders.

But while the legal aspects of receiving refugees (providing legal avenues to seek asylum in signatory countries) might be straightforward, we often underestimate the complexity of "protection" beyond the legal documentation that qualifies refugee newcomers to stay within the receiving country when civil, social, and political rights of the majority of the citizenry is in fact extremely curtailed. In such context, what role does the nation-state hosting the refugees as well as the international community have in intervening in cases where refugee-native relations involve competition and violence? Can the alleviation of refugee suffering be divorced from that of the locals in a context where marginalization and violence define daily reality of a large segment of the citizenry? As will be illustrated in the next section, discussions on refugee and suffering in the South African context often decouple this experience from that of the local population, a practice that I argue is counter to alleviating the violence and conflict.

Contradictions in Citizenship: Suffering in Post-apartheid South Africa

After the fall of Apartheid in 1994 and the triumph of the liberation movement represented by Nelson Mandela's presidential election, South Africa pursued a major reform to its immigration policies and drafted its first ever refugee act in 1998, subsequently finalized in 2001 (Handmaker 2001). Unlike the migration policies under apartheid which viewed whites as the only desirable migrant group able to integrate well into the dominant "white" ruler group, Africans were historically allowed to come into South Africa as temporary labor migrants, with the expectation that they would eventually return to their home countries (Crush 2008; Siddique 2004; Adepoju 2003). Within the span of less than two decades since the migration and refugee policy reforms, however, South Africa emerged as a major migrant and refugee magnet, in fact remaining "the leading destination country of new asylum-seekers worldwide between 2008 and 2012" and still remains in the top ten asylum-providing countries, now superseded only by European countries and Turkey as a result of the Syrian refugee crisis (UNHCR 2015:53).

What does asylum mean in the post-apartheid context of South Africa? Asylum in essence connotes a safe haven, a place where social, economic, and political security might be achievable, contrary to the place from which refugees fled. Asylum is thus the first step in the alleviation of refugee suffering. In the South African case, however, the persistence of economic, physical, and psychological insecurities of the majority Black population whose lives remain curtailed by extreme levels of exclusion requires attention in light of hundreds of thousands of refugees seeking safe haven. Any research in South Africa has to grapple with persistent structural violence, the result of apartheid legacy but also as an outcome of neoliberal economic policies in post-apartheid regimes and the slow pace of reforms (Abdi 2015, 2011; Marais 2011). This structural violence remains deeply entrenched despite great efforts to transform this nation from its apartheid condition, with governments since 1994 delivering millions of homes for the poor, increasing educational expenditure for Black pupils, and opening employment opportunities in all sectors in the public and private sphere for those previous excluded (Møller 1998, 2007; The Economist 2010). This is to say that it is undeniable that the fall of apartheid ushered a multiracial nation, where legal forms of segregation and discrimination were eliminated from the books. Despite these legal reforms, however, extreme levels of suffering remain as a result of persistent structural violence that the majority Black South African population experience in their daily lives. The data on poverty, unemployment, homicide, rape, and housing all indicate acute suffering experienced by a large portion of South Africa's Black (and colored) populations.

For example, South Africa remains a "high crime society" (Berg and Scharf 2004), with its population suffering from what some called "murderous intolerance" (Nedcor Project 1997, cited in Louw 1997:151). The fact that 28% of men in South Africa admitted to have raped at least once in their life time renders this violence concrete (*The Economist* 2010:12). These extreme levels of gender violence unfortunately occur in a context where the prevalence of HIV and AIDS for those aged 15–49 years is 18%–20% (UNAIDS 2014). And while rates of violent crime go and up and down, they remain exceptionally high for South Africa. As the South African Institute for Security concludes: "The most notable aspect of the crime statistics for 2012/13 is that the violent crimes that cause the most fear and trauma amongst the public have increased." (Africa Check 2013) Some argue the crime statistics in South Africa are similar to what might be expected from a country at war (ibid).

Moreover, the economic gap between the haves and the have-nots continues to widen. This persistent economic chasm led a leading economist-Thomas Piketty-to decry in a Guardian article that "[o]f course now we are 25 years after the fall of apartheid ... [but] inequality is not only still very high in South Africa, but has been rising and in some ways income inequality is even higher today than 20 years ago." (Allison 2015). In addition to debilitating poverty and unemployment and underemployment, however, the physical insecurity experienced by a large segment of the population living with inadequate shelter and protection is what most characterized social suffering in this country (*The Economist* 2010). The extremes of wealth and deprivation found in this country are concurrent with its place in the African continent as an exceptionally wealthy nation, thus a magnet for refugees and migrants from around Africa and beyond. The then South African -Deputy President Thabo Mbeki stated in 1998 that a "major component part of the issue of reconciliation and nation-building is defined by and derives from the material conditions in our society which have divided our country into two nations, the one [B]lack and the other [W]hite." (International Relations Cooperation 1998). Though some Blacks have now joined what Mbeki called the White camp of the division in economic terms, the sense of two nations, unequal and separate, remains in South Africa.

The magnet pulling refugees and migrants thus includes first-class infrastructure and economies of Cape Town and Johannesburg. But the majority of refugees and migrants to South Africa join the "black" nation, a majority that is marginal and at the bottom of the food chain. This majority never enters the glittering high rises in the financial districts as they remain segregated within the omnipresent shacks and underdeveloped informal settlements and townships that house millions of poor and black citizens.

For these local citizens, unemployment is often estimated to be between 25–40%, (Kingdon and Knight 2004; IDASA 2008). As such, a recent World Bank report stated that "[T]he country is plagued by one of the highest levels of unemployment and economic inactivity for middle-income countries. More than one-third of its labor force is out of work or has stopped searching for jobs. The unemployment rate for young people is close to 50 percent, and many more of them are neither employed nor in the education system (World Bank 2015:3). Economic deprivation and marginalization translates to lives lived on the margins, in residential areas where those most vulnerable rarely benefit from law and order and suffering is omnipresent. Abject poverty and constant fear of victimization translates to denial of dignity. New refugees and migrants seek their livelihoods in this environment, a pursuit that becomes complicated given the levels of turmoil that already prevail in this setting.

In Search of Economic Prosperity

The majority of refugees seek asylum in the countries bordering their birth place. As such, 86% of the global refugee population lives in the developing countries, with Syria, Afghanistan and Somalia producing the highest numbers over the past few years (UNHCR 2014). Turkey for Syrians, Pakistan for Afghanis, and Kenya and Ethiopia for Somalis are the destinations hosting these large refugee populations. But as the case of Somali refugees in South Africa illustrates, many migrants and refugees undertake secondary migrations following their initial flight from conflict zones. Somalis in South Africa, for example, have crossed five to six borders to get to their destination (Abdi 2015).

Between 20,000 and 30,000 Somalis have sought asylum in South Africa since 1994, with the majority arriving since the early 2000s. Many of these Somalis had already lived in Kenya or Ethiopia before traveling farther afield in search of better opportunities than they were able to secure in their first country of asylum. This is to say that these refugees had many opportunities to submit asylum applications in any of the countries that they came through, including Kenya, Tanzania, Malawi, Zambia, Zimbabwe, or Mozambique, but chose South Africa as their country of choice given the economic opportunities deemed to be available for them there. The categories of refugees and economic migrants in South Africa, similar to most places around the world, are thus a bit more complex and often harder to detangle as these Somalis are both refugees whose initial displacement was the result of the generalized violence and absence of law and order in Somalia, but their secondary movements are driven by a concerted search for economic advancement absent to them in the first places of asylum (Abdi 2015).

The majority of Somalis thus seek their livelihoods in the midst of the acute deprivation that is the reality for a large segment of the Black South African population. As I detailed elsewhere, Somalis bring with them social networks and entrepreneurial skills that they developed either in Somalia or other places of settlement (Abdi 2011, 2015). They also benefit from and become anchored in business networks that they cultivate with the Indian Muslim minority in Mayfair, Bellville, and Kosten among other towns. Such networks allow Somalis to progressively expand their economic pursuits, from hourly wage workers in the warehouses and stores owned by Indian Muslims, to peddlers on the trains and buses all over the country, to finally expanding and even dominating the smaller corner stores (spazas) in informal settlements or slums and on the margins of the townships. Thus economic pursuit involves extreme hard work and sacrifice. For example, many of the Somali men running these stores stay away from their wives and children for weeks on end, as their families' residential areas often differ from the places where they find work opportunities (Abdi 2011, 2015). Also, refugees achieving economic success in areas where structural conditions curtailed skills development and financing opportunities for local potential entrepreneurs heightens resentment and conflict between these two groups. In the following section, I juxtapose the shared suffering expressed by Somalis and native poor South African Blacks in South African townships and informal settlements followed by the divergent readings of this indignity and insecurity.

Agency, Empathy, and Hierarchies of Suffering: Somali Refugees and Poor Black South African Citizens

A 46-year-old Black South African woman who lives in Khayelitsha and whom I interviewed in 2009 decried the constant insecurity that she and her neighbors confront in their daily lives.

> Oh, the crime is so high! If you are sleeping, you are scared—maybe someone will open your door and like I told you last time, there was a man who opened my daughter's shelter and he stuck something in her. It was a screwdriver. So we are not safe in our community—we are not safe at all.

Others I interviewed supported this pervasive insecurity, with another woman repeatedly emphasizing that it is both the daytime and the night time when violence and victimization can occur. Also there is a sense that "one does not care about the other" in South Africa as a 21-year- old in Langa put it. So while South Africa is not a war zone comparable to Somalia, the daily insecurities and psychological and physical dangers, or suffering, which the native poor confront is no less acute, no less real. Worthy of mention is that this danger is classed and racialized, as South African spend the most in private security in the world, with private security personnel of 300,000–400,000 far exceeding the 150,000 or so in the national police force (Blackmore 2003: 439–40; *The Economist* 2010:12). Thus security for citizens is up for sale, and that remains out of reach for those whose housing conditions make it impossible to have secured electric fences and private armed guards.

It is within what I call generalized violence among the poor Black residential areas where attacks against migrants and refugees drew international attention over the past decade or so. In the now 2008 iconic image of a Zimbabwean man in flames with his torso sticking out from a burning tire, and the subsequent death of more than sixty people in what have been dubbed "xenophobic" attacks against foreigners in many parts of South Africa, violence against migrants and refugees drew the international media gaze. But the attention constructed two contrasting images: that of the demonized "South African" Black and poor who is xenophobic, and that of the victimized "other," whose blackness and foreignness drew the wrath of the angry local. This image appears not only in media analysis of the violence but also in academic literature on this topic. Further distinguishing the two groups are the claims that South Africans owe gratitude to other Africans, whose countries have sheltered liberation movement exiles during the apartheid era. For example, Sinclair, referring to the violence subjected to African migrants and refugees, writes that "these stand as a sad reflection of the inability of South African people to acknowledge the contributions and inevitability of foreigners in the new South Africa…" (Sinclair 1999: 466).

While the majority of migrants and refugees also struggle on the margins in South Africa, it is my contention that most migrants are faring better economically when compared to the native poor, whose residential areas were shut out from economic development under apartheid, and whose potential entrepreneurial skills development as well as access to capital and investments continues to be highly restricted. In these residential areas, highly organized and entrepreneurial migrants such as Somalis and Ethiopians enter and often place pressure on the small number of locally owned businesses. Searching livelihoods in areas where basic safety is absent for the locals, as well as places where gangs terrorize the local population, inevitably exposes refugees and migrants to new forms of persecution similar to and even worse than that which drove them outside their own countries.

Economic success of the newcomers triggers resentment which renders the latter targets. In the case of Somalis, for example, I found that their prices often remain lower than those offered by South African black competitors. The ability of Somalis to buy in bulk, often pooling the resources of a number of co-ethnic store owners, and their relations with Indian wholesalers, gives them the upper hand over the local business owners who have much more curtailed social and economic capital. The case of a Somali woman who runs a medium-sized store in the Western Cape region with her husband and two other salaried employees highlights the success that migrants and refugees can achieve in the midst of South African communal crises. Discussing her income, Shukria stated:

> I make about R5000[1] per month. My labor accounts for R2000 and R3000 is from my share of the profit from the store. The income from my labor is constant, but the profits fluctuate. I may get R4000, R4500, R5000 depending on how well the business is doing.

To put this monthly income into context, we need to compare it to the data on South African born wages. South African earning less than R30,164 per year in 2005/2006 included 72.5% of Black Africans, 45% of Colored, 17.6% of Indians and 3.3% of Whites (Statistics South Africa 2011). Racial disparities clearly account for the two extremes. If we assume that Shukria's husband made about the same income as she did, though in reality his share of the investment in the store was larger, then their household income would place them in the upper quintile (those earning more than R68,528 per year), a position only 7.9% of Blacks, 25.6% of Colored, 50% of Indians and 83% of Whites occupied in 2005/2006 (ibid). As such an individual monthly income ranging from R4000 to R5000 for this Somali woman, adding up to about R48,000 to R60,000 yearly, placed her in the higher end of the income bracket for Blacks in South Africa. In fact the median income for South Africans in 2011 was only R3033 per month, lower than what Shukria was making in 2009. Even those Somali refugees at the bottom of the income bracket—maids or young men who are waged employees for other Somali business owners—were paid monthly wages that were often double what Somalis pay to their South African, Zimbabwean and Malawian employees (R2000 compared to about R800–R1000 Rand to non-Somali workers). Here we see discrimination on the basis of co-ethnic preferences by Somalis as these are viewed to be more trustworthy than the local non-Somali workers (Abdi 2015).

It is important to highlight the hard work and sacrifices that allowed Shukria and other migrants and refugees to succeed in their work. She left two children with her mother in Somalia so that she can work in South Africa. She also reported confronting daily verbal abuse from the locals who view her as taking the economic opportunities that the locals should have occupied. It is hence this context of competition but also resentment and ultimately violence that migrants and refugees confront. The slow progress of the promises of liberation include the absence or the inadequate service provisions (housing, sanitation, security etc.) for many who live on the margins of townships. Riots triggered by anger against the local and national government often transmute to targeted wrath against those most vulnerable in these areas: migrants, refugees, and their properties. As such, I suggest that poorer foreigners who escaped from suffering in their home countries end up being "embraced"

[1] The Rand has fluctuated much over the past two decades as clear from its value to the American dollar in 1994 (R3.55), in 2000 (R6.94), in 2009 (8.41) and at its lowest in 2016 (R15.34) (UKForex 2016).

into the lot of the South African poor: a generalized violence that is omnipresent for the locals, many of whom remain resigned to their condition—killings, robberies, and rapes. As this suffering is concentrated in areas inhabited by the mostly poor and Black citizens, it rarely draws attention at national and international levels.

Violence against migrants has led to the deaths of hundreds of Somalis in South Africa since the late 1990s (personal communication, The Somali Association of South Africa). As such, Somalis and many other African refugees express their horror of leaving a war zone and settling in a war zone. But the targeted violence against migrants and refugees often dubbed as xenophobic means that these attacks draw extensive attention from rights organizations. Unlike Kenya, Ethiopia and other countries that isolate refugees into closed refugee camps, South Africa through its asylum process grants renewable resident permits to those who successfully petition their case. With these permits, refugees join many of their compatriots around the country and seek their livelihoods in the informal sector, as the formal sector is shut out to them due to their low educational skills and their non-citizen status.

Newcomers who escaped from political and economic strains in their own countries enter the most underdeveloped areas of South Africa, where the first-class economic infrastructure found in central Pretoria, Johannesburg or Cape Town are non-existent, where tea, diapers, and tomatoes are retailed and sold by the piece. Cognizant of the great livelihood opportunities on the edges of townships, a Somali who hailed South Africa as a wonderful place described how insecurity is making him and many in his community strive and strategize for further migration, as the levels of violence are intolerable. Talking about his views on migration to the Western world [there], he concluded:

> If you compare there and here at the economic level, it is better here. But there is no security here whereas there is peace there. Here, you are not safe and you don't have legal documents. I don't have documents I can use if I decide to visit my mother in East Africa. When you have legal documents, life becomes easier … One of the main reasons why I want to migrate relates to security, to a place where I can wake up in peace. I am scared when I am sleeping and the phone rings. Even if I am not sleeping at the store, whenever the phone rings, you fear that someone will tell you that your brother was killed or your cousin or someone you know was killed. If you are at the store, you get scared at every crack or sound you hear because you are frightened and thinking, someone will break into the store right now. What can be worse than being afraid of every customer? Whenever someone enters your store, you are asking yourself "does he have a gun? Is he the one who will kill you?" You always have this feeling that you are going to be killed or that you will receive news of someone's death. I don't think that people in the U.S. or Europe are walking in the streets thinking that someone will kill them (Asad, interview Bellville 2009).

In addition to the uncertainly of securing legal documentation, which in the South African context has become harder and harder as the Home Office is now mired in corruption scandals, the psychological stress of fearing every customer that he serves illustrates the acute nature of the suffering that Somalis and other refugees and migrants in poorer areas in South Africa confront. But the above assessment of the reality of violence in South Africa is also aligned with the earlier statement made by the South African woman who said "no one is safe in our community."

"No one is safe in our community" showcases the normalized suffering and insecurity in a highly underdeveloped and unpoliced area where the majority of the people live in abject poverty. But it also shows that new migrants and refugees coming into this setting, whose language, nationality and social networks are disconnected from that of the locals, also become very vulnerable (just like local women, children and the elderly in these volatile settings). Such vulnerability, or the suffering shared by many of the local Black population and the African unskilled Black migrants and refugees, is however not represented as deserving of the same outcry, empathy, and intervention

A whole body of global bureaucratic agencies and agents and conventions dealing with refugees produce a reductive category of the "refugee," eternally victim, eternally an object of technological and humanitarian intervention and management (Hyndman 2000; Malkki 1992). This, I argue, comes to the fore when refugees are attacked in these townships and informal settlements. International outcry to the suffering of the refugees and migrants in South Africa pressure the South African government to take steps to try to deal with the violence against migrants and refugees. The U.N. General Secretary Ban Ki-moon added his voice to this outcry, calling the South African government to protect migrants and refugees from xenophobic violence while Amnesty International called the African Union to pressure South Africa to protect migrants and refugees (Human Rights Watch 2008; UN 2015; Amnesty International 2015)

Arthur Kleinman (1997: 321) writes that.

> … suffering is social, not only because social force breaks networks and bodies, but also because social institutions respond with assistance to certain categories of sufferers (categories that institutions have constructed as authorized objects for giving help), while denying others or treating them with bureaucratic indifference. Thereby social institutions, through their policies and programs, frequently deepen certain forms of social suffering and become obstacles to their alleviation.

In the South African case, Nobel laureate Archbishop Desmond Tutu captures the problem of blaming individuals and communities for entrenched structural violence, which in part explains the crisis and conflict between newcomer poor African migrants and refugees and local, marginalized citizens. In reaction to recent attacks against migrants and refugees, he said that: "Our rainbow nation that so filled the world with hope is being reduced to a grubby shadow of itself, more likely to make the news for gross displays of callousness than for the glory that defined our transition to democracy under Nelson Mandela" (Mail and Guardian 2015). Or as Tutu's foundation phrased it in this same article. "The fabric of the nation is splitting at the seams." (Ibid). While the call for the South African government to protect refugees and migrants is laudable, rarely do we hear a call for the South African government to protect its own citizens whose reality of suffering remains acute and whose living conditions can never serve as a safe haven for newcomers.

Hope: Initiatives to Alleviate Conflict and Violence

Human agency is key to resolving communal violence. Such agency can be state-led or can emerge from civil society. In the South African case, religious organizations remain significant actors in efforts to alleviate the suffering of refugee and migrants who have been displaced and dispossessed by the violence in townships and informal settlements (Evans 2015). For Somali refugees for example, Islamic charities provided Halal food to those who found themselves in temporary shelters after being chased from their stores in various parts of the country.

Churches also continue to provide various spiritual and economic support for those subjected to this violence (Phakathi 2010; Evans 2015). While this is an integral part of the need to alleviate suffering, the discourses of violence against migrants continue to separate the communal crisis confronted by locals from that of the newcomers. I would argue that alleviating suffering in these settings should be an urgent priority. This would involve work with these communities beyond when tensions reach a boiling point, with national and international media attention broadcasting riots, lootings, killings, and expulsions. As commendable as the work of religious organizations is then, more sustained attention and intervention to the invisible and normalized violence that is omnipresent in many areas in the townships and informal settlement by religious charities and other civil society organizations can aid in alleviating violence targeting newcomers as well as locals.

Unlike civil society and religious organizations' approach above, the South African state's treatment of violence against migrants and refugees often highlights the criminal elements in attacks against migrants and refugees. As such, the solution that has been used thus far involves police arrests and increased involvement of these communities within the criminal justice system. This unfortunately is occurring in a country that has one of the highest incarceration rates in the world (Wicks 2016). Whether this is effective in protecting refugees and migrants, and whether this appeases the sense of dispossession and the generalized insecurity that is the norm in townships and informal settlements, is of course questionable. By criminalizing the most marginalized groups in the country, I argue that the local and national political leadership cedes responsibility for some of the underlying and often real challenges that these citizens confront. The state thus abdicates for the need to alleviate suffering of its marginalized citizens. This is of course problematic and leads to a vicious cycle that perpetuates conflict and violence.

Refugees and migrants are also aware of the above failure of the state and the justice system to protect them. They are also aware of the extreme corruption that prevails in the courts and police force (The Economist 2012; Steyn 2015). Many of those I interviewed highlighted refugee-initiated efforts that strive to diminish the conflict and resentment that they encounter in their settlements. As such, many of the more successful Somali businessmen in both Gauteng and Western Cape sponsor soccer tournaments of local youth, while they also contribute to any fundraising efforts that the local communities initiate. One particular businessman discussed how he paid for cows that were used for ceremonial purposes in the community following a major attack and looting against migrants and their businesses. He viewed this investment as holding out an olive branch to the community where his store is located, hoping that this would lead to alliance-building with the community leaders.

Many other Somali store owners also put local community leaders on their payroll, often giving a small stipend of R500-R1000 Rand. Though these leaders were not employees of the stores in the official sense, this payment served as an appeasement so that these leaders might diffuse any resentment that might exist for the foreign storeowners, but also act as advocates for them. As such, refugee store owners underscored the need to engage with the local population to diffuse conflict, cognizant of the need to alleviate their suffering while also recognizing the extreme suffering the local population often confronts.

Asked why they deem such initiatives important, a 44-year-old Somali store owner that I interviewed in 2009 stated:

> When they talk about us negatively and decide to do bad things to us, I want to create people who will say in their meetings, "Is that not the guy who did this or that for us? What do we want from him?"

Such initiatives are part of other locally driven negotiations that aim to diminish the competition between foreign and native business owners. Initiatives aimed to cement the building of local-foreign trust include a recent agreement to form partnerships between the South African Spaza Shop Co-operative (SASSCO) and the Somali Business Community Organization in the Khayelitsha township on the edge of Cape Town in May 2016 (Mahashe 2016). These partnerships can alleviate some of the tensions and distrust that persists between these communities. They can also potentially enhance a transfer of skills by the refugees and migrants to the local entrepreneurs, as the former often hold a competitive edge over local businessmen and women, whose training, networks, and options for investment are highly constrained.

Conclusion

The suffering of African refugees and migrants in South Africa does matter, but so does the suffering of the Black poor who remain victims of daily structural violence. The suffering of migrants and refugees is framed to be the outcome of "xenophobia" whereas that of the South African poor is viewed as the norm. But as Anderson rightly argues, "[S]uffering ranks high on the list of what it means to be human, yet the desire and action to alleviate our suffering, and that of others, ranks even higher." (Anderson 2015:3). This paper argues that the alleviation of human suffering should be pursued at all costs, irrespective of the migration status, race, gender and nationality of those suffering. This South African case demonstrates the consequences of failing to do so. The two groups whose suffering is outlined in this paper have more in common through their suffering than the South African state, the civil society, and international organizations who support refugees and migrants are willing to admit. Unfortunately, the failure to prioritize the alleviation of suffering for all produces the current stalemate, where a protracted inter- communal crisis of South African natives as well as intra-communal conflict between natives and newcomers persists, often culminating in deadly attacks against the latter. In addition to advocating for the protection of refugees and migrants in times of violence in the townships, international human rights organizations and religious organizations are required to hold the South African government accountable for its role in the sense of despair experienced by a large segment of its population.

What we see in South Africa should serve as a cautionary tale. Seeking protection for refugees in a context where extreme violence affects the majority of the population can only lead to an incorporation of newcomers into generalized suffering that prevails in the context. Disfranchised locals direct their anger towards those least able to defend themselves, refugees, and migrants, women, children, the elderly. But ultimately the social, economic, and racial crisis in South Africa which persists in the post-apartheid era and the communal suffering that is normalized should anchor any efforts to alleviate suffering for all. As Paul Farmer wrote: "Tacitus is credited with the aphorism "they created a desert and called it peace." Erasing history is perhaps the most common explanatory sleight-of-hand relied upon by the architects of structural violence. Erasure or distortion of history is part of the process of desocialization necessary for the emergence of hegemonic accounts of what happened and why." (Farmer 2004: 308). To neglect to even acknowledge the suffering of the South African poor, in relation to the suffering of the refugees and migrants, undermines the efforts that might be pursed to alleviate refugee and migrant suffering, leading to the current vicious cycle of violence that confronts both these groups. A new approach that acknowledges the interdependence of the fate of all those in our communities requires a holistic strategy that rejects a bandage approach to multi-faceted crises.

References

Abdi, C. M. (2011). Moving beyond xenophobia: Structural violence, conflict and encounters with the "other" Africans. *Development Southern Africa, 28*(5), 691–704.

Abdi, C. M. (2015). *Elusive Jannah: The Somali Diaspora and borderless Muslim identity*. Minneapolis: University of Minnesota Press.

Adepoju, A. (2003). Continuity and changing configurations of migration to and from the Republic of South Africa. *International Migration, 41*(1), 3–28.

Africa Check. (2013). *South Africa's official crime statistics for 2013/14*. Researched by the Institute for Security Studies and Africa Check. Factsheet. https://africacheck.org/factsheets/factsheet-south-africas-official-crime-statistics-for-201314/#sthash.sp7sgDVS.dpuf. Accessed 7 July 2016.

Allison, S. (2015). "Black economic empowerment has failed": Piketty on South African inequality. News Article. *The Guardian*. http://www.theguardian.com/world/2015/oct/06/piketty-south-africa-inequality-nelson-mandela-lecture. Accessed 7 July 2016.

Amnesty International. (2015). African Union should call on South Africa to protect refugees and migrants from xenophobic attacks. *News Article*. https://www.amnesty.org/en/latest/

news/2015/06/african-union-should-call-on-south-africa-to-protect-refugees-and-migrants-from-xenophobic-attacks/. Accessed 7 July 2016.
Anderson, R. E. (2015). Implications of World suffering for human progress. In R. E. Anderson (Ed.), *World suffering and quality of life* (pp. 3–29). New York: Springer.
Bass, L. E. (2014). *African immigrant families in another France*. Basingstoke: Palgrave MacMillan.
Berg, J., & Scharf, W. (2004). Crime statistics in South Africa 1994–2003. *Journal of Criminal Justice, 1*(17), 57–78.
Blackmore, F. (2003). A panel data analysis of crime in South Africa. *South African Journal of Economic and Management, 6*(3), 439–458.
Crush, J. (2008). *South Africa: Policy in the face of Xenophobia*. Resource Document. Migration Policy Institute. http://www.migrationpolicy.org/article/south-africa-policy-face-xenophobia. Accessed 7 July 2016.
Evans, S. (2015). Not in our name: Religious leaders plan march to end xenophobia. News Article. *Mail and Guardian*. http://mg.co.za/article/2015-04-15-not-in-our-name-religious-leaders-plan-march-to-end-xenophobia. Accessed 7 July 2016.
The Economist, 2010. The price of freedom: A special report on South Africa, 5 June, pp. 1–16.
Farmer, P. (1996). On suffering and structural violence: A view from below. *Daedalus, 125*(1), 261–283.
Farmer, P. (2004). An anthropology of structural violence 1. *Current anthropology, 45*(3), 305–325.
Frost, L., & Hoggett, P. (2008). Human agency and social suffering. *Critical social policy, 28*(4), 438–460.
Handmaker, J. (2001). No easy walk: Advancing refugee protection in South Africa. *Africa Today, 48*(3), 91–113.
Herbst L. (2015). Zuma Blasts press for making South Africa look bad. News Article. *Record*. https://www.newsrecord.co/zuma-blasts-press-making-south-africa-look-bad/. Accessed 7 July 2016.
Holmes, S. M. (2007). "Oaxacans like to work bent over": The naturalization of social suffering among berry farm workers. *International Migration, 45*(3), 39–68.
Human Rights Watch. (2008). South Africa: Punish attackers in xenophobic violence. Government should protect victims to ensure justice. *News Article*. www.hrw.org/en/news/2008/05/22/south-africa-punish-attackers-xenophobic-violence. Accessed 4 Sep 2009.
Hyndman, J. (2000). *Managing displacement: Refugees and the politics of humanitarianism*. Minneapolis: University of Minnesota Press.
International Relations Cooperation. (1998, May 29). *Statement of Deputy President Thabo Mbeki at the opening of the debate in the National Assembly, on "Reconciliation and Nation building, National Assembly Cape Town"*. Government Document. http://www.dfa.gov.za/docs/speeches/1998/mbek0529.htm. Accessed 7 July 2016.
IDASA (Institute for Democracy in Africa), 2008. *Background report on recent xenophobic violence in Gauteng: Preliminary investigation*. Institute for Democracy in Africa, 28 May. www.idasa.org.za/. Accessed 11 August 2009.
Keaton, T. D. (2006). *Muslim girls and the other France: Race, identity politics, & social exclusion*. Bloomington: Indiana University Press.
Kingdon, G. G., & Knight, J. (2004). Unemployment in South Africa: The nature of the beast. *World Development, 32*(3), 391–408.
Kleinman, A. (1997). "Everything that really matters": Social suffering, subjectivity, and the remaking of human experience in a disordering world. *Harvard Theological Review, 90*(3), 315–333.
Kleinman, A., Das, V., & Lock, M. M. (1997). *Social suffering*. Berkeley: University of California Press.
Koinange, J. (2006). Katrina: When New Orleans went from developed world to Third World. News Article. *CNN*. http://www.cnn.com/2006/US/08/30/btsc.koinange/index.html?eref=aol. Accessed 7 July 2016.
Louw, A. (1997). Surviving the transition: Trends and perceptions of crime in South Africa. *Social Indicators Research, 41*(1–3), 137–168.

Mahashe, M. (2016). Somali traders in Khayelitsha joins with locals for fair trade. News Article. *News 24*. http://www.news24.com/SouthAfrica/Local/City-Vision/somali-traders-in-khayelitsha-joins-with-locals-for-fair-trade-20160525. Accessed 7 July 2016.

Mail and Guardian. (2015). No end in sight to S. African xenophobic attacks; Tutu says fabric of the nation "splitting at the seams". *News Article*. http://mgafrica.com/article/2015-04-17-no-end-in-sight-safrican-anti-immigrant-attacks-spread-to-downtown-johannesburg. Accessed 7 July 2016.

Malkki, L. (1992). National geographic: The rooting of peoples and the territorialization of national identity among scholars and refugees. *Cultural anthropology, 7*(1), 24–44.

Marais, H. (2011). *South Africa pushed to the limit: The political economy of change London*. London: Zed Books.

Medicine Sans Frontier. (2010). *The lives of survival migrants and refugees in South Africa*. Resource Document. http://www.unhcr.org/556725e69.html. Accessed 7 July 2016.

Møller, V. (1998). Quality of life in South Africa: Post-apartheid trends. *Social Indicators Research, 43*(1–2), 27–68.

Møller, V. (2007). Quality of life in South Africa: The first ten years of democracy. *Social Indicators Research, 81*(2), 183–201.

Phakathi, S. (2010). The response of Churches to the May 2008 Xenophobic attacks. News Article. *City-Region Observatory (GCRO)*. http://www.atlanticphilanthropies.org/app/uploads/2010/07/11_Church_c.pdf. Accessed 7 July 2016.

Siddique, M. A. B. (2004). *South African migration policy: A critical review*. Crawley: University of Western Australia, Business School.

Sinclair, M. R. (1999). "I know a place that is softer than this…"–Emerging migrant communitites in South Africa. *International Migration, 37*(2), 465–483.

Statistics South Africa. (2011). *Income and expenditure of households: 2005/2006: Analysis of results, Report No. 01–00-01*. Resource Document. https://www.statssa.gov.za/publications/Report-01-00-01/Report-01-00-012005.pdf. Accessed 7 July 2016.

Steyn, L. (2015). South Africa: The land where the corrupt go free. News Article. *Mail & Guardian*. http://sa-monitor.com/south-africa-land-corrupt-go-free-mail-guardian-14-september-2015/. Accessed 7 July 2016.

The Economist, 2010. *The price of freedom: A special report on South Africa*, 5 June, pp. 1–16.

The Economist. (2012). South Africa's police: Something very rotten. News Article. *The Economist*. http://www.economist.com/node/21557385. Accessed 7 July 2016.

UKForex. (2016). *Foreign exchange services: Yearly average rates*. Reference Document. http://www.ukforex.co.uk/forex-tools/historical-rate-tools/yearly-average-rates. Accessed 7 July 2016.

UN. (2015). *Ban condemns deadly xenophobic violence in South Africa*. Reference Document. United Nations. http://www.un.org/apps/news/story.asp?NewsID=50660#.V0ri7SMrK2w. Accessed 7 July 2016.

UNAIDS. (2014). *South Africa*. Reference Document. UNAIDS. http://www.unaids.org/en/regionscountries/countries/southafrica. Accessed 7 July 2016.

UNHCR. (2011). *The 1951 Convention Relating to the Status s of Refugees and its 1967 Protocol*. UNHCR.

UNHCR. (2014). *Global trends: Forced displacement in 2014*. Reference Document. UNHRC. http://www.unhcr.org/556725e69.html. Accessed 7 July 2016.

UNHCR. (2015, December 8). *UNHCR statistical yearbook 2014* (14th ed). United Nations High Commissioner for Refugees (UNHCR).

Wicks, J. (2016). UN rights body releases damning report on SA prisons. News Article. *News 24*. http://www.news24.com/SouthAfrica/News/un-rights-body-releases-damning-report-on-sa-prisons-20160411. Accessed 7 July 2016.

World Bank. (2015). *Jobs and South Africa's Changing Demographics*. Reference Document. http://wwwwds.worldbank.org/external/default/WDSContentServer/WDSP/IB/2015/08/14/090224b08307421f/1_0/Rendered/PDF/South0Africa0e0hanging0demographics.pdf. Accessed 7 July 2016.

Chapter 14
Dignity and Rule of Law: Governance and the Alleviation of Social Suffering

Mark P. Lagon and Ryan T. Kaminski

Introduction

Starting from the premise that social suffering marks the qualities of suffering that most need alleviation, Mark Lagon and Ryan Kaminski (2015) place their greatest hope in human survival in conceptions of human dignity and the rule of law. *Human dignity*, they argue, consists primarily in (1) promoting human beings' agency to apply their gifts as they so choose, (2) recognizing equal value across all groupings of human beings—irrespective of gender, ethnicity, caste, or race, and (3) supporting institutions that make agency and equality deep and lasting. Their thesis is that the *rule of law* is needed to guarantee human dignity and to empower the world to alleviate social suffering including universal eradication of poverty, violence, injustice and disrespect. They find comfort in the fact that the new Sustainable Development Goals (SDGs) not only support their conception of human dignity but has an explicit goal, Goal 16, that includes advancing rule of law as a priority. Finally, their conclusion is that the alleviation of social suffering cannot occur without both human dignity and the rule of law broadly defined. And they call for mobilizing a pluralistic array of actors in dialogue on dignity and partnering to see it realized.

Suffering as a concept extends far beyond its traditional association with physical pain (Anderson 2014, p. 5). Other categories include "mental" and "social" suffering. Ronald Anderson defines the latter as "suffering whose sources are social collectivities and/or social institutions" (2014, p. 6). Arthur Kleinman, Venna Das,

M.P. Lagon (✉)
Walsh School of Foreign Service, Georgetown University, Washington, DC 20057, USA
e-mail: marklagon@gmail.com

R.T. Kaminski
United Nations Foundation, Washington, DC 20006, USA
e-mail: rykaminski@gmail.com

R.E. Anderson (ed.), *Alleviating World Suffering*, Social Indicators Research Series 67, DOI 10.1007/978-3-319-51391-1_14

and Margaret Lock (1997, p. ix) observe, "social suffering results from what political, economic, and institutional power does to people, and reciprocally from how these forms of power themselves influence response to social problems." Social suffering then includes individual or collective suffering stemming from institutions, policies, and governance.

Social suffering crisscrosses national boundaries, impacting the global north and south across a wide spectrum of individual circumstances and national situations. Corruption, gender inequality, lack of access to education, extreme poverty, criminal violence, trafficking, internal conflict, interstate war, environmental degradation, and epidemics contribute to varying degrees of social suffering across the world. Social suffering can also seed or amplify physical or mental suffering.

Alleviating social suffering demands a profound cultural shift in both attitudes and policy (Anderson 2014, p. 91). Effective global institutions that can concretize the implementation of human rights norms are a necessary condition for this shift, but for too long the keystone role of rule of law has gone underemphasized due to lack of will and constructed divisions within the human rights community (Lagon and Kaminski 2015). This demands a push to realize rights beyond rhetoric and a corresponding means for assessing outcomes.

A strategy focused on the new Sustainable Development Goals (SDGs) of the 2030 Agenda for Sustainable Development and a conception of "human dignity" can present a mutually reinforcing, medium- to long-term opportunity to alleviate social suffering, spanning borders as well as diverse political and economic orientations. The new SDGs, accepted by the UN General Assembly in September 2015, include a powerful international consensus on the role of rule of law for alleviating human suffering. The new sustainable development agenda also establishes a potentially transformative institutional basis for tracking progress and outcomes. In tandem, promotion of a global dialogue on human dignity emphasizing agency and social recognition can reinforce this ambition by expanding opportunities for human-rights coalition building while also informing an inclusive review and measurement framework.

The Global Goals and Social Suffering

Accepted by acclamation in the UN General Assembly in September 2015, the SDGs of the 2030 Agenda for Sustainable Development, present a political blueprint for combatting social suffering on two interrelated levels (United Nations 2014b). First, they do so procedurally, by relying upon the principle of inclusion and universality. Second, and interrelated, is the historic commitment of the new sustainable development agenda to advancing good governance and rule of law on a universal basis.

Inclusion and Universality

Despite the helpful international agenda-setting role of the original Millennium Development Goals (MDGs) for development priorities such as extreme poverty, gender equality, and maternal health, the predecessor 15-year development agenda to the SDGs agreed to by world leaders in 2000 was not without controversy (McArthur 2013). A common critique of the original eight MDGs concerns process. The effort to craft the MDGs was largely perceived as an internal UN technical exercise that primarily reflected the priorities of the developed world, lacking both genuine consultations with relevant diverse stakeholders as well as a commitment to transparency (Tran 2012). As a result, many within the development community expressed concern that the MDGs were too limited in focusing on a particular grouping of nations of the developing world, sidestepping the reality and intricacy of cross-border challenges central to achieving baseline development outcomes (Glennie 2010).

In marked contrast, a core driving theme of the new 2030 Agenda for Sustainable Development reflects an acknowledgement of Anderson's (2014, p. 30) observation that "some trivialize suffering because they are unaware of how pervasive suffering has become even in wealthy societies." Adopting the SDGs in September 2015, the 193 member states of the UN laud the principle of universality as well as a foundational role for dignity for achieving sustainable development, declaring:

> We pledge that no one will be left behind. Recognizing that the dignity of the human person is fundamental, we wish to see the Goals and targets met for all nations and peoples and for all segments of society. (United Nations 2014b, p. 2.)

The pledge for a sustainable development agenda where "leave no one behind" refers not only to the implementation of the agenda, but also the process how the new SDGs were debated, refined, and ultimately endorsed. This includes an unprecedented degree of transparency and inclusion in developing the SDGs among a diversity of international actors extending far beyond just governments and traditional institutions. For the new sustainable development agenda, the focus on inclusion took many forms over a more than 2-year process extending far beyond UN headquarters in New York. An online portal allowed millions of people around the globe to fill out a simple ballot to voice what issues should be covered in the new post-2015 development agenda. The portal, MyWorld2015, is still available at http://vote.myworld2015.org/ as is real-time data analysis at http://data.myworld2015.org/. Eighty-eight national-level consultations were also launched in combination with other thematic dialogues on what should follow the original MDGs. For a synthesis of these consultations see the United Nations Development Group's 2013 document, "A Million Voices; The World We Want" (2013a). Similarly, countless official dialogues and side events at UN headquarters sought to provide a pipeline for input from the private sector, various UN agencies, philanthropic groups, faith communities, civil society organizations, academic institutions, and other issue-area experts. UN member states and hundreds of representatives from the private sector and civil society also convened in Addis Ababa, Ethiopia to finalize a comprehensive framework, the Addis Ababa Action Agenda, for financing the ambitious new sustainable development agenda (United Nations 2015).

Governance and Rule of Law

In addition to process differences regarding the *how* between the MDGs and SDGs, there are also transformational differences concerning the *what*. Quantitatively, the number of SDGs is more than double the MDGs. As to the number of targets falling under goals—or more specific actions crucial to realizing each broad goal—the SDGs also include 169 targets, compared to just 21 linked with the MDGs. While some in the development community have hailed the evident ambition of the SDGs, others worry this expansive agenda may be too aspirational. William Easterly (2015), for example, has warned the 17 goals and 169 targets a part of the post-2015 development agenda too closely resembles a laundry list of development priorities that, as a package, prioritizes nothing.

Nevertheless, outright dismissing the inherent ambition of the post-2015 development framework for alleviating global human suffering is equally, if not more, risky. Among many qualitative differences, a critical feature of the new SDGs includes focus on good governance, a cross-cutting development concern conspicuously missing from the original eight MDGs (Harris 2015). As the UN Development Program (UNDP) has concluded that states undergoing "widespread fragility or conflict" have struggled to make even marginal progress on the original MDGs, the role of governance for achieving baseline development outcomes cannot be overstated (2013, p. 3–4).

Specifically, Goal 16 of the SDGs calls for advancing peaceful and inclusive societies, ensuring access to justice for all through accountable and inclusive institutions, as well as promoting the rule of law.[1] This reflects a unequivocal political acknowledgement of a devastating 2008 UNDP estimate that places four billion persons around the world living outside the scope of rule of law protections. As such, Stacey Cram and Vivek Maru (2016) celebrate the adoption of Goal 16 as "a milestone, a recognition that people cannot improve their lives without the power to exercise their rights." Terra Lawson-Remer (2015) goes further regarding the enabling role of Goal 16, observing "Without good governance, the other efforts to improve human well-being outlined in the other 16 SDGs will be impossible to realize."

Despite this apparent consensus from experts within the development community, some influential governments, particularly from the developing world, expressed skepticism about Goal 16 as negotiations on finalizing the SDGs unfolded. From the perspective of these countries, Goal 16 presented a risk of politicizing the new sustainable development agenda and repeating the mistakes of the MDGs in

[1] Goal 16 of the 2016 of the 2030 Agenda for Sustainable Development reads: "Promote peaceful and inclusive societies for sustainable development, provide access to justice for all and build effective, accountable and inclusive institutions at all levels."

focusing too much on development challenges solely in the global south. (Cram and Maru 2016).

The counterargument was repeatedly made that no country can boast a perfect record on rule of law and that the then-proposed Goal 16 actually strengthened the principle of universality of the SDGs. Goal 16 advocates also voiced the urgency of ensuring that all individuals, especially those within vulnerable populations, have equitable access to justice. Backing for this overarching theme of Goal 16 is also reflected as a top priority for millions of individuals around the world—from both the global north and south—who used the "My World2015" portal along with other advocacy channels to call for a new sustainable development agenda that encompasses good governance. For instance, an "honest and responsible government" was rated as the fourth highest priority among seventeen potential issue areas on the online platform.[2] As evidence in the global north, there is an emerging bipartisan consensus in the United States on addressing increasingly apparent racial disparities in sentencing within the U.S criminal justice system.

Acknowledging gaps even in those institutions charged with ensuring access to justice, then UN Secretary-General Kofi Annan (UN Security Council 2004, p. 4) defined rule of law in 2004 as "a principle of governance in which all persons, institutions and entities, public and private, including the State itself, are accountable to laws that are publicly promulgated, equally enforced and independently adjudicated, and which are consistent with international human rights norms and standards." This interpretation demands that rule of law not stop with crafting laws and regulations on the books, but ensuring that all segments of a population have access to justice, including vulnerable populations. Anderson (2014, p. 95) clarifies:

> While many governments have systems of justice that administer criminal punishment to individuals as a means to hold them accountable for the suffering of their victims, little progress has been made toward holding organizations and governments responsible for suffering created by their policies and practices. Often when an organization is taken to court, the sentence received is not commensurate with the human suffering produced by their actions. This may be a sign that appropriate laws are not in place or that politics has produced a biased, unfair justice system.

Consequently, rule of law is inextricably linked to alleviating social suffering in establishing the conditions for all segments of societies to realize human rights, whether in developing or developed countries. According to the International Development Law Organization, effective rule of law can empower vulnerable groups—including women children, children, and minorities—as "agents of development" or rights claimers (2014, p. 17). During the 2014 UN High-Level Summit on Rule of Law, then UN Secretary-General Ban Ki-moon (UN 2014a) reiterated, "Realizing the rights of every man, woman and child for well-being, security and justice will require coherent and effective rule of law."

With strong and responsive legal systems international human international rights standards can be better imbedded and implemented through domestic

---

[2] The platform, MyWorld2015, is available at http://vote.myworld2015.org/. Real-time data analysis is also available at MyWorld2015 Analytics at http://data.myworld2015.org/.

legislation. At the same time, individuals can become better aware of rights commitments made by governments as well as channels for pursuing justice and accountability. Observance of binding human rights treaties can also be better tracked, making it easier for rights advocates to advance reform as well as 'name and shame' governments in cases of violations. Analyzing the evolution of the human rights movement of the lesbian, gay bisexual and transgender community, Ryan Thoreson (2014, p. 199) underscores the importance of the ability for rights groups to vocalize rights claims at international rights mechanisms like treaty bodies, even when tangible shifts in policy do not immediately materialize.

Empirical data and several case studies have also indicated a relationship between effectively rule of law and institution-building for advancing the economic empowerment of individuals and, ultimately, agency. Anoop Singh (2014, p. 103) clarifies:

> The global surge in public protests against perceptions of bad governance and lack of inclusive growth are a reminder of the importance of developing strong institutions on the one hand and expanding the benefits of the formal economy to encourage economic growth and opportunities on the other … [T]he presence of large underground economies and weak domestic institutions lead to unequal opportunities and thereby hinder the freedom of individuals to thrive based on their capabilities …

A World Bank regression study *Where is the Wealth of Nations?* also found that investments in intangible capital, such as rule-of-law institution building, account for the vast majority of economic development within states relative to other factors (quoted in Haugen and Boutros 2014, p. 155). Others within the financial services sector have linked advancements within the rule of law with the potential to unlock trillions of dollars in nascent capital for sustainable development outcomes (Buckley 2015). Irene Kahn (2013) summarizes it simply: "You cannot fight poverty and cannot promote sustainable development without the rule of law."

From Guarantees to Outcomes: The Role of Human Dignity

It is commonplace for public officials to reference dignity and pervasive human suffering in conversations regarding the urgency of the international community rising to meet the expansive ambition of the new SDGs (United Nations 2016b). Yet few unpack "human dignity" in terms of a component of a strategy for concretizing norms, global institution-strengthening, as well as supporting implementation of the new sustainable development agenda's focus on governance and rule of law.

Agency, Social Recognition, and Outcomes

Examining myriad cross-cultural philosophical, religious, academic, and political texts stretching from the ancient to the contemporary period, Lagon and Arend define human dignity as: "the fundamental agency of human beings to apply their gifts to thrive" as well as "social recognition of a person's inherent value and claim to equal access to opportunity." They add a third element, "to be meaningful, human dignity must be institutionalized in practice and governance" (Lagon and Arend 2014a. p. 16). Social suffering stemming from extreme poverty, gender inequality, or other varied manifestations naturally restrains individuals from reaching their full potential. Similarly, lack of respect for the equal value of human life is a time-tested prerequisite for seeding social discrimination, violence, and conflict. While treaties, declarations, and rhetorical commitments can establish a necessary normative blueprint for promotion of human dignity and combatting social suffering, effective institutions simultaneously present the bricks and mortar for the project.

This interpretation of dignity is helpful in advancing the global consensus on rule of law and combatting social suffering for several reasons. In terms of the assessment of outcomes, both human dignity and social suffering as concepts emphasize an individual's ability to thrive—or agency—and the assessment of quality of life (Anderson 2014, p. 27). As Anderson (2014, p. 26) notes:

> When you are relieving another's suffering, you are also improving their quality of life. This frame is uniquely justified by its emphasis on quality of life as a concrete human need and its emphasis on social suffering as a qualitatively different type of suffering.

Mirroring the role of rule of law in advancing sustainable development, prioritizing agency straddles the need for improvements in both socioeconomic as well as civil and political rights. Anderson highlights the relevance of both of these baskets of rights in defending the need for an inclusive conceptualization of suffering that incorporates social suffering. "At a minimum, the concept [social suffering] is likely to lead to a fuller acknowledgement of what happens to the humanity of those who suffer, whether under the extremes of economic hardship, social injustice, or political oppression," he offers (2014, p. 27).

Relatedly, the "social recognition" component of human dignity reinforces the necessity of a broad interpretation of suffering as to include social suffering. For example, Wilkinson contends that one benefit of a focus on social suffering is to establish a basis for humanizing and connecting with distant others as global citizens (2005). A report at a key juncture of the SDGs process of UN Secretary General Ban Ki-moon, "The Road to Dignity by 2030" also seeks to synthesize the gargantuan scale of inputs from different actors for the new sustainable development agenda explicitly under the umbrella of human dignity (United Nations 2014b).

Overall, focus on the interrelationship between human dignity, rule of law, and alleviating social suffering stands to advance the realization of human rights beyond rhetoric or guarantees on paper. Anderson, for example, cites the human rights sector as a "critical partner" for alleviating suffering. He continues, "No other social movement tackles social suffering as directly as human rights organizations, which work hand-in-hand with other social justice movements" (2014, p.92). Indeed since the adoption of the Universal Declaration of Human Rights in 1948, an impressive array of global human rights mechanisms, tools, and accompanying institutions have developed. The latter address many facets of social suffering around the world while acting as enabling and engagement platforms for human rights globally.

These human rights instruments include a growing list of legally binding human rights conventions, ranging from protecting the rights of disabled persons to banning torture. It is indicative of a global consensus—at minimum at a normative level—on human rights and alleviating social suffering that 80 percent of UN member-states have ratified at least four core binding human rights treaties (United Nations n.d.). The UN Human Rights Council as a political organ that includes member countries from all major world regions, has established more than 55 special rapporteur mandates concerning challenges spanning from the pernicious health impacts of toxic waste to ensuring the rights to the freedom of peaceful assembly and of association.

At the regional level, human rights institutions with varying capacities and mandates have emerged. This includes the Organization of American States Inter-American Commission on Human Rights, African Union Commission on Human and People's Rights, Association of Southeast Asian Nations Intergovernmental Commission on Human Rights, European Court of Human Rights, as well the Organization of Islamic Cooperation Independent Permanent Human Rights Commission, among others. Hybrid institutions like the Global Fund to Fight Aids, Tuberculosis, and Malaria; private sector organs like the Microsoft Technology and Human Rights Center; as well as a growing concert of civil society groups promoting human rights are also key actors.

Bridging Gaps

Despite the impressive growth of the human rights system at global, regional, and local levels, significant clashes between those prioritizing civil and political rights versus those favoring elevation of economic and social rights persist (Lagon and Arend 2014a, p. 6). The impact of this debate has often been an unhelpful clash between those human rights norms critical to alleviating social suffering and the cultivation of political will to build institutions with the requisite capacity to execute implementation, support rule of law capacity-building, and address human suffering on the ground (Lagon and Kaminski 2014).

This constructed binary has a colorful history, with the clash visibly evident during the Cold War (Lagon and Arend 2014a, p. 7). One manifestation of this conflict is the bifurcated progeny of the Universal Declaration of Human Rights in the form of two legally binding treaties, the International Covenant on Civil and Political Rights (ICCPR) and the International Covenant on Economic, Social and Cultural Rights (ICESCR). Debates have also continued in prominent international settings well beyond the end of the Cold War era. At the UN, for example, arguments are common between member states along predictable ideological lines regarding the so-called "right to development" (U.S. Mission in Geneva 2015). Recently, several grassroots U.S. human rights advocates were dismayed to see economic and social rights relegated to the euphemistic term, "measures," within the U.S. 2015 Universal Periodic Review (UPR) national stakeholder report (Dawkwar 2015). Lagon and Arend (2014a, p. 7) find this longstanding debate may actually represent a "false dichotomy".

In fact, a closer examination reveals significant connections between what many would consider disparate camps of thinking. A 2015 McKinsey Global Institute report *The Power of Parity* concluded that establishing the conditions for gender equity and facilitating the empowerment of women could pump more than twenty trillion dollars into the global economy (Woetzel et al. 2015). Similarly, a preliminary World Bank Group study estimated the economic cost of the social exclusion of lesbian, gay, bisexual, and transgender individuals (LGBT) in India at $32 billion per year (Badgett 2014).

Promoting a global normative and political dialogue on human dignity—a "dignitarian dialogue"—stands to highlight and build upon these often-understated intersections. Such a dialogue could provide transformative opportunities for expanding coalitions within the human rights community, whether grassroots advocates or entrepreneurs committed to social justice, with the overarching goal of better equipping rights advocates to understand and address challenges related to social suffering (Lagon and Arend 2014b, p. 323).

Coalition and Institution-Building

Like the process to develop the new SDGs, a genuine dialogue on dignity centered on agency and the social recognition of the equality of others can advance conceptual consensus, then political will, and then meaningful interventions that can catalyze overdue transitions from human rights norm building to realizing implementation. This includes an operational role for what Cass Sunstein (1996) labels "norm entrepreneurs" through forums ranging from conferences, the university, regional organizations, global institutions, and the Internet. For example, Pakistan's Malala Yousfazi's is a prominent norm entrepreneur who has played a catalytic role in elevating the issue of girl's access to education on the international agenda. Paula Ettelbrick (quoted in Thoreson 2014, p. 187–188) discusses the logic of norm-building from the bottom up:

> At heart, it's about the old-fashioned word "consciousness-raising." … Once you're conscious of something, one you're aware of a problem, once you're aware of a situation, you begin to start seeing things. Have you ever had that situation where you read something and it's like, oh, I never knew that, and then all of a sudden, everywhere you look, it seems like you're seeing things in a different way? … I think that's very much the human rights process…

In terms of forums for dignitarian dialogue, social media platforms have emerged as powerful new force multiplier instrument for norm entrepreneurs, including bringing global attention to cases of social suffering. In September 2015, for instance, a virally shared photo of a dead child on a beach in Turkey galvanized world attention on the plight of those fleeing Syria (Smith 2015).

Emphasis on human dignity also holds a proven political will-building and mobilization capacity. The UN Charter, Universal Declaration of Human Rights, ICCPR, CESCR, and most recently the 2030 Agenda for Sustainable Development outcome document all reference human dignity as a mobilizational premise (Lagon and Arend 2014b, p. 321). As Thomas Banchoff (2014, p. 271) notes, "Appeals to human dignity and of the inviolable worth of each and every human person have helped to mobilize national and international coalitions in support of diverse human rights agendas". In early 2016, Pope Francis made human dignity a centerpiece of his remarks to the Vatican diplomatic corps that focused on need to compassionately and conclusively address the historic wave of refugees from the Middle East (Pullella 2015).

A dignitarian dialogue should be no panacea for alleviating social suffering worldwide, but it offers the basis for a universal approach to a universal challenge, including supporting the institutionalization of the fledging SDGs, as Lagon and Kaminski (2015) insist as essential to dignity). Lagon and Arend (2014b, p. 325), however, caution that "true dialogue" will require time and careful deliberation among myriad international actors in varying forums to solidify a consensus about the meaning of dignity in practice. There is also need for continued conversations on effectively balancing tradeoffs between the "agency" and "social recognition" pillars of dignity, as well as negotiation on what these pillars entail for effective measurement of outcomes. (Lagon and Arend 2014b, p. 325). But difficult as this dialogue will be, it would immeasurably advance the implementation of the SDGs, and its key enabler, Goal 16.

Metrics

Finally, a robust strategy to combat suffering requires what Anderson (2014, p. 98) refers to as "development and operationalization of compassion." As simultaneously both preconditions and outputs for assessing the impact of human rights efforts on the ground, human dignity's three pillars of agency, recognition, and institutionalization are instructive regarding effective measurement of efforts to alleviate social suffering.

Indicators for Sustainable Development

Assessing progress in this regard should meld both the comparative advantages of the emerging institutional framework to measure the new SDGs, including Goal 16, as well as the three core pillars of a global dignitarian dialogue. In practice, this presents a complex undertaking, necessitating cooperation among and input from various sectors in a process that is formalized yet also dynamically adaptable to innovation. The principle of universality key to the SDGs also demands the institutional capacity to track and assess rule-of-law outcomes, whether in the United Kingdom or United Arab Emirates.

To develop requisite indicators to support the considerable breadth of the SDGs, a multi-stakeholder process has emerged, involving the UN system, national statistics offices, individual statisticians, data-tracking organizations, and other actors. An initial official proposal for global-level metrics, namely a set of baseline indicators applicable to all countries to annually track progress on the SDGs, has yielded a list of over 220 indicators under the new 17 SDGs (United Nations 2016b, p. 26-47). Importantly, however, a window has been left open for refinement of the global-level indicators to assimilate technological advancements and other best practices over the 15-year timeline linked with the SDGs (United Nations 2016b, p. 3).

Interpreting Goal 16, Rule of Law and Access to Justice

For Goal 16 and the advancement of rule of law, a robust data collection and analysis effort emphasizing individual agency and social recognition is essential. As U.S. Ambassador to the UN, Samantha Power (U.S. Mission to UN 2016) outlined the stakes:

> …promoting the rule of law and ensuring equal access to justice for all is the sine qua non of so many of the Sustainable Development Goals. And if we cannot agree on ways to measure whether we are making progress toward meeting this crucial target – as you all are aiming to do today and beyond – we risk undermining the effectiveness of the entire enterprise.

Asserting that "Goal 16 belongs to the people," Cram and Maru (2016) assert the need for global-level indicators, or indicators applying to all countries irrespective of circumstance, that can address the full spectrum of challenges related to individuals' access to justice, instead of indicators focused solely on criminal violence. A 2016 expert-level meeting on indicators for Goal 16 convened by UNDP and the Oslo Peace Research Institute also reiterates the need for a broad interpretation of rule of law and access to justice under Goal 16. It also cites the need to track access to justice related to *both* criminal and civil disputes (United Nations 2016a).

UN member states and development practitioners alike have also acknowledged the benefits of reinforcing global-level indicators with other more localized measures, relevant to regional and national level contexts (UN 2016b, p. 5–6). UNDP, for example, has stewarded a cross-sector, expert-level process to develop a

Goal 16 indicator "sourcebook" that contains not only recommendations for global-level indicators pertaining to peace, justice, and institutions, but also hundreds of other benchmarks more applicable to national-level contexts for governments to voluntarily track and report (Milante et al. 2015). This additional basket of indicators would keep the SDGs relevant to highly-particularized national circumstances, acting to embed more political will to address the new sustainable development agenda, and ensure access to justice by vulnerable populations (Denney 2016).

Methods and Partnerships

Two key priorities for advancing the agency and social recognition components of human dignity are (1) disaggregating indicator data under the new SDGs, and (2) integration of experiential and survey data.

Disaggregation according to sex, race, age, ethnicity, migratory status, and other factors can aid in understanding challenges facing specific populations that could otherwise be overshadowed.[3] While some governments have justifiably noted there are challenges associated with breaking data down in this manner, disaggregation should nonetheless remain a core element distinguishing the new SDGs from the MDGs for two reasons. First, disaggregation supports the standard of "no one left behind." Second, it serves to amplify the social recognition aspect of human dignity. Similarly, while integrating survey or experiential data is demonstrably more challenging relative to relying exclusively on administrative data, there are many instances of successful employment of these methods across a wide range of country contexts and local situations.

Governments' national statistical offices need not face this enterprise alone. Capitalizing on the concept of an ongoing "data revolution," third-party data partnerships can help integrate capacity of a diverse cast of actors in information-sharing as well as seed innovation in reporting and analysis (United Nations 2013b, p. 23). Among many new approaches, these partnerships should include crowdsourcing data gathering, in effect transforming local communities into active data agents.[4] Emerging global coalitions and newly empowered institutions focused on the advancement of human dignity will be well-positioned to assist in this process.

Several case studies exhibit promise for successful measurement of governance and rule of law. From Freedom House's (2015a, b) annualized global reporting on

[3]The UN Inter-agency and Expert Group on Sustainable Development Indicators agreed on "an overarching principle" of data disaggregation to include "income, sex, age, race, ethnicity, migratory status, disability, and geographic location, or other characteristics in accordance with the Fundamental Principles of Official Statistics."

[4]See Freedom House (2016). Also see: "Measuring Peace: A Discussion Paper on the measurement of Peace in the post-2015 indicator framework." (March 2015). SaferWorld.

the status of civil and political liberties and freedom of expression, to the "Strategy for the Harmonization of Statistics in Africa" (also known as SHaSA) initiative, best practices should be dynamically identified and scaled. Partnerships among the private sector, civil society, and other institutions can also assist in facilitating an overdue transition away from reliance on purely administrative data and, importantly, on *datasets* lacking specificity relevant to vulnerable populations.

Conclusion

Anderson (2014, p. 98) reminds one that the stakes cannot be higher, noting that suffering "generates social disorder, threatening the survival of individuals, communities, and societies. Genocide epidemics are the most vivid examples." Adopting a broad perception of suffering encompassing the concept of "social suffering" is beneficial to recognizing ineffective or repressive institutions, and suitable solutions. Advancing the attitudinal culture shift necessary to alleviate social suffering in what has been cited as "the age of megacrises" demands elevating rule of law and human dignity.

The new SDGs offer a basis for addressing social suffering at its source. In particular, Goal 16 of the new SDGs represents an overdue international accord on the need for rule of law and access to justice for all, in many cases a requisite for development outcomes, notably economic empowerment. Commitments to meaningful data gathering and analysis are essential to gauging progress on the 2030 Agenda for Sustainable Development. Like the effort to develop the SDGs, multi-stakeholder participation is not only helpful in assessment, but also a critical catalyst for implementation.

Similarly, a focus on a conception of human dignity emphasizing agency and the social recognition as preeminent normative values stands to strengthen the international human rights system in helping move more from aspirations to outcomes. Such a focus would go far toward tangibly alleviating social suffering. Promoting a focus on individuals' ability to thrive and emphasizing the equality of others, human dignity also offers yardsticks for measuring outcomes and identifying bottlenecks related to good governance and rule of law.

In short, the massive scope of social suffering worldwide today necessitates a multi-tiered approach threading norm-building, international public policy, and an inclusive, cross-sector effort to measure outcomes. While change is unlikely overnight, both policymakers and advocates alike have the tools and momentum to move forward. Change will come if they recognize social suffering as the problem, Goal 16 as a vehicle, and enhancing people's dignity as both a measurable, tangible, and critical goal.

References

Anderson, R. (2014). *Human suffering and quality of life: Conceptualizing stories and statistics*. New York: Springer.

Badgett, M. V. (2014). *The economic cost of stigma and the exclusion of LGBT people: A case study of India*. World Bank Group. http://documents.worldbank.org/curated/en/2014/10/23952131/economic-cost-stigma-exclusion-lgbt-people-case-study-india. Accessed 19 April 2016.

Banchoff, T. (2014). Religion and the global politics of human dignity: The Catholic Church and beyond. In M. P. Lagon & A. C. Arend (Eds.), *Human dignity and the future of global institutions* (pp. 257–276). Washington, DC: Georgetown University Press.

Buckley, J. (2015). *Rule of law: Enabling social finance and sustainable development*. BNY Mellon. https://www.bnymellon.com/us/en/newsroom/news/expert-voices/rule-of-law-enabling-social-finance-and-sustainable-development.jsp. Accessed 19 April 2016.

Cram, S., & Maru V. (2016). Access to Justice for all? Now that would be a measurably good thing. *Guardian*. http://www.theguardian.com/global-development/2016/jan/01/access-to-justice-for-all-sustainable-development-goal-16-indicators. Accessed 19 April 2016.

Dawkwar, J. (2015). *The United States considers itself a human rights champion. The world begs to differ*. ACLU: Speak Feely. https://www.aclu.org/blog/speak-freely/united-states-considers-itself-human-rights-champion-world-begs-differ. Accessed 19 April 2016.

Denney, L. (2016). Providing access to justice for all? Four lessons for the SDGs from past rule of law assistance. *SaferWorld Blog*. http://www.saferworld.org.uk/news-and-views/blog-post/32-providing-access-to-justice-for-all-four-lessons-for-the-sdgs-from-past-rule-of-law-assistance. Accessed 19 April 2016.

Easterly W. (2015). The SDGs should stand for senseless, dreamy, and garbled. *Foreign* Policy. http://foreignpolicy.com/2015/09/28/the-sdgs-are-utopian-and-worthless-mdgs-development-rise-of-the-rest/. Accessed on 19 April 2016.

Ettelbrick, P. qtd. in Thoreson, R. (2014). *Transnational LGBT activism: Working for sexual rights worldwide* (pp. 187–188). Minneapolis: University of Minneapolis Press. /2015/sep/02/shocking-image-of-drowned-syrian-boy-shows-tragic-plight-of-refugees. Accessed 19 April 2016.

Freedom House. (2015a). Freedom on the net-privatizing censorship, eroding privacy. *Freedom House*. https://freedomhouse.org/article/privatizing-censorship-eroding-privacy-freedom-net-2015-new-findings-released. Accessed 19 April 2016.

Freedom House. (2015b). Freedom of the press 2015-Harsh Laws and violence drive global decline. *Freedom House*. https://freedomhouse.org/sites/default/files/FOTP%202015%20Full%20Report.pdf.

Freedom House. (2015c). Freedom on the net-privatizing censorship, eroding privacy. *Freedom House*. https://freedomhouse.org/article/privatizing-censorship-eroding-privacy-freedom-net-2015-new-findings-released. Accessed 19 April 2016.

Freedom House. (2016). Freedom in the world 2016-anxious dictators, wavering democracies: Global freedom under pressure. *Freedom House*. https://freedomhouse.org/report/freedom-world/freedom-world-2016. Accessed 19 April 2016.

Glennie, J. (2010). After 2015, we need a new set of Millennium Development Goals that apply to all countries. *Guardian*. http://www.theguardian.com/global-development/poverty-matters/2010/nov/03/millennium-development-goals-inequality. Accessed 19 April 2016.

Harris A. (2015). Agenda 2030: Recognition for the role of justice and governance in sustainable development. Open Society Foundations: Voices: https://www.opensocietyfoundations.org/voices/agenda-2030-recognition-role-justice-and-governance-sustainable-development. Accessed 19 April 2016.

Haugen, G., & Boutros, V. (2014). *The Locust effect: Why the end of poverty requires the end of violence* (p. 155). New York: Oxford University Press.

International Development Law Organization. (2014). *Doing justice to sustainable development: Integrating the rule of law into the post-2015 development Agenda*. Rome: IDLO.
Khan, I. (2013). Remarks made during Global Dialogue on the Rule of Law and the Post 2015 Development Agenda (conference). http://www.worldwewant2015.org/file/417694/download/454285. Accessed 19 April 2016.
Kleinman, A., Das, V., & Lock, M. (1997). *Social suffering* (p. ix). Berkeley: University of California Press.
Lagon, M. P., & Arend, A. C. (2014a). Introduction: Human dignity in a neomedieval world. In M. P. Lagon & C. A. Arend (Eds.), *Human dignity and the future of global institutions* (pp. 1–24). Washington, DC: Georgetown University Press 16.
Lagon, M. P., & Arend, A. C. (2014b). Constructing a dialogue on dignity: The path ahead. In M. P. Lagon & A. C. Arend (Eds.), *Human dignity and the future of global institutions* (pp. 319–337). Washington, DC: Georgetown University Press P. 321.
Lagon, M. P., & Kaminski, R. (2014). The global rights regime: Assessing and renovating the architecture. In M. P. Lagon & A. C. Arend (Eds.), *Human dignity and the future of global institutions* (pp. 123–150). Washington, DC: Georgetown University Press.
Lagon M. P. & Kaminski R. (2015). *A new multilateralism for Atrocities prevention: A global fund and development Agenda for advancing the rule of law*. Stanley Foundation Policy Analysis Brief. http://www.stanleyfoundation.org/resources.cfm?id=546. Accessed 19 April 2016.
Lawson-Remer, T. (2015). *How can we implement sustainable development goal 16 on institutions*. Brookings Institution. http://www.brookings.edu/blogs/future-development/posts/2015/10/01-global-goals-institutions-lawson-remer. Accessed 19 April 2016.
McArthur, J. (2013). Own the goals: What the Millennium Development Goals have accomplished. *Foreign Affairs*. https://www.foreignaffairs.com/articles/2013-03-01/own-goals. Accessed 19 April 2016.
Measuring peace: A discussion paper on the measurement of peace in the post-2015 indicator framework. (2015, March). *SaferWorld*. http://www.saferworld.org.uk/resources/view-resource/891-measuring-peace-from-2015-an-indicator-framework-at-work. Accessed 19 April 2016.
Milante, G. et al. (2015). *The indicators we want: Report of the virtual network of stakeholders for the development of indicators on peaceful societies, justice and effective institutions for SDG 16*. http://www.undp.org/content/dam/undp/library/Democratic%20Governance/Virtual%20Network%20on%20Goal%2016%20indicators%20-%20Indicators%20we%20want%20Report.pdf. Accessed 19 April 2016.
Mission of the United States in Geneva. (2015). *U.S. explanation of vote with regard to the right to development*. United States Department of State. https://geneva.usmission.gov/2015/03/27/u-s-explaination-of-vote-with-regard-to-the-right-to-development/. Accessed 19 April 2016.
Mission of the United States to the UN. (2016). *Ambassador Samantha Power remarks on access to legal aid as a measure of access to justice*. Geneva: US Mission to UN.
Pullella, P. (2015). Pope criticizes nations that close door to migrants. *Reuters*. http://www.reuters.com/article/us-europe-migrants-pope-idUSKBN0OX0XN20150617. Accessed 19 April 2016.
Singh, A. (2014). Inclusive growth, institutions, and the underground economy. In M. P. Lagon & A. C. Arend (Eds.), *Human dignity and the future of global institutions* (pp. 103–122). Washington, DC: Georgetown University Press.
Smith, H. (2015). Shocking images of drowned Syrian boy show tragic plight of refugees. *Guardian*. http://www.theguardian.com/world. Accessed 19 April 2016.
Sunstein, C. (1996). Social norms and social roles. *Columbia Law Review, 96*(4), 903–968.
Thoreson, R. (2014). *Transnational LGBT activism: Working for sexual rights worldwide* (p. 199). Minneapolis: University of Minneapolis Press.
Tran, M. (2012). Mark Malloch-Brown: Developing the MDGs was a bit like nuclear fusion. *Guardian*. http://www.theguardian.com/global-development/2012/nov/16/mark-malloch-brown-mdgs-nuclear. Accessed 19 April 2016.

United Nations. (n.d.). *The foundation of international human rights law*. http://www.un.org/en/sections/universal-declaration/foundation-international-human-rights-law/index.html. Accessed 19 April 2016.

United Nations. (2013a). *A million voices; the world we want*. United Nations. http://www.worldwewant2015.org/bitcache/9158d79561a9de6b34f95568ce8b389989412f16?vid=422422&disposition=inline&op=view. Accessed 19 April 2016.

United Nations. (2013b) *Report of the high-level panel of eminent persons on the post-2015 development Agenda* (p 23). United Nations. http://www.post2015hlp.org/wp-content/uploads/2013/05/UN-Report.pdf Accessed 19 April 2016.

United Nations. (2014a). *Ban Ki-moon, remarks made during contributions of human rights and the rule of law in the post-2015 development Agenda (conference)*. United Nations. http://www.un.org/News/Press/docs/2014/sgsm15918.doc.htm. Accessed 19 April 2016.

United Nations. (2014b). *The road to dignity by 2030: Ending poverty, transforming all lives and protecting the planet*. UN Secretary General Synthesis Report. http://www.un.org/disabilities/documents/reports/SG_Synthesis_Report_Road_to_Dignity_by_2030.pdf. Accessed 19 April 2016.

United Nations. (2015). *Addis Ababa action agenda of the third international conference on financing for development*. United Nations. pp. 113, 51. http://www.un.org/esa/ffd/wp-content/uploads/2015/08/AAAA_Outcome.pdf. Accessed 19 April 2016.

United Nations. (2016a, January) *Report of the conveners-executive summary: UNDP/PRIO Expert Meeting on Measuring SDG 16: "Targets 16.1 on Peace, 16.3 on Justice, 16.7 on Inclusion and 16.10 on Freedom"*. UNDP and Peace Research Institute Oslo.

United Nations. (2016b). *Report of the inter-agency and expert group on sustainable development goal indicators* (pp. 15–62). UN Economic and Social Council. http://unstats.un.org/unsd/statcom/47th-session/documents/2016-2-SDGs-Rev1-E.pdf. Accessed 19 April 2016.

United Nations Development Program. (2013). *Rule of law and development: Integrating rule of law in the post-2015 development framework*. http://www.worldwewant2015.org/node/341332. Accessed 19 April 2016.

United Nations General Assembly. (2015). *Transforming our world: The 2030 Agenda for sustainable development*. United Nations: A/RES/70/1. https://sustainabledevelopment.un.org/post2015/summit. Accessed 19 April 2016.

United Nations Security Council. (2004). *The rule of law and transitional justice in conflict and post-conflict societies*. UN S/2004/616. http://www.unrol.org/files/2004%20report.pdf. Accessed 19 April 2016.

Wilkinson, I. (2005). From the sociology of risk to a critical sociology of suffering. In *Presentation at the SCARR Network Conference*. http://www.kent.ac.uk/scarr/events/finalpapers/wilkinson.pdf. Accessed 19 April 2016.

Woetzel, J. et al. (2015). *The power of parity: How advancing women's equality can add $12 trillion to global growth*. McKinsey Global Institute: http://www.mckinsey.com/insights/growth/the_power_of_parity_advancing_womens_equality_in_india. Accessed 19 April 2016.

Chapter 15
Dysfunctional Population Growth: The Links to Human Suffering

J. Joseph Speidel

Reproductive Health and Suffering

Providing access to health care to avoid death and relieve the pain and suffering caused by disease and disability is an important way to alleviate human suffering. Access to reproductive health, including family planning and safe abortion services, is a key preventive measure that avoids the suffering of unsafe abortion or unwanted childbirth that often leads to medical complications and premature death. In the developing countries, the lifetime risk of dying in childbirth is about 1 in 75 compared to about 1 in 7300 in developed countries (Smith et al. 2009). In poor countries the suffering caused by a death in pregnancy or childbirth goes far beyond the pain of a death because of the disruption of family life that frequently includes deepening poverty, and illness and death among surviving children. Family planning makes possible a much safer pattern of childbearing. Avoiding pregnancies among women who are adolescent or over age 35 and a 2-year or longer spacing between births is associated with a 30% reduction in maternal deaths and a 10% decrease in newborn and infant mortality (Cleland et al. 2006; Rustein 2008).

Because contraceptives are not always used or sometimes fail, abortion is needed to achieve fertility goals and avoid the social and economic suffering caused by an unintended pregnancy. Of the estimated 56.3 million annual abortions worldwide in 2014 about half were carried out under unsafe conditions (Sedgh et al. 2016b). Medically safe abortion only rarely causes fatalities—it is about ten times safer than childbirth—whereas unsafe abortion results in an estimated 47,000 deaths worldwide each year (Shah and Ahman 2010).

In addition to the benefits of preventing unintended pregnancies, contraception contributes to a pleasurable and anxiety free sexual life, and some methods of family

J.J. Speidel (✉)
Bixby Center for Global Reproductive Health, University of California, San Francisco,
3333 California Street, Suite 335, Box 0744, San Francisco, CA 94118, USA
e-mail: joe.speidel@ucsf.edu

R.E. Anderson (ed.), *Alleviating World Suffering*, Social Indicators Research Series 67, DOI 10.1007/978-3-319-51391-1_15

planning have direct health benefits. For example, oral contraceptives help to alleviate heavy, irregular and painful menstrual bleeding and protect women against ovarian, endometrial and colorectal cancer, endometriosis, benign breast disease and anemia. And progestin-releasing IUDs can reduce heavy menstrual bleeding, improve anemia and decrease the likelihood of pelvic infections and uterine cancer. Use of condoms is an effective way for sexually active women and men to prevent transmission of sexually transmitted infections, including HIV (Hatcher et al. 2011).

Social and Economic Development

An estimated three billion people live on $2.50 a day or less, and poverty is closely associated with human suffering (World Poverty 2016). Slow progress on measures to increase economic growth and eliminate poverty has a population dimension. After the Second World War, better worldwide availability of medical technologies such as antibiotics, together with public health measures, such as better access to clean water and immunization, brought about a rapid reduction of death rates. But without simultaneous strong efforts to provide birth control in developing countries, birth rates remained high and many countries experienced rapid population growth (McFalls 2007). Between 1950 and 2015 world population more than doubled, from 2.6 billion to 7.3 billion. Almost all of this past growth occurred in developing countries, and current population growth, estimated at 83 million per year, is largely confined to developing countries (UN 2015a).

Rapid population growth makes needed expansions of agriculture, schools, infrastructure and jobs much more difficult or impossible as is evident by the crowded dilapidated schools and burgeoning slums without adequate power or sanitation found in many developing countries. In rapidly growing regions about half of the population is under age 20 with youth unemployment high and competition for jobs intense. Large numbers of unemployed and frustrated young men lead to social tensions, high crime rates and political unrest.

Families with fewer children direct more resources toward the health and education of each child and slowing population growth improves the economic well being of entire countries as well as individuals (Bongaarts et al. 2012). Well-managed, high-quality voluntary family planning programs in Thailand, South Korea, Malaysia, Taiwan, and Singapore were an important factor in their emergence from poverty. Rapid declines in average family size reduce the dependency ratio—the number of children, youth, and elderly who are not as economically productive, compared to the number of workers in the labor force. Fewer nonworking dependents provided a temporary window of opportunity, a demographic dividend, that contributed to the East Asian economic miracle that occurred in these countries (Bloom et al. 2003).

Preserving the Environment

Studies of the status of natural systems make it clear that human over-consumption is depleting the earth's natural resources and harming life-supporting ecosystems (Barnosky et al. 2013). The UN-sponsored Millennium Ecosystem Assessment, carried out by 1300 scientists from 95 countries, concluded that humans have degraded ecosystems more rapidly and extensively over the past 50 years than ever before, primarily to meet increasing demands for food, fresh water, timber, fiber, and fuel (Millennium 2005).

The Assessment found that 60% of ecosystem services—the benefits people obtain from ecosystems—are being degraded or used unsustainably (Millennium 2005). Biodiversity loss has increased rapidly due to human impacts, such as habitat depletion, pollution, introduction of diseases and invasive species, and exploitation of commercially desirable species. Global forest cover has declined by 50% since pre-agricultural times and wildlife populations have been halved in the past 40 years (McLellan 2014).

The impact of humans on their environment is related to their numbers, their per capita consumption, and the environmental impact of the technology used to produce what is consumed (Ehrlich and Holdren 1971). The lifestyle of each person in a rich country has a greater detrimental impact on the environment than each person in a poor country. Surely people deserve to emerge from poverty, but when they do so their consumption increases, and five times as many people live in developing countries as live in developed countries.

In 1998 the noted biologist E. O. Wilson summed up the environmental challenge of increasing consumption by the large number of people living in developing countries as follows:

> *Homo sapiens* is approaching the limit of its food and water supply. Unlike any species that lived before, it is also changing the world's atmosphere and climate, lowering and polluting water tables, shrinking forests, and spreading deserts. Most of the stress originates directly or indirectly from a handful of industrialized countries. Their proven formulas for prosperity are being eagerly adopted by the rest of the world. The emulation cannot be sustained, not with the same levels of consumption and waste. Even if the industrialization of developing countries is only partly successful, the environmental aftershock will dwarf the population explosion that preceded it (Wilson 1998, p. 314).

This aftershock is vividly illustrated by China where per capita consumption, as measured by GNI per capita, is only 24% of that of that of the U.S. ($13,130 vs. $55,860), but China's population is more than four times larger (1.37 billion vs. 321 million) (2015 World Population Data Sheet, 2015). With the exception of petroleum products, China is now the number one consumer of almost all commodities such as steel, grain and meat and the largest greenhouse gas emitter (Brown 2009).

Lester Brown has described the interaction between life-supporting ecosystems and population growth as follows:

> As land and water become scarce, competition for these vital resources intensifies within societies, particularly between the wealthy and those who are poor and dispossessed. The

> shrinkage of life-supporting resources per person that comes with population growth is threatening to drop the living standards of millions of people below the survival level, leading to potentially unmanageable social tensions (Brown 2009).

In 1992, over 1700 of the world's leading scientists—including a majority of Nobel laureates in the sciences—warned:

> If we do not stabilize population in voluntary, humane ways, it will be done for us by Nature; it will be done brutally, relentlessly and whether we wish it or not (Kendall 1992).

Food Security, Climate Change, Family Planning and Population

By reducing unintended pregnancies and slowing population growth, strengthened family planning programs would also powerfully and relatively inexpensively contribute to improvements in food security and slow the buildup of the greenhouse gas emissions that cause climate change. According to the UN Food and Agriculture Organization, the suffering of hunger affects about 800 million people or 13% of people living in developing countries, and in 20 countries in protracted crisis, 39% are hungry (FAO 2015). Poverty is a fundamental reason there are millions of chronically undernourished people, but their situation is being made worse by a confluence of long-term population and environmental trends that are undermining world food availability. Every week, population growth is adding an estimated 1.6 million people to the planet who need food. The most rapid growth of population is occurring in Sub-Saharan Africa, a region with weak family planning programs that is projected to more than double in population size in just 35 years, from 949 million in 2015 to 2.1 billion in 2050 (2015 World Population Data Sheet, 2015).

Other factors at work that threaten future progress toward elimination of hunger include increased diversion of grains for biofuels, more use of grain for livestock and poultry feed, and the declining productive capacity of croplands and fisheries. Eighty percent of global fisheries have been over-fished or are at their biological limit, and the loss of half the world's mangroves and coral reefs has reduced the breeding grounds of many fish species that humans consume (FAO 2009b, Burke et al. 2001).

Climate change is leading to increasingly unstable weather and the hotter temperatures that cut crop yields. Cropland is shrinking because of soil erosion and desertification, and crop yields are threatened by inadequate water supply—perhaps the most important threat to food security. By 2025, three out of four people worldwide will face some degree of water scarcity (UN Environment 2006). Water tables are falling as 15 countries containing nearly half of the world's people, a total of 3.5 billion, are over pumping aquifers (Brown 2012). And this depletion of aquifers threatens production of grains in the three largest producing countries—China,

India, and the U.S. Any decline in world production of food grains will have a serious impact on the 50 countries that import half of their grain and especially on the 15 countries that import all of their grain (Worldwatch Institute 2016).

These trends are an important reason that food in developing countries has become more expensive, and the UN Food Price Index has doubled over the past decade. In addition to these long-term trends, short-term food security is under constant threat by surges in food prices driven by crop failures caused by bad weather, for example, a recent weak monsoon in India, and a crop-withering drought in Ethiopia and Zimbabwe.

The important relationships between population, agriculture and climate are increasingly recognized. The Intergovernmental Panel on Climate Change considers population growth and economic development the two most important drivers of increasing carbon dioxide emissions. Clearly the developed nations of the world bear much of the responsibility for curbing greenhouse gas emissions, but as current low-income countries become more populous and more successful in reducing poverty, consumption and greenhouse gas emissions from these countries will increase as they have in India, Brazil, Indonesia and especially in China—now the country emitting the largest amount of greenhouse gasses (see Fig. 15.1).

If climate change were to cause the projected 10-meter (32.8 foot) rise in sea level it would displace more than 600 million people and flood large areas of cropland (McGranahan et al. 2007). Agriculture, livestock and poultry production currently account for 30% of greenhouse gas emissions (See Fig. 15.2). The largest sources of agricultural greenhouse gas emissions are carbon dioxide from tropical deforestation, methane from livestock and rice production, and nitrous oxide from

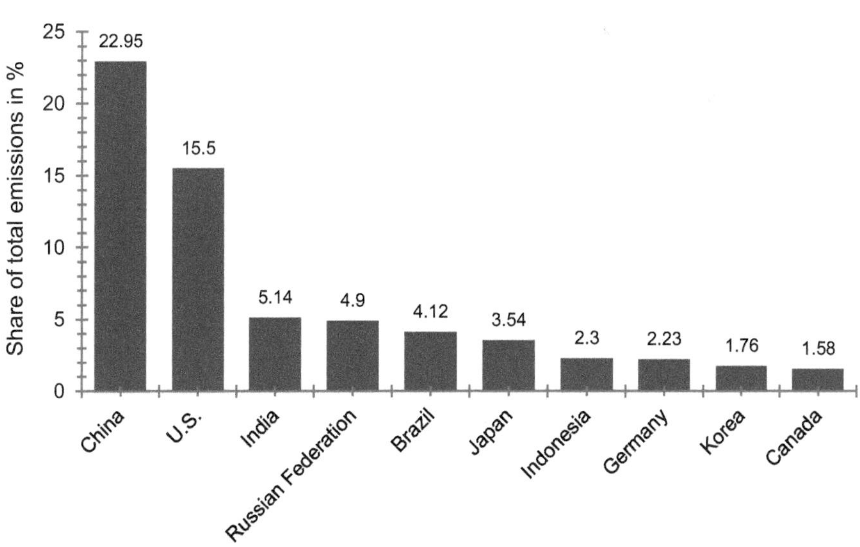

Fig. 15.1 Largest emitters of carbon dioxide worldwide by country, 2013 (Burck et al. 2014)

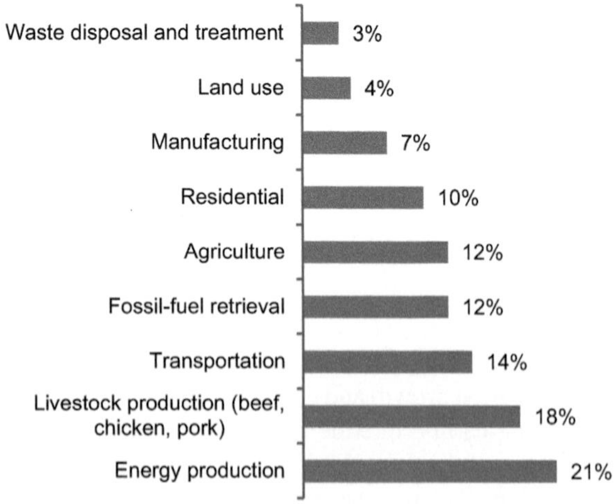

Fig. 15.2 Greenhouse gases emissions, as a percent of the total from each source (Data are from Fiala 2009)

nutrient additions to croplands (Vermeulen et al. 2012). Worldwide meat production alone emits more greenhouse gases than all forms of global transportation or industrial processes. This is one reason many environmentalists advocate moving toward a plant-based diet. Since agriculture, and especially production of meat, is the largest single contributor to greenhouse gas emissions, avoiding the need to intensify agriculture to feed a growing population will help address climate change (Fiala 2009).

Although the previous very low UN population projections now seem unlikely, in 2010, O'Neil estimated that reaching what was then the lowest UN fertility scenario could contribute 16% to 29% of the reduction in greenhouse gas emissions needed by 2050, and, if world population were to decline according to the UN low projection to below six billion, 37% to 41% of the reduction needed by 2100 to avoid global warming of 2 °C (O'Neill et al. 2010).

Better reproductive health care and decreased population pressures are essential but insufficient to alleviate present and future human suffering from climate change and degradation of life-supporting ecosystems. There is an urgent need for people everywhere, and especially in high-consuming developed countries, to adopt a new sustainable economic regimen that reduces consumption, waste and pollution, ends the profligate and ecologically unsustainable exploitation of natural resources and preserves and restores natural systems. It would be beneficial to minimize meat consumption; replant forests to sequester carbon; conserve soils; restore fisheries; preserve water resources; and transition from a fossil fueled economy to an electric economy, powered by renewable energy sources, while simultaneously decreasing per capita energy use through energy-efficiency (Speidel et al. 2009).

Human Rights and Reproductive Justice

Lack of autonomy and control over sexual behavior, childbearing and reproductive health shapes human suffering. Unintended childbearing generates suffering by harming the physical and mental health of women and their children, straining family relationships, and perpetuating poverty by closing off opportunities for education and employment. Conversely, ability to control reproductive decisions, including whether to be sexually active and with whom, whether to bear children, the ability to determine family size and the timing of births by preventing or terminating a pregnancy, all provide an enhancement of human rights, reproductive justice, and serve to empower women. Although The United Nations' Universal Declaration of Human Rights states that everyone has the right to health and well-being, and the United Nations Population Fund (UNFPA) has declared that access to family planning is a fundamental human right, these rights are still not available to many people (UN 1948).

In recent years advocates of reproductive rights have called for an expanded vision of rights under the rubric of reproductive justice, a framework that focuses attention on the social, political, and economic inequalities among different communities. Reproductive justice is defined as: …the complete physical, mental, spiritual, political, economic, and social well-being of women and girls, and will be achieved when women and girls have the economic, social, and political power and resources to make healthy decisions about our bodies, sexuality, and reproduction for ourselves, our families, and our communities in all areas of our lives (Asian Communities for Reproductive Justice 2005)

Surveys in many countries, and especially in developing countries, reveal substantial deficiencies in access to family planning with up to a quarter of women who want to either stop childbearing altogether or delay the birth of their next child lacking access to modern contraception. A recent study estimates that in 2014, 225 million women in developing countries who wanted to avoid a pregnancy were not using an effective contraceptive method because they lack access or face other barriers to using contraception (Singh et al. 2014). Access to safe abortion services is even more constrained with many impediments to access ranging from total bans to a broad variety of unnecessary legal barriers that make access difficult or unobtainable.

The Sustainable Development Goals and Human Suffering

Demography and reproductive health are highly relevant to many of the goals of the recently adopted 2030 Agenda for Sustainable Development (UN 2015c). Targets under SDG Goal 3. *Ensure healthy lives and promote well-being for all at all ages* and SDG Goal 5. *Achieve gender equality and empower all women and girls* calls for strengthening access to reproductive health and rights:

- *By 2030, ensure universal access to sexual and reproductive health-care services, including for family planning, information and education, and the integration of reproductive health into national strategies and programmes.*

- *Ensure universal access to sexual and reproductive health and reproductive rights as agreed in accordance with the Programme of Action of the International Conference on Population and Development and the Beijing Platform for Action and the outcome documents of their review conferences.*

Several of the SDGs call for protection of the environment: Goal 12, *Ensure sustainable consumption and production patterns;* Goal 13, *Take urgent action to combat climate change and its impacts;* Goal 14, *Conserve and sustainably use the oceans, seas and marine resources for sustainable development*; and, Goal 15, *Protect, restore and promote sustainable use of terrestrial ecosystems, sustainably manage forests, combat desertification, and halt and reverse land degradation and halt biodiversity loss.*

Population and Family Planning: A Report on Progress

Population Policies

The 1994 International Conference on Population and Development (ICPD) adopted a broad strategy for population work that in addition to basic family planning and other reproductive health services, included poverty eradication, women's empowerment, gender equity, human rights, environmental protection, male responsibility in sexual behavior and family welfare, adolescent reproductive health, and safe abortion (UNFPA 1995). The ICPD addressed urgent issues relating to human welfare in the developing world, but in the years following the ICPD there was not a concomitant increase in development assistance or locally available funds for this broader array of activities except for HIV/AIDS and modest increases for general reproductive health.

Population: Family Planning Programs and Other Influences on Fertility

The forces at work that heighten demand for small families are likely to become increasingly widespread globally. They include lower mortality rates, increased urbanization, better education, the high cost of childrearing, and improvements in the status, employment, education and economic independence of women.

Support for family planning from national governments and foreign aid donors has been inconsistent and inadequate to meet the family planning needs of all individuals and couples. However, even with this less than optimal support, great progress has been made. In many countries provision of modern contraceptives through organized family planning programs has gone a long way toward successfully meeting much of the demand for small families, decreasing fertility and slowing population growth (Bongaarts et al. 2012).

Table 15.1 Population size, total fertility rates and annual growth of population in more developed and less developed regions by year

	1950	1970	1990	2015
TFR, developed	2.8	2.27	1.74	1.67
TFR, less developed	6.2	5.6	3.65	2.65
Population, developed	0.5 b	0.8 b	1.0 b	1.25 b
Population, less developed	1.1 b	1.7 b	2.7 b	6.1 b
Annual population growth	15 m	48 m	75 m	83 m

Source: (UN 2015a)
TFR average lifetime number of children per woman, *b* billion, *m* million

Between 1960 and 2014, contraceptive usage in less developed countries increased from about 9% of married women of reproductive ages, or 30 million users, to 57%, or 652 million users, and the lifetime average number of children per woman, or total fertility rate (TFR) declined by more than half, from 6.0 to 2.65. A TFR of 2.1 will, over time, result in a stable population size (Cleland et al. 2006, UN 2015b). The Guttmacher Institute and UNFPA estimate that in 2014, use of modern contraception in developing countries prevented 231 million unintended pregnancies, 1.1 million newborn deaths, and 100,000 maternal deaths (Singh et al. 2014). But even with declines in fertility, between 1970 and 2015 the developing countries added 4.4 billion people. In contrast, the developed countries grew by only 450 million (UN 2015a). Although family planning programs have made remarkable progress in reducing fertility rates, the annual increment of population growth in the world has increased substantially, with nearly all growth still occurring in the developing countries. (See Table 15.1)

Developing Country Family Planning Success Stories

The impact of organized family planning programs on population growth is clear: such programs have been responsible for much of the fertility decline in both developed and developing countries. No fertility decline has been observed in a poor and largely illiterate country in the absence of a strong family planning program (Jain and Ross 2012). The experiences of Thailand and Iran demonstrate how quickly well-designed government supported family planning programs can bring the benefits of family planning to a country and curb rapid population growth. Thailand's government launched its population program in 1970 and by the late 1980s, Thailand's TFR had dropped from about seven births per woman to below the "replacement-level" of TFR 2.1. A cost-benefit analysis projected that Thailand's program would save the government $16 for every dollar invested in the program (Chao and Allen 1984).

Recognizing an impending imbalance between available natural resources and population size, the Iranian government, with the support of Muslim religious leaders, reinvigorated its national family planning program in 1989 (Aghajanian and Merhyar 1999). From a TFR of 6.8 in 1984, the TFR declined to 2.8 by 1996 and is currently below replacement-level at 1.8 births per woman (UN 2015a). The long list of additional developing countries with successful voluntary family planning programs and low fertility includes Brazil, Bangladesh, Columbia, Indonesia, Tunisia, Turkey, and Vietnam. China with its one-child policy is a special case in that its family planning program, while effective in reducing fertility, is not voluntary. The experience of many other countries shows that coercion is not necessary.

Lessons Learned

International surveys reveal substantial unmet demand for birth spacing and family-size limitation in virtually all countries. This is the main reason why well-managed voluntary family planning programs offering counseling and high quality services can go a long ways toward meeting the demand for family planning and lowering fertility. The experience of many countries has taught us the keys to effective family planning programs (Cleland et al. 2006):

- High-level political commitment, especially from governments, is important.
- Broad support from leadership groups is needed.
- Smaller families & modern contraception should be legitimized through mass media, for example through serial dramas (soap operas).
- It is essential to offer a broad choice of contraceptive methods including the most effective methods, sterilization and long-acting reversible contraceptive (LARC) methods, the IUD and implant.
- Provide woman-centered counseling, information and services through a variety of convenient sources, e.g., medical facilities, social marketing, and outreach services through field workers.
- Ensure access to affordable safe abortion care.
- Adequate funding is needed to ensure family planning availability at an affordable cost.

However, as John Bongaarts has noted, family planning service programs alone are not enough to eliminate unintended pregnancies.

> Among the reasons for unwanted and unplanned pregnancies are low levels of female education, a lack of knowledge about and access to contraception, insufficient supplies and services, cost and fear of side effects. Just as problematic are opposition from spouses and other family members and traditional gender roles that support a desire for large families. To reduce unintended pregnancies, family-planning programmes must go beyond simply providing supplies and services; they must also reduce or eliminate these other obstacles. (Bongaarts 2016)

Population and Family Planning: The Future

The Remaining Challenge

As is shown in Table 15.2, three-quarters of the population of the developing world is found in six large countries and Sub-Saharan Africa. Their demographic future will largely shape the future of world population size.

Table 15.3 shows that there are profound differences in the expected contribution of eight of the largest countries and Sub-Saharan Africa to population growth between 2015 and 2050, depending to a large extent on the quality and strength of their family planning programs, but also on addressing misinformation about contraceptive side effects and safety, opposition to family planning by spouses and family members and the sway of cultural norms that support high fertility (Sedgh et al. 2016a). Much improvement is needed in the family planning programs where rapid population growth is occurring: in Africa, some middle-eastern countries such as Iraq and Afghanistan, and in Pakistan and parts of India. Because in Sub-Saharan Africa many women and men still want to have large families, communication about the individual and family benefits of family planning is of particular importance.

Unless family planning services in Africa are strengthened, this rapidly growing region could nearly quadruple in size, from today's 1.2 billion to 4.4 billion by 2100 (UN 2015a). Longer-term projections are even more alarming. If the birth rates and death rates at the time of a UN projection in 2011were to remain unchanged, Africa would reach a population of three trillion in 2300! (UN 2011). Clearly this is not possible. So the current levels of birth and death rates in Africa are not sustainable. Either fertility will fall or the demographic transition to low birth and low death rates will be reversed as death rates rise.

Table 15.2 Population is concentrated in a few developing countries & regions

Country	Population in 2015 (millions)	% of all developing countries
China	1372	23
India	1314	22
Sub-Saharan Africa	949	16
Indonesia	256	4.2
Brazil	205	3.4
Pakistan	199	3.3
Bangladesh	160	2.6
Countries & regions listed	4455	73
All developing countries	6082	100

Source: 2015 World Population Data Sheet (2015)

Table 15.3 High growth will occur where family planning is weak

Country	Family planning program	TFR in 2014	Population in 2015	Population in 2050	Growth 2015–2050	Percent change
China	Very strong	1.7	1372	1366	−6	−0.4%
India	Moderately strong	2.3	1314	1660	346	26%
Sub-Saharan Africa	Very weak	5.0	949	2081	1132	119%
Indonesia	Moderately strong	2.6	256	367	111	43%
Brazil	Strong	1.8	205	226	30	10%
Pakistan	Weak	3.8	199	344	121	64%
Bangladesh	Moderately strong	2.3	160	202	42	26%
Philippines	Weak	2.9	103	157	54	52%
All developing countries	Various	2.6	6082	8495	2410	40%
All developed countries	Very strong	1.7	1254	1310	56	4.5%

Population in Millions
Source: 2015 World Population Data Sheet (2015)

Abortion is Essential to Family Planning Success

Although contraception decreases the need for abortion, under typical conditions of use many contraceptive methods fail. Women with unintended pregnancies turn to abortion to attain their childbearing goals regardless of its legal status. Worldwide eighty-five million pregnancies, representing 40% of all pregnancies, were unintended in 2012. Of these, 50% ended in abortion, 13% ended in miscarriage, and 38% resulted in an unplanned birth. Most unintended pregnancies are occurring in developing countries—nearly 80 million each year (Sedgh et al. 2014). Almost all countries with low fertility rely on extensive use of abortion. As Malcolm Potts has noted:

> All societies with unconstrained access to fertility regulation, including abortion, experience a rapid decline to replacement levels of fertility, and often lower. (Potts 1997)

Although controversial and opposed by many people and conservative religions, access to safe abortion is necessary for women to fully control their fertility. Safe abortion should be an integral part of the services provided by family planning programs and is essential to meeting many of the SDG goals (Crane and Hord Smith 2006, p. 5–9).

Developing Country Family Planning Funding and Population Growth

In 2014, the UN projected that with an 80% probability, world population size would increase from 7.2 billion to between 9.6 and 12.3 billion in 2100, with almost all growth occurring in developing countries (Gerland et al. 2014). World population growth of 2.4 billion (a 33% increase) rather than 5.1 billion (a 70% increase) is unlikely without increased investment in family planning.

An increase from an estimated $4.1 billion from all sources to $9.4 billion annually is needed to provide family planning to all women in developing countries who want to end or delay childbearing (Singh et al. 2014). An annual expenditure of $9.4 billion is less than 5% of the $209 billion annual expenditure estimated to be necessary to meet the need for food in developing countries between now and 2050 (FAO 2009a).

Many large countries, including China, India and Indonesia, are able to fund family planning programs for their citizens with their own resources. But the countries that are categorized as least developed often lack both the political will and financial resources to mount strong programs. They must rely heavily on donor assistance. Funds provided by foreign aid donors exclusively for family planning were lower in 2008 ($572 million) than they were in 1994 at the time of the ICPD ($723 million). Since then, annual donor assistance for family planning has increased to $882 million in 2010, $1.1 billion in 2012 and $1.4 billion in 2014 (UN 2013, Wexler et al. 2015).

One important impetus for increased funds for family planning came from the 2012 London Summit on Family Planning (since renamed Family Planning 2020), an initiative to strengthen world commitment to and funding for family planning. Led by Melinda Gates, of the Bill and Melinda Gates Foundation, and British Prime Minister David Cameron, the Summit set a goal of providing 120 million additional women in the 69 poorest countries with family planning by 2020. Donors pledged to provide an additional $2.6 billion and developing countries an increase of $2 billion over the next 8 years (Family Planning 2020 2016).

Very Low Fertility: A Problem or a Benefit?

About half of the world population lives in some 80 countries with fertility at or below the replacement level of TFR=2.1 (Population Reference Bureau 2015). They include China, most European nations, the U.S., Russia, Brazil and Japan. Only a few countries, including Germany and Japan, have had sufficiently sustained sub-replacement fertility to be experiencing population decline. Most low-fertility countries still have growing populations because of immigration and population momentum based on an age structure with large numbers of young men and women of reproductive ages. For example, birth and death rates in the U.S. are about the same and do not drive either population growth or decline, but immigration is high and immigrants tend to have large families. So immigration is the main source of a projected increase in U.S. population from the current 315 million to 398 million by 2050 (Population Reference Bureau 2015; Kent and Mather 2002).

With a few exceptions, such as the U.S., compared to high developing-world birth rates, most people living in wealthy developed countries are on the other side of a "demographic divide"—where birth rates are so low that population decline and rapid aging is almost inevitable (McFalls 2007). A smaller population in high-consumption wealthy countries could benefit the environment. Paul Ehrlich estimates that the planet could sustainably support only two billion people at the standard of living and consumption pattern of people in the U.S. and Europe (Ehrlich and Ehrlich 2013). However population decline is a cause for concern with regard to the resilience of economies and the adequacy of support for generous but often poorly funded health and pension systems. A shrinking proportion of workers compared to elderly dependents may already be a problem for people living in some European countries and Japan. So far, pro-natalist child and family-friendly government policies, programs and incentives, including reduced taxes, subsidized care for children and bonuses, have done little to increase birth rates (Chamie and Mirkin 2015).

Conclusion

The global challenges of unintended pregnancy, high maternal and infant mortality, rapid population growth, poverty, hunger, climate change and devastation of essential ecosystems are all inter-connected. Reducing the human suffering linked to each of these challenges depends considerably on improving reproductive health rights and services and reducing population growth rates. Many countries have already made remarkable progress in meeting reproductive health challenges. With sound policies and adequate funding their success can be emulated elsewhere including in high-fertility countries such as those in Sub-Saharan Africa.

Fortunately, when given the opportunity through provision of reproductive health information and services, women and men usually chose to limit reproduction enough to slow and eventually halt population growth. Family planning and reproductive health programs are affordable, practical and low cost, especially compared to the cost of inaction. There is reason for optimism about the further success of family planning programs: In the volume *Global Family Planning Revolution* Stephen Sinding commented:

> In my view, the family planning movement has been one of the most successful examples of development cooperation in history. For all the underlying cultural and political conflict that attended it, the movement stands alongside the Green Revolution in agriculture as a demonstration of what collective political will and strong international cooperation can achieve. As such, it should serve as a beacon of hope to those who despair about the prospects for effective global action to reverse such pressing contemporary problems as global warming or the AIDS pandemic. (Robinson and Ross 2007)

And as Jared Diamond has observed:

> To save ourselves we don't need new technology: we just need the political will to face up to our problems of population and the environment. (Diamond 2005)

This chapter has presented the case for alleviating suffering arising from reproductive risks and over population. It also demonstrated linkages of reproductive health to other global challenges. Hopefully as people become committed to the ethic of alleviating the suffering of others, commitment to address all of the grand challenges defined by the new Agenda for Sustainable Development will take on a higher priority and we will collectively work toward reducing major suffering arising from all sources, both now and in the future.

References

Aghajanian, A., & Merhyar, A. H. (1999). Fertility, contraceptive use and family planning program activity in the Islamic republic of Iran. *International Family Planning Perspectives, 25*, 98–102.

Asian Communities for Reproductive Justice. (2005). *A new vision for advancing our movement for reproductive health, reproductive rights, and reproductive justice.* Oakland: Asian Communities for Reproductive Justice. http://strongfamiliesmovement.org/assets/docs/ACRJ-A-New-Vision.pdf. Accessed 19 July 2016.

Barnosky, A.D., et al. (2013). *Scientific consensus on maintaining humanity's life support systems in the 21st century.* http://consensusforaction.stanford.edu/see-scientific-consensus/consensus_english.pdf. Accessed 19 July 2016.

Bloom, D. E., Canning, D., & Sevilla, J. (2003). *The demographic dividend: A new perspective on the economic consequences of population change.* Santa Monica: Rand.

Bongaarts, J. (2016). Slow down population growth. *Nature, 530*, 409–412. http://www.nature.com/polopoly_fs/1.19415!/menu/main/topColumns/topLeftColumn/pdf/530409a%20%28corrected%29.pdf. Accessed 19 July 2016.

Bongaarts, J., Cleland, J., Townsend, J., Bertrand, J., & Das Gupta, M. (2012). *Family planning programs for the 21st century: Rationale and design.* New York: Population Council.

Brown, L. R. (2009). *Plan B 4.0: Mobilizing to save civilization.* New York: W.W. Norton & Company.

Brown, L. R. (2012). *Full planet, empty plates: The new geopolitics of food scarcity.* New York: W.W. Norton & Company.

Burck, J., Marten, F. & Bals C. (2014). *The climate change performance index 2014. A comparison of the 58 top CO2 emitting nations.* Bonn: Germanwatch. https://germanwatch.org/en/download/8599.pdf. Accessed 19 July 2016.

Burke, L., Kura, Y., Kassem, K., et al. (2001). *Pilot analysis of global ecosystems: Coastal ecosystems.* Washington, DC: World Resources Institute.

Chamie, J, & Mirkin, B. (2015, November 17). Analysis: More countries want more babies. *Inter Press Service News Agency.* http://www.ipsnews.net/2015/11/analysis-more-countries-want-more-babies. Accessed 19 July 2016.

Chao, D. N. W., & Allen, K. B. (1984). A cost-benefit analysis of Thailand's family planning program. *International Family Planning Perspectives, 10*, 75–81.

Cleland, J., Bernstein, S., Ezeh, A., Faundes, A., Glasier, A., & Innis, J. (2006). Family planning: The unfinished agenda. *The Lancet Sexual and Reproductive Health Series, 368*(9549), 1810–1827. doi:10.1016/S0140-6736(06)69480-4.

Crane, B. B., & Hord Smith, C. E. (2006). *Access to safe abortion: An essential strategy for achieving the millennium development goals to improve maternal health, promote gender equality, and reduce poverty* (pp. 5–9). New York: NYP Millennium Project. http://www.unmillennium-project.org/documents/Crane_and_Hord-Smith-final.pdf. Accessed 19 July 2016.

Diamond, J. (2005, January 1). The ends of the world as we know them. *The New York Times.*

Ehrlich, P. R., & Ehrlich, A. H. (2013, January 9). Can a collapse of global civilization be avoided? *Philosophical Transactions of the Royal Society B,* 280, rspb 2012.2845. http://dx.doi.org/10.1098/rspb.2012.2845

Ehrlich, P., & Holdren, J. (1971). The impact of population growth. *Science, 171*, 1212–1217.

Family Planning 2020. (2016). http://www.familyplanning2020.org/. Accessed 19 July 2016.

Fiala, N. (2009). The greenhouse hamburger: Producing beef for the table has a surprising environmental cost: It releases prodigious amounts of heat-trapping greenhouse gases. *Scientific American, 300*(2), 72–75.

Food and Agriculture Organization of the United Nations. (2009a, October 12–13). *High-level expert forum on how to feed the world in 2050.* Rome: FAO. http://www.fao.org/wsfs/forum2050/wsfs-background-documents/hlef-issues-briefs/en/. Accessed on 26 July 2016.

Food and Agriculture Organization of the United Nations. (2009b). *The state of world fisheries and aquaculture 2008.* Rome: United Nations Economic and Social Council.

Food and Agriculture Organization of the United Nations, IFAD, & WPF. (2015). *The state of food insecurity in the world 2015. international hunger targets: Taking stock of uneven progress.* Rome: FAO. http://www.fao.org/3/a-i4646e.pdf. Accessed 19 July 2016.

Gerland, P., et al. (2014). World population stabilization unlikely this century. *Science, 346*(6206), 234–237. doi:10.1126/science.1257469.

Hatcher, R. A., et al. (2011). *Contraceptive technology*, twentieth revised. New York: Ardent Media.

Jain, A. K., & Ross, J. A. (2012). Fertility differences among developing countries: Are they still related to family planning program efforts and social settings? *International Perspectives on Sexual and Reproductive Health, 38*(1), 15–22. doi:10.1363/3801512.

Kendall, H. (1992). *World scientists' warning to humanity.* Cambridge, MA: Union of Concerned Scientists.

Kent, M. M., & Mather, M. (2002). *What drives U.S. population growth?* Washington, DC: Population Reference Bureau.

McFalls, J. A. (2007). *Population: A lively introduction, Population Bulletin, 62*. Washington, DC: Population Reference Bureau.

McGranahan, G., Balk, D., & Anderson, B. (2007). The rising tide: Assessing the risks of climate change and human settlements in low elevation coastal zones. *Environment and Urbanization, 18*, 17–37.

McLellan, R. (Ed.). (2014). *Living planet report.* London: Zoological Society of London; Global Footprint Network; World Wildlife Fund.

Millennium Ecosystem Assessment. (2005). *Ecosystems and human well-being: Synthesis.* Washington, DC: Island Press.

O'Neill, B. C., et al. (2010). Global demographic trends and future carbon emissions. *PNAS, 107*, 41. http://www.pnas.org/content/107/41/17521.full. Accessed 26 July 2016.

Population Reference Bureau. (2015). *2015 world population data sheet.* Washington, DC: Population Reference Bureau.

Potts, M. (1997). Sex and the birth rate. *Population and Development Review, 23*, 1–39.

Robinson, W. C., & Ross, J. A. (Eds.). (2007). *The global family planning revolution: Three decades of population policies and programs.* Washington, DC: The International Bank for Reconstruction and Development, The World Bank.

Rustein, S. O. (2008). *Further evidence of the effects of preceding birth intervals on neonatal, infant, and under-five-years mortality and nutritional status in developing countries: Evidence from the demographic and health surveys* (p. 41). Washington, DC: USAID, DHS Working Papers.

Sedgh, G., Singh, S., & Hussain, R. (2014). Intended and unintended pregnancies worldwide in 2012 and recent trends. *Studies in Family Planning, 45*(3), 301–314.

Sedgh, G., et al. (2016a). *Unmet need for contraception in developing countries: Examining women's reasons for not using a method.* New York: Guttmacher Institute. http://www.guttmacher.org/report/unmet-need-for-contraception-in-developingcountries. Accessed 26 July 2016.

Sedgh, G., et al. (2016b). Abortion incidence between 1990 and 2014: Global, regional, and subregional levels and trends. *Lancet, 388*(10041), 258–267. http://dx.doi.org/10.1016/S0140-6736(16)30380-4
Shah, I., & Ahman, E. (2010). Unsafe abortion in 2008: Global and regional levels and trends. *Reproductive Health Matters, 18*(36), 90–101.
Singh, S., Darroch, J. E., & Ashford, L. S. (2014). *Adding it up: The costs and benefits of investing in sexual and reproductive health 2014*. New York: Guttmacher Institute and United Nations Population Fund.
Smith, R., Ashford, L., Gribble, J., & Clifton, D. (2009). *Family planning saves lives* (4th ed.). Washington DC: Population Reference Bureau.
Speidel, J. J., Weiss, D. C., Ethelston, S. A., & Gilbert, S. M. (2009). Population policies, programmes and the environment. *Philosophical Transactions of the Royal Society B, 364*, 3049–3065.
UNFPA. (1995). *Summary of the ICPD programme of action*. http://www.unfpa.org/icpd/summary.cfm. Accessed 26 July 2016.
United Nations. (1948) *Universal declaration of human rights*. United Nations, Paris, General Assembly resolution 217(III). http://www.un.org/en/universal-declaration-human-rights/. Accessed 19 July 2016.
United Nations (2011, January). World demographic trends, report of the secretary general to the commission on population and development. E/CN9/2011/6, 21. UN Economic and Social Council New York.
United Nations. (2013, April). *The flow of financial resources for assisting in the implementation of the programme of action of the international conference on population and development, report of the secretary-general*. Commission on Population and Development, Forty-sixth session, 22–26, Item 3 of the provisional Agenda.
United Nations. (2015a). *World population prospects: The 2015 revision*. New York: Population Division of the Department of Economic and Social Affairs of the United Nations Secretariat.
United Nations. (2015b). *Trends in contraceptive use worldwide 2015, ST/ESA/SER.A/349*. New York: Population Division United Nations, Department of Economic and Social Affairs.
United Nations. (2015c, September 25). *70/1 Transforming our world: The 2030 Agenda for sustainable development*. Resolution adopted by the General Assembly. http://www.un.org/sustainabledevelopment/. Accessed 26 July 2016.
United Nations Environment Program. (2006). *Challenges to international waters: Regional assessments in a global perspective*. Nairobi: United Nations Environment Program.
Vermeulen, S. J., Campbell, B. M., & Ingram, J. S. I. (2012). Climate change food systems. *Annual Review of Environment and Resources, 37*, 195–222.
Wexler, A., Kates, J., & Leif, E. (2015). *Donor government assistance for family planning in 2014*. Washington, DC: The Henry J. Kaiser Family Foundation. http://kff.org/global-health-policy/report/donor-government-assistance-for-family-planning-in-2014/. Accessed 19 July 2016.
Wilson, E. O. (1998). *Consilience: The unity of knowledge* (p. 314). New York: Alfred A. Knopf.
World Poverty Statistics. (2016). http://www.statisticbrain.com/world-poverty-statistics/. Accessed 19 July 2016.
Worldwatch Institute. (2016). *State of the world 2015: Confronting hidden threats to sustainability* (p. 73). Washington, DC: Island Press.

Chapter 16
Reproductive Health and Justice in Alleviating World Suffering

Andrzej Kulczycki

Introduction

Health is a major contributor to development and is intertwined with such fundamental goals as reducing poverty, improving education, assuring gender equality, achieving sustainable economic growth and mitigating climate change. The role of reproductive health is an often under-appreciated part of this dynamic, yet it is pivotal to achieving these internationally agreed-upon goals and to reducing world suffering. Reproductive health helps assure quality of life, dignity, and opportunity for individuals, couples, and communities. However, humanity faces major challenges in assuring reproductive rights and well-being due to a host of socio-cultural and political sensitivities and the difficulties of operationalizing reproductive health programs. These challenges are compounded by increasing world demographic size and diversity, as well as pronounced socio-economic inequalities.

The world's population has seen unprecedented growth since the mid-twentieth century. It reached 7.4 billion in 2016, twice its number in 1969. This growth reflects former high birth rates and great progress in combating infectious and childhood diseases, and in reducing the burden of premature and avoidable deaths, including maternal mortality. Despite fertility levels declining recently in virtually all regions, the world's population is projected to grow by another billion people to 8.4 billion by 2030 and then to 9.7 billion by 2050 (UN 2015a). This poses great challenges for making the prompt adjustments needed to accommodate a significantly larger population eager to achieve improved health and living standards, while minimizing environmental impact and world suffering. Moreover, the world's population is becoming more demographically diverse as growth rates decline further, which implies that many population and health policies need to be reframed.

A. Kulczycki (✉)
Department of Health Care Organization & Policy, University of Alabama at Birmingham (UAB), 320 Ryals Public Health Bldg, Birmingham, AL 35294-0022, USA
e-mail: andrzej@uab.edu

R.E. Anderson (ed.), *Alleviating World Suffering*, Social Indicators Research Series 67, DOI 10.1007/978-3-319-51391-1_16

There were 1.9 billion women of reproductive age alive in 2016. Although the total number of women of reproductive age is projected to drop 10% or more in a number of European countries by 2030, it will increase in all other major areas and by 45% in Africa (UN 2015a). Securing their reproductive rights, along with universal access to sexual and reproductive health care, is crucial to allowing women and couples to exert control over the number and spacing of their children. Further, achieving gender equality in education, in the labor force and in political processes is associated with better relationships, lower fertility, improved opportunities, and protection from abuse and exploitation. However, maternal deaths, mortality of children younger than 5 years, and adolescent deaths still account for 37% of the global burden of premature mortality (Kassebaum et al. 2014; You et al. 2015), despite almost all these deaths being preventable. Growing numbers of women of reproductive age and increased use of contraception will raise demand for family planning services, much of which is currently not met. Moreover, high rates of unintended pregnancy imply continued high rates of abortion.

Achieving universal access to maternal, sexual, and reproductive health care and improving service quality is critical to fulfilling the human rights of women, improving development prospects, and alleviating suffering. To take the most graphic example of such suffering, each maternal death is an individual tragedy that constitutes an unacceptable public health and ethical problem. Furthermore, it significantly disrupts the health, survival, and wellbeing of children and families. Data from Bangladesh shows that whereas a father's death has negligible effects on a child's odds of dying, a mother's death was associated with a ten-fold increase on children's chances of survival (Ronsmans et al. 2010). While reductions in maternal mortality are to be applauded, they can mask other maternal disabilities that can also have intergenerational repercussions, because the children of these women face an increased risk of serious morbidity or mortality.

Additionally, international estimates suggest that for every maternal death, approximately another 20 women face serious morbidity which is often underreported. For example, obstetric fistula disables millions of women and girls in the world's poorest nations, primarily in sub-Saharan Africa (SSA) and South Asia (Miller et al. 2005). Most fistula occur among women living in poverty in societies where a woman's status and self-esteem may depend almost entirely on her marriage and ability to bear children. This is a highly stigmatizing and preventable complication of inadequate obstetrical care for prolonged obstructed labor, thus it is a prototypical example of social suffering. It can largely be avoided by delaying the age of first pregnancy, ending harmful traditional practices, and providing timely access to quality obstetric care. It can also be repaired surgically. Obstetric fistula has both physical and social consequences, including premature death associated with social isolation, poverty, and malnutrition. Women who experience obstetric fistula suffer constant incontinence, other health problems, shame, and social segregation. Obstetric fistula still exists because health care systems fail to provide accessible, quality maternal health care including family planning, skilled care at birth, basic and comprehensive emergency obstetric care, and affordable treatment of fistula. This serious childbirth injury has been relatively neglected, despite the devastating impact it has on the lives of girls and women.

In the current era of rapid demographic, epidemiological, and socioeconomic change, it is important to take stock of recent reproductive health trends and prospects. Such an assessment will show that despite significant improvements, huge disparities remain with major threats to progress posed by inequities of access to services and poor quality care. This results in continued suffering. The response should involve an increased focus on health systems, comprehensive reproductive health programming, and ensured inclusion of populations that are most vulnerable in the delivery of such services. Moreover, the response must go beyond the health sector and address the social determinants of reproductive health.

Realizing the Pillars of Reproductive Health and Rights

Soon after many less developed countries began to be confronted by rapid population growth, vanguard family planning efforts during the 1960s were expanded into major programs, particularly in South and East Asia. Despite the diversity of local political and economic agendas, by the 1970–1980s, there emerged considerable policy harmonization in efforts to control rapid population growth (Finkle and McIntosh 1994). Some of these policies led to well-documented human rights abuses, notably during India's emergency period (1975–1977) and China's one-child policy, that were subsequently abandoned. Others failed due to poor design and implementation (e.g. Pakistan), prompting further soul-searching about the value of family planning by itself in reducing rapid population growth, notwithstanding major policy successes in Thailand, Bangladesh, and elsewhere (Robinson and Ross 2007; May 2012). Many gradually realized that family planning services were insufficient to reduce fertility and that other changes, such as improved female educational attainment and gender equity, were potentially as important. Moreover, the long-running debate about the complexity of population-development interrelations and their implications, and the changing rationales for population policies and interventions, meant that dialogue between technocrats, policymakers, and publics about population policy needed to be strengthened (Kantner 2014).

At the same time, reproductive rights began to be slowly articulated in international forums and declarations, co-opting the language of human rights approaches. Reproductive rights groups coalesced with the transnational women's movement to push through adoption of the Cairo Program of Action at the 1994 International Conference on Population and Development (ICPD) (McIntosh and Finkle 1995). The Cairo agenda was much criticized for being too broad and ill-defined, but it was also a political push that facilitated the extension of legal rights and freedoms to human reproduction and reproductive health. Further, it represented a major advance by broadening the parameters of family planning to include other important pillars of reproductive health. These can be summarized as:

- Gender equality
- Family planning
- Maternal and newborn care
- Safe abortion
- Sexually transmitted and other reproductive tract infections
- Infertility
- Adolescent sexuality and reproductive health
- Sexual behavior and harmful sexual practices

Sexual and reproductive health includes certain aspects of human experience beyond the purview of morbidity and mortality data. These include harmful traditional behaviors and sexual practices. For example, studies suggest that about 100 million to 125 million girls and women have been subjected to female genital cutting (FGC) in the 28 African countries and Yemen where this customary practice has been documented and for which reasonably reliable estimates exist (Yoder et al. 2013; UNICEF 2013a). FGC is nearly universal in Somalia, Guinea, Djibouti, and Egypt. This violation of the rights of children and women causes much silent suffering. Societal pressures prevent many individuals who oppose FGC from being able to abandon the practice, but there is evidence from some countries that the practice is slowly becoming less prevalent among younger cohorts (see chapter by Boyle and Svec (2017, Chap. 21) in this volume).

Another harmful behavior concerns child marriage, which disproportionately affects girls. Child marriage has decreased globally but is still widespread in South Asia (notably India, Pakistan, and Afghanistan) and many African countries, notably in the Sahel region (including Mauritania, Mali, Burkina Faso, Niger, Central African Republic, and Sudan), as well as Liberia, Sierra Leone, Nigeria, and Somalia. The practice is especially common in impoverished rural areas and is deeply grounded in cultural, social, and economic structures. These are difficult to overcome (Lee-Rife et al. 2012), even though international conventions (notably the Convention on the Rights of the Child adopted by the UN General Assembly in 1989) establish the legal age of consent to marriage as 18 years. Worldwide, more than 250 million women alive today were married as children before age 15, with the highest rates found in South Asia and (UNICEF 2013b). Child marriage can lead to a lifetime of disadvantage and social isolation. Its effects include health problems related to premature pregnancy such as increased risks of maternal and infant mortality, stillbirth and obstetric fistulae (Raj and Boehmer 2013), as well as sexual abuse. However, in countries where child marriage remains common, many governments have tended to overlook the problems that it causes.

A more widespread and previously underreported global health problem concerns domestic violence, the most common form of violence against women. Worldwide, 35% of women aged 15 or older have experienced physical and/or sexual intimate partner violence (IPV) or non-partner sexual violence, based on estimates from 81 countries (WHO 2013). The highest prevalence (65%) is found in parts of central SSA, a level exacerbated by poverty and conflict, but prevalence is also high elsewhere; from 36 to 42% of ever-partnered women report lifetime experience of such violence in West and East Africa, the Middle East and North Africa (MENA), and South Asia. In these regions, the status of women is relatively lower than in other world regions, but reports by women worldwide indicate that IPV is all too common a behavior. Moreover, honor killings continue to occur in many, if not all, MENA countries, where mostly young females are murdered by their male kin for supposed inappropriate female sexuality and modesty (Kulczycki and Windle 2011).

The reproductive health consequences of IPV often include unintended pregnancies and poor pregnancy outcomes, as well as more hospitalizations, greater use of outpatient care for acute problems, and less preventive care (Pallitto et al. 2013). Physical violence has also been associated with a range of common gynecological disorders such as fibroids, decreased libido, chronic pelvic pain, pain on intercourse, urinary tract, vaginal, and sexually transmitted infections (STIs). Although violence screening protocols, counseling and referral services, treatment and rehabilitation programs can be implemented, ending such abuse requires changing attitudes that permit it, developing legal and policy frameworks to prohibit it, and improving women's access to education and economic opportunities.

Greater attention is now being paid to these widespread and earlier neglected practices. Nevertheless, both in the U.S. and internationally, a political backlash ensued against the expanded reproductive health agenda, and the Western feminist and liberal attitudes that were seen to inform it (Kulczycki 1999, 2007). By the turn of the century, conservative political administrations reduced global aid flows for family planning and reproductive health issues, a loss compounded by the greatly escalated response to the dramatic health and development crisis of the HIV/AIDS epidemic, particularly in SSA (van Dalen and Scharf 2014). These shifting policy approaches reduced the urgency attended to global reproductive rights, with the implications particularly serious for the least developed countries found primarily in Africa. In 2010–2012, UN agency reports indicated that SSA, with 12% of the world's population, accounted for 57% of its pregnancy-related deaths, 49% of its infant mortality, and 67% of all HIV infections (Kulczycki 2014).

Meanwhile, the potential vision for reproductive rights continued to be articulated by advocates applying human rights principles to sexuality and reproductive health concerns beyond reducing fertility. The International Planned Parenthood Federation (IPPF), which links more than 150 national member family planning associations and works to improve women's sexual and reproductive health worldwide, published in 1996 the first full "Charter on sexual and reproductive rights" (IPPF 2008). Although this and similar declarations have not become legally binding as part of international human rights law, they have helped improve reproductive justice by highlighting a broader set of reproductive health concerns, their linkages, and the need for their respect by individuals, groups, communities and governments. The IPPF's Charter recognized the freedoms to manage reproductive health and rights, as well as family and gender relationships, among its 12 basic rights. The Charter also sought to connect women's sexual and reproductive health and rights with the concepts and conventions of basic human rights. It includes access to health care and information, civil and political liberties, with the right to equality in the face of all forms of discrimination, as listed below:

- The right to life
- The right to liberty and security of the person
- The right to equality, and to be free from all forms of discrimination
- The right to privacy
- The right to freedom of thought
- The right to have access to information and education
- The right to choose whether or not to marry and to found and plan a family
- The right to decide whether or when to have children
- The right to health care and health protection
- The right to the benefits of scientific progress
- The right to freedom of assembly and political participation
- The right to be free from torture and ill treatment

Owing to political pressure and expediency, the Millennium Development Goals (MDGs)—the United Nations' blueprint for developmental goals over the 2000–2015 period—initially neither included reproductive health, nor demographic considerations. Target 5b, which sought to "Achieve universal access to reproductive health," was added only in 2007. This broad target covered a wide range of issues, making it difficult to agree on a manageable set of appropriate indicators, but four specific indicators were set: adolescent birth rate; antenatal care visits; contraceptive prevalence rate; and unmet need for family planning. Reproductive health is recognized in the UN's successor Sustainable Development Goals (SDGs) as part of the health and gender goals. Also, the 2014 London Summit gave rise to the Family Planning 2020 (FP2020) initiative, funded primarily by the Bill & Melinda Gates Foundation, whose ambitious goal is to have an additional 120 million users of modern contraceptives in the world's poorest 69 countries by the year 2020 (Brown et al. 2014). Although estimated increases in the number of modern contraceptive users are still below the benchmarks of new users, these new initiatives are expected to better address the acute reproductive health needs found particularly in low- and middle-income countries (LMICs).

Maternal Health and Ill-Health

Health must be considered an urgent right to be fought for and is increasingly seen as a cornerstone of sustainable development and even good business. Reproductive health is central to these concerns, with the right to good quality maternal health care being universal. However, we are far from reaching the goal of safe pregnancy and childbirth for all women and girls, in all countries. Worldwide, about 220 million women become pregnant and 135 million babies are delivered each year (UN 2016), but about 40% of all pregnancies are unintended (Sedgh et al. 2014). This leads to more than 50 million abortions occurring annually with about 20 million of

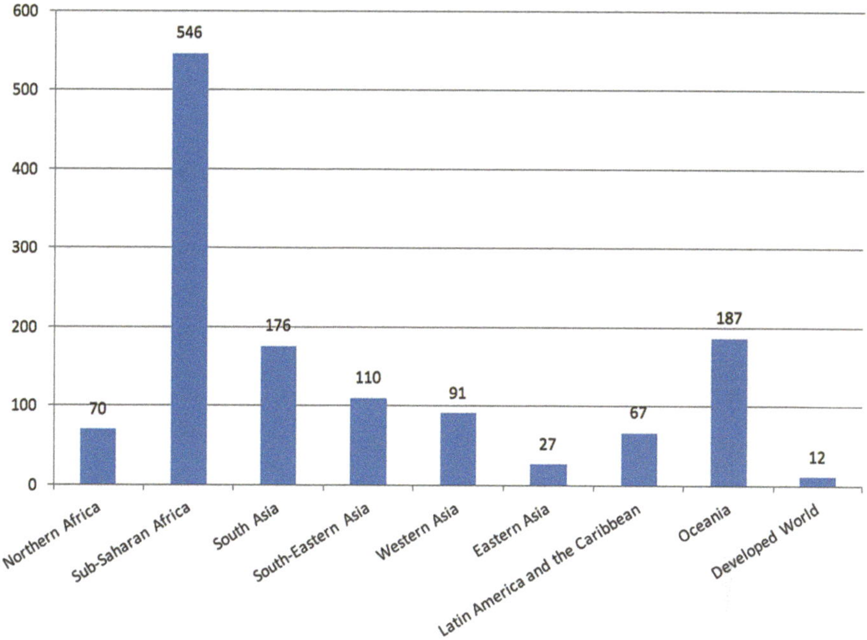

Fig. 16.1 Maternal mortality rates (maternal deaths per 100,000 live births) by World Regions – Data source: WHO (2015)

these considered unsafe, that is, carried out by persons lacking the necessary skills, or in an environment that does not conform to minimal medical standards (WHO 2011). An estimated 303,000 maternal deaths occurred in 2015, with rates of maternal mortality 19 times higher in developing countries than in developed ones (Fig. 16.1). Globally, 45% (2.7 million) of all under-age-5 deaths happen during the neonatal period (the first 28 days of life), the vast majority of which are preventable through many of the same investments in health systems that are needed to improve maternal health outcomes (UNICEF et al. 2015).

During 1990–2015, maternal deaths fell by 44% (from 385 women of childbearing age per 100,000 live births to 216/100,000), child mortality decreased by 53%, and use of maternity services increased markedly (WHO 2016). A range of factors help explain the significant progress made during the Millennium Development Goals (MDGs) era, including funding increases, invigorated country actions, global partnerships, and scale-up of interventions. However, the maternal mortality ratio (MMR) was still far short of the MDG 5a target of a 75% reduction and many challenges to equity remain.

The new global target (SDG 3.1) for 2030 is 70 per 100,000 live births by 2030, requiring a further 68% reduction, and to have no country with an MMR above 140. This is significantly below the current average MMR of 546/100,000 in SSA, the highest regional average among major world regions (Fig. 16.1). Expressed another way, an African woman has a lifetime risk of dying from maternal causes of 1 in 37,

Table 16.1 Poor quality maternal care in all countries

Regional grouping	Major common problems in maternal health care
A. Low- and middle-income countries	
Care for the most vulnerable:	
Too little, too late	Lack of evidence-based guidelines
	Lack of equipment, supplies and medicines
	Insufficient number of skilled providers
	Women delivering alone
	Lack of emergency medical services
	Delayed inter-facility referrals
Care for the wealthy and those in private care:	
Too much, too soon	Unnecessary caesarean section
	Routine induced or augmented labor
	Routine continuous electronic fetal monitoring
	Routine episiotomy
	Routine antibiotics postpartum
B. High-income countries	
	Medical liability costs are often very high
	Fear of litigation
	Weak data and surveillance systems
	Human resource shortages

Source: Adapted from Miller et al. (2016)

compared with 1 in 4900 in high-income countries (WHO 2015). In SSA, 63% of total years of life lost occur among pregnant women and children under 15 years of age. Clearly, many countries and groups of women have seen little or no progress, despite significant global political attention devoted to maternal health.

More effort is needed to guarantee access to quality care for every woman and every newborn. Some women using services receive excellent care, but too many experience one of two extremes: too little, too late, where women receive care that is not timely or sufficient, or too much, too soon, marked by over-medicalization of normal pregnancy and birth with excessive use of unnecessary interventions (Table 16.1).

Both extremes represent maternal health care that is not grounded in evidence. Also, a growing number of low- and middle-income countries (LMICs) now straddle the two extremes of maternal health care, with too much, too soon care among the wealthy and those in private care, and too little, too late care among the most vulnerable (Koblinsky et al. 2016; Miller et al. 2016). Women in sparsely populated rural areas, dense urban centers, and in poorer regions invariably risk receiving poor quality care that is too little, too late.

Recent increases in maternity care coverage mean that three-quarters of women now deliver with assistance from a skilled birth attendant and two-thirds receive at least four antenatal care visits. And yet worldwide, an estimated 53 million women (or about a quarter of all pregnant women) still receive no skilled assistance at birth, almost all in the poorest countries. These births often occur in low-quality health care facilities (Campbell et al. 2016), such that although facility-based births continue to rise, the current strategy of encouraging women to give birth in health facilities ("birth at any clinic") may be misguided because many such clinics continue to lack emergency obstetric care, reliable water supply, and even the most basic capability to manage uncomplicated deliveries and provide respectful evidence-based routine care. Thus, poor quality is undermining the goal of reducing maternal and newborn mortality around the world.

This awkward reality is underscored by nationally representative survey data from five African countries with high maternal mortality (Kenya, Namibia, Rwanda, Tanzania, and Uganda). In these countries, over 40% of health facility births occur in poor-quality facilities with crucial deficiencies in staffing, infrastructure, referral systems, and routine and emergency care practices (Kruk et al. 2016). Quality of basic maternal care functions was assessed at 1715 health care facilities using an index of 12 indicators, including the availability of skilled providers, a functional ambulance, electricity, clean water, and antibiotics. Further, almost 90% of these facilities did not have the capacity to perform cesarean births, but these clinics delivered 44% of all babies born in a health care facility. Small primary care clinics scored, on average, only 3.8 out of 10 on the index of quality, whereas facilities with surgical capability had nearly double this score.

In contrast, evidence from high-income countries indicates that neonatal and obstetric care is of highest quality in facilities that handle a high volume of births and have the capacity to perform cesareans. This implies that larger, better health care facilities may be better equipped to deliver babies and that lower-income countries, global donors and health care agencies would best pivot from promoting access alone to improving quality of care for childbirth.

Wider adoption of more effective maternal and reproductive health interventions and equitable policies is needed to improve quality of care and reduce inequities and world suffering. However, efforts to boost women's and children's health remain fragile, often shrouded in rhetoric, with inadequate domestic country resources. Al-though the MDG era galvanized widespread political commitment to improving women's and children's health that can be expected to continue under the SDGs, the real causes of maternal and child deaths—poverty, inequality, lack of financing, and poor governance—remain largely ignored. Indeed, this is true of much of the reproductive health agenda, which offers a particularly striking example of a pervasive failure to change local and international governance to improve health care and its priorities for greater justice.

One guide for the global health community to potentially follow is the UN Secretary General's *Global Strategy for Women's, Children's and Adolescents' Health* Report (UN 2016). This has the three major objectives of survive, thrive, and transform, for the three groups of women, children, and adolescents. It also emphasizes the reduction of inequalities. By late 2016, over 50 countries and 120 organizations had pledged more than $25 billion to women's, children's, and adolescents' health toward implementation of the Global Strategy under the *Every Woman Every*

Table 16.2 Actions needed to improve quality care for every woman and newborn in all countries

Action	Key components
Quality	Good quality, evidence-based maternal health services, responsive to local needs and emerging challenges. Services start with prevention (e.g. family planning), are context-appropriate and interlinked along the continuum of care, and address increasing diversity in the burden of poor maternal health.
Equity	Maternal health services and the overall health system need to promote equity (e.g. through investments in universal health coverage) to reach all women with good quality care everywhere and without causing undue economic burden.
Health systems strengthening	Strengthening all dimensions including data and surveillance systems, facility capability, health workforce skills, and linkages, to help ensure adequate response to changing contexts of women's lives and resilience to threats to maternal and newborn health.
Financing and political buy-in	Ensuring adequate and sustainable financing to maintain maternal health gains and accelerate progress, building and presenting the case for investing in maternal, newborn, and reproductive health to secure political attention and support.
Better evidence	Routine audits, strengthened health management information systems, and smarter metrics to provide evidence for improving quality maternal care for all and to help build a platform to advocate for resources, learn from programmatic successes and failures, strengthen laws and policies, and promote accountability.

Source: Adapted from UN (2016); and Koblinsky et al. (2016)

Child movement banner. However, it remains unclear how much financial and political buy-in the Strategy will actually receive. Without adequate financial and human resources, it risks falling by the wayside in some 5 years' time as empty rhetoric. Also, at the start of the SDG era, there remains an overwhelming focus on mortality reduction, with insufficient attention paid to preventing stillbirths, early child development, advancing adolescent reproductive health, or gender equity.

Strategies that have improved outcomes for women and their newborn babies in many contexts include midwifery-led care, adoption of evidence-based guidelines and health surveillance systems, and ensuring health facilities are capable of providing evidence-based routine childbirth care and basic emergency obstetric care (Table 16.2). However, access to evidence-based care remains inadequate across all settings. Team-based care in maternity hospitals and increased midwifery care may be effective in addressing staff shortages, excessive interventions, and high costs. However, their use is very limited in the U.S., where the maternal mortality ratio actually increased from 2000 to 2014, leaving it now far behind other industrialized nations in efforts to improve maternity care for the four million U.S. women giving birth each year (MacDorman et al. 2016). This situation reflects systemic and political failures to improve health care access and population health. Deep inequities in underlying health and quality of care across race, socioeconomic status, and geography contribute to these dismal numbers (Handler et al. 2011). Racial-group differences in the U.S. are among the most-cited examples of differentials of maternal mortality in high-income settings, with the risk for maternal death among black women (39/100,000 live births) over three times higher than for white women (12/100,000). This differential has remained largely unchanged more than six decades and also reflects the uneven quality of care, especially for uninsured and underinsured women.

Health systems in high- and middle-income countries face challenges in supporting quality reproductive health care, as illustrated by the tendency of women to receive maternity care that is too much, too soon. This may cause harm, raise health costs, and contribute to a culture of disrespect and abuse. Additionally, medical liability costs are often very high and fear of litigation is common, particularly in the U.S. Other challenges to continued progress in all countries may come from a diluted focus on reproductive health, weak data and surveillance systems, and common human resource shortages.

Contraceptive Use and Family Planning Services

Access to contraception is transformative for women, couples and communities, and is a fundamental right. Giving women the means to prevent unintended pregnancy helps achieve health and well-being, and is linked to gender equity, educational attainment and economic development. The case for investing in family planning is particularly strong and includes averted deaths (maternal, newborn, and stillbirth), reduced maternal morbidities and unsafe abortions, and improved child outcomes, in addition to economic and environmental benefits (Bloom et al. 2003). For example, one recent study suggests that each additional dollar spent on contraceptive services reduces the cost of pregnancy-related care by $1.47 (Guttmacher Institute and UNFPA 2014). This is in addition to its various other benefits at multiple levels. Closing the gap between fertility preferences and contraceptive use would help to avoid unwanted pregnancies, abortion, maternal and child morbidity, and mortality.

Awareness and use of family planning has improved in recent years. Globally, contraceptive prevalence rose from 55% of married or in-union women of reproductive age in 1990 to 64% in 2015, although contraceptive use was much lower in the least developed countries (40%) and was particularly low in Africa (33%). Modern contraceptive use increased from 48% to 57% among married or in-union women aged 15–49 over the same period, constituting 90 per cent of contraceptive users, with the increase in use driven by a 10 percentage point rise in developing countries (Alkema et al. 2013; UN 2015b). However, all countries still show large socioeconomic differences in overall and modern method contraceptive use among couples who want to prevent pregnancy.

The recent gains in contraceptive prevalence have led to corresponding modest declines in the level of unmet need for family planning and in the rate of unintended pregnancies (from 43% to 40% of all pregnancies between 1995 and 2012) (Alkema et al. 2013; Sedgh et al. 2014). Worldwide in 2015, 12% of married or in-union women were estimated to have had an unmet need for family planning; that is, they wanted to stop or delay childbearing but were not using any method of contraception. In the least developed countries, the level was much higher (22%), with unmet need highest (22%) in SSA where only 60% of demand for family planning was satisfied. The aforementioned FP2020 initiative aims to accelerate meeting unmet needs in contraception.

Substantial gaps persist in the proportion of total demand for family planning satisfied with modern methods in countries where overall contraceptive use is low or where many couples rely on traditional contraceptive methods. In 2015, less than half of total demand for family planning was being met with modern methods in 54 countries (34 of them in Africa). When users of traditional methods are counted as having an unmet need for family planning, 18% of married or in-union women worldwide were estimated to have had an unmet need for modern methods in 2015 (UN 2015b). Nevertheless, levels of unmet need for family planning were estimated to have fallen across educational groups within many countries.

The two most widely used contraceptive methods by married or in-union women worldwide are female sterilization (19%) and the IUD (14%). Globally, long-acting or permanent methods (female and male sterilization, IUDs and implants) accounted for 56% of contraceptive prevalence, with more than one in three married or in-union women using these methods in 2015. Women report less frequent reliance on short-term methods such as the pill (9%), male condoms (8%) and injectables (5%).

However, many family planning programs do not offer an adequate method mix. A limited choice of contraceptive options tends to be associated with increased method discontinuation and non-use, leading to more unintended pregnancies than would otherwise be expected. It is estimated that in at least one out of every four countries, a single method accounts for over half of all contraceptive use among women of reproductive age. Moreover, countries where contraceptive practice is heavily concentrated on one or two methods can be found in all regions and at all levels of overall contraceptive prevalence (UN 2015b).

For African women, the increase in the met demand for family planning with a modern method that has occurred has led to a drop in the unintended pregnancy rate (from 69 per 1000 women of reproductive age to 53/1000 women). Primary infertility (or non-voluntary childlessness) also declined over this time in SSA (the region where it is most common) and in South Asia, although there was little change in other regions (Mascarenhas et al. 2011). However, large inequalities still remain in all areas, underscoring the need for an increased focus on equity and service quality, as well as on continued improvements in access to family planning services and contraceptive use.

Abortion and Postabortion Care

Approximately 56 million abortions are estimated to be performed annually worldwide, with the overwhelming majority (88%) occurring in developing countries (Table 16.3). Expressed another way, more than one-fifth of all known pregnancies end in abortion, which is now one of the safest procedures in medicine when performed by a trained professional in hygienic conditions using modern methods. Nevertheless, about half of all abortion procedures performed annually are considered unsafe, causing some 47,000 maternal deaths (WHO 2011). These deaths and injuries are almost entirely preventable, as are the high associated levels of morbidity that are strongly stigmatized and overlooked. Abortion is stigmatized not only because of legal sanctions, but because it violates the three cherished feminine ideals of perpetual fecundity, the inevitability of motherhood, and instinctive nurturing (Kumar et al. 2009). The stigma tends to be strongest for young and unmarried sexually active women. Unsafe abortion and abortion-related maternal mortality and morbidity are far more frequent in countries where restrictive abortion laws prevail, or where relatively permissive statutes are not implemented. Africa accounts for most abortion-related mortality, largely because the vast majority of abortions are clandestine and unsafe.

Data on abortion are often incomplete and vary greatly in both quantity and quality (Kulczycki 2015). Two-thirds of nations do not collect data and obtaining accurate data is especially challenging in countries where abortion is illegal; most unsafe abortions go undocumented because they are performed clandestinely, so that figures are therefore estimates. Nevertheless, estimates suggest that induced abortion

Table 16.3 Global and regional estimates of induced abortions, 1995–2014

Region	Estimated number of abortions (in millions)				Estimated Abortion rate[a]			
	1995–1999	2000–2004	2005–2009	2010–2014	1995–1999	2000–2004	2005–2009	2010–2014
World	49.7	49.9	52.4	56.3	37	35	34	35
Developed countries	10.2	8.7	7.7	6.7	40	34	31	27
Developing countries	39.5	41.2	44.7	49.6	36	35	35	37
Africa	5.4	6.2	7.20	8.3	33	33	33	34
Asia	30.7	30.8	32.7	35.8	37	34	34	36
Europe	7.1	6.0	5.2	4.4	45	38	34	30
Latin America	4.9	5.4	6.1	6.5	40	41	44	44
Northern America	1.5	1.4	1.3	1.2	22	20	19	17
Oceania	0.1	0.1	0.1	0.1	21	21	20	19

Source: Sedgh et al. (2016), based in part on analyzes conducted by WHO researchers
[a]Abortions per 1000 women aged 15–44

rates were between 20 and 40 per 1000 women of reproductive age in regions with legal restrictions on induced abortion. They are highest in Latin America (Table 16.3), where the procedure is illegal nearly everywhere (Kulczycki 2011). Contraceptive prevalence rates have risen in many countries, thereby preventing many abortions (Ahmed et al. 2012). New technologies have become available to allow women to obtain earlier and safer abortions, but these still need to be made more widely accessible.

The incidence of abortion may be reduced through good access to a range of effective contraceptive methods, but women and couples often need better access to contraceptive services, and sex education and abortion are controversial in many countries. In particular, too many women who seek unsafe abortions lack adequate access to family planning and other reproductive health services that could help them avoid unintended pregnancies. The primary methods for preventing unsafe abortion are more permissive abortion laws and more effective contraceptive use, but there exists a range of socio-cultural, legal, political and institutional barriers to realizing such improvements. For example, safe abortion services are often unavailable to many poor, rural women in India, where many women remain unaware that the procedure is legal and few primary health centers provide it. Consequently, many desperate women, confronting an unwanted pregnancy and believing they have no other option, will continue to risk their lives by undergoing unsafe abortions.

In settings where abortion is legally restricted or access to safe services is limited, women often resort to unsafe abortions and then require emergency medical attention to treat incomplete abortions or severe complications such as hemorrhage, infection, sepsis, and genital trauma. Worldwide, five million women are estimated to be hospitalized each year for treatment of such abortion-related complications (Singh 2006), but many women who suffer abortion complications do not obtain needed medical care. Data on non-fatal long-term health complications are also deficient, but document poor wound healing, internal organ injury and their consequences, and infertility. The burden of unsafe abortion falls not only on women and families, but also on health care systems. Hospitalized abortion patients typically require blood products, antibiotics, oxytocics, anesthesia, operating rooms, and surgical specialists. However, postabortion care (PAC) services are often deficient in terms of emergency medical treatment and provision of family planning and other reproductive health services.

Postabortion care (PAC) is a multi-pronged strategy to prevent deaths and injury from unsafe abortion. A comprehensive public health model for PAC services should include treatment, counseling, provision of family planning to prevent future unwanted pregnancies, and other services to respond to women's sexual and reproductive health needs and concerns as needed. For example, these should integrate screening for STIs and gender-based violence which also result from unprotected sex, the same source of vulnerability as unintended pregnancy. Partnerships should also be built with service providers and communities to help generate acceptance and support (Table 16.4).

Table 16.4 Five essential elements of Postabortion care

Element	Objective/Definition
Community and service provider partnerships	To prevent unwanted pregnancies and unsafe abortion; to mobilize resources to help women receive appropriate and timely care for complications from abortion; and to ensure that health services reflect and meet community expectations and needs
Counseling	To identify and respond to women's emotional and physical health needs and other concerns
Treatment	To treat incomplete and unsafe abortion and potentially life-threatening complications
Contraceptive and family planning services	To help women practice birthspacing or prevent an unwanted pregnancy
Reproductive and other health services	To provide on-site (preferably, or via referrals) to other accessible facilities in providers' networks

Source: Corbett and Turner (2003)

Many PAC clients want and need family planning, and postabortion family planning (PAFP) uptake is generally good if a range of contraceptives is offered at the point of treatment, with uptake higher than if a woman is referred elsewhere for FP counseling. The return to fertility after abortion can be rapid (as little as 10 days), and almost all contraceptive methods are suitable for postabortion use. There is clear evidence that the provision of no-cost contraception and promotion of more effective, long-acting methods prevents more unintended pregnancies (Peipert et al. 2012). Further, male involvement in counseling—always with the woman's concurrence—can increase family planning uptake and support (Huber et al. 2016). PAFP can help women limit and space their pregnancies, prevent unintended pregnancies and subsequent unsafe and repeat abortions, and reduce maternal morbidity and mortality.

However, the integration of family planning services with postabortion treatment continues to be challenging in too many settings. All too often, contraceptive services are offered in a separate place, by different service providers, and often during limited hours. More effort is needed to overcome such impediments to more effective service delivery so as to reduce suffering further. High quality PAC services should be accessible and available to all women who experience an incomplete abortion, whether it is spontaneous (miscarriage) or induced. It is now also clear that PAC services can be provided at lower-level, rural health facilities so long as these are equipped with the necessary equipment, drugs, and supplies. Additionally, mid-level providers can safely provide PAC services, including treatment of complications (WHO 2012).

The Continuing Struggle for Reproductive Justice

Substantial gains have been made in reducing unsafe abortions and preventable maternal mortality, as well as in expanding contraceptive use. These gains are not to be underestimated, but poor access to services, limited resources and political will, and numerous other factors preclude greater reproductive justice. High rates of unintended pregnancy and deficiencies in maternity care are still found in all settings, with unsafe abortions widespread in many countries. As noted above, at least 1 in 10 married or cohabitating women worldwide are believed to have an unmet need for family planning services, and about 53 million women annually still received zero childbirth care in 2015. Multiple socio-cultural and political sensitivities pose major challenges to improving reproductive health and well-being, as do the difficulties of operationalizing reproductive health programs. Tremendous suffering prevails worldwide due to the continued failure to achieve further gains.

Efforts to alleviate world suffering and to improve the quality of life of the world's population must be far-reaching and inclusive, without compromising the ability of future generations to meet their needs. Accomplishing these goals depends in part on the ability of countries and the international community to ensure the reproductive health and rights of their populations.

The returns on investment in reproductive health care are very good as a result of the improved health and wellbeing of women, their children and families. Such gains could be realistically attained by additionally funding critical sexual and reproductive health services in developing regions at an annual average cost of $25 per woman of childbearing age. Although this amount equates to doubling current funding for reproductive health to $39.2 billion annually, the long-term gains for women, society and the economy far outweigh the costs. This essential package of services would include providing modern methods of contraception for all women aged 15–49 who want them, offering the recommended levels of maternal and newborn healthcare, and effective care and support for women whose pregnancies end in miscarriage, stillbirth or abortion. It also includes HIV testing for pregnant women and antiretroviral treatment for those who are HIV-positive, as well as treatment for major curable sexually transmitted infections (STIs). The payback would equate to: a 70% drop in unintended pregnancies annually, from 74 million to 22 million (which would in turn reduce abortion incidence and suffering from unsafe abortions); a 67% decline in maternal deaths, from about 300,000 to 96,000; a 77% decline in newborn deaths, from almost three million to 660,000; and a 93% reduction in mother-to-child HIV transmissions (Guttmacher Institute and UNFPA 2014).

Reproductive health problems are more acute in LMICs, particularly in sub-Saharan Africa, which has greater poverty, weaker health systems, and relatively low gender equity. Although services for different components of reproductive health can be readily integrated with others even where health systems are weak, this is rarely achieved. Most reproductive health services in LMICs, and even in more affluent societies, continue to be delivered vertically or offer at most partial integration of services, often only for particular groups.

Health systems in high-income countries also face challenges in supporting good quality, woman-centered care, as discussed in the case of the over-medicalization of normal pregnancy and birth with routine use of interventions unsupported by evidence. Indeed, access to evidence-based care remains inadequate across all settings. Moreover, disparities in outcomes between and within all countries highlight shared needs to improve healthcare capacity, quality, and equity.

The burden of poor reproductive health is concentrated among vulnerable populations who in poorer countries often include women affected by humanitarian crises, or who live in fragile states or areas prone to natural disasters. These women are more likely to face high fertility, higher-risk pregnancies, and difficulties in accessing services and in asserting their rights. But everywhere, vulnerable groups include adolescents, poor women, marginalized ethnic/racial and religious minorities, and often, women living in informal urban settlements or in sparse rural areas. For example, youth are frequently denied access to reproductive health services because health care providers have little accountability to youth clients, and consider sex education as the responsibility of parents and adolescent sexual activity as unacceptable. Adolescent females are particularly vulnerable for poor sexual and reproductive health outcomes. Women (and men) living with HIV/AIDS are often bereft of family planning and other reproductive health services, notwithstanding significant declines in HIV incidence and prevalence, and gains in antiretroviral therapy (ART) and prevention to mother-to-child transmission (PMTCT) coverage and adherence.

The persistence of disparities and vulnerable populations underscores that while a central goal of the reproductive health agenda should continue to be increased provision and access to services, this now has to be expanded to include greater equity, dignity, and quality of care to increase reproductive justice and reduce world suffering. This requires the adoption of effective and equitable reproductive health interventions and models of care, including promising new approaches. It also requires continued advocacy and ensuring that women's rights and agency are acknowledged, which includes involving adolescents and women in defining priorities at local and national levels, and for their voices to be a starting point and not an afterthought.

Other factors contributing to success include increased global and country-level consensus and commitment, expansion of education, improvements in legislation and measurement. For example, it is widely believed that the recent enhanced ability to more regularly monitor intervention coverage has helped sharpen the focus on reproductive health. Better data and more investment in implementation research are still needed to evaluate different programmatic solutions in a range of situations and contexts.

There has also been some progress in the adoption of policies and laws to increase recognition of reproductive health and rights. For instance, there has been a modest decline in the prevalence of FGC from the mid-1990s to 2010 (Yoder et al. 2013; see also Boyle and Svec (2017, Chap. 21) in this volume) as the issue has gained recognition as a human rights violation. Over this period, at least 24 of the 29 countries that practice FGC passed anti-FGC laws or decrees (UNICEF 2013a), although implementation remains a problem.

Also, between 1975 and 2010, 119 countries enacted 260 changes in legislation to address intimate partner violence (IPV), with 95% of these changes enacted since 1995 (Pierotti 2013). However, survey reports indicate that IPV remains a widespread problem in all regions. Indeed, there remain numerous obstacles to ending child marriage, FGC, and IPV, let alone curtailing the incidence of STIs which remains high for many pathogens.

Conclusion

Securing reproductive rights and universal access to sexual and reproductive health care are vital development goals. Reproductive rights are critical to health, particularly for women, but they are shaped by powerful social, political, and other determinants. Also, they are often neglected because of their sensitive and intimate nature, and complex cultural and social ramifications. Significant gains have been recently made in implementing the reproductive health and rights agenda, but major disparities remain and aggregate gains mask glaring inequalities that entail much avoidable human suffering and lost opportunities for realizing better individual well-being and societal development. Achieving further progress and reproductive justice requires continued advocacy for reproductive and sexual rights and sound public health programming.

More effort is needed to address the unfinished agenda for reproductive health to improve the quality of reproductive health care for all and access to care for those left behind. These goals are vital to improving reproductive justice and reducing world suffering. The enactment and implementation of sound policy and laws can have a major impact on reproductive health, but policy development and program implementation have often fallen short of realizing international commitments. Aggregate gains mask stark inequalities, especially low service coverage for the poor and those otherwise marginalized and underprivileged. Achieving greater reproductive justice and reducing world suffering will require strengthening health systems and substantially increasing investment in comprehensive and integrated reproductive health services, especially to reach the poor and underserved.

References

Ahmed, S., Li, Q., Liu, L., & Tsui, A. (2012). Maternal deaths averted by contraceptive use: an analysis of 172 countries. *Lancet, 380*(9837), 111–125.

Alkema, L., Kantorova, V., Menozsi, C., & Biddlecom, A. (2013). National, regional, and global rates and trends in contraceptive prevalence and unmet need for family planning between 1990 and 2015: A systematic and comprehensive analysis. *Lancet, 381*(9878), 1642–1652.

Bloom, D. E., Canning, D., & Sevilla, J. (2003). *The demographic dividend: A new perspective on the economic consequences of population change*. Santa Monica: Rand.

Boyle, E. H., & Svec, J. (2017). Success in reducing female genital cutting: A multilevel framework of social change. In R. E. Anderson (Ed.), *Alleviating world suffering* (pp. XX–XX). Dordrecht: Springer.

Brown, W., Druce, N., Bunting, J., et al. (2014). Developing the '120 by20' goal for the global FP2020 initiative. *Studies in Family Planning, 45*(1), 73–84.

Campbell, O. M. R., Calvert, C., Testa, A., et al. (2016, September 15). The scale, scope, coverage, and capability of childbirth care. *Lancet.* Published online. http://dx.doi.org/10.1016/S0140-6736(16)31528-8

Corbett, M., & Turner, K. (2003). Essential elements of postabortion care: An expanded and updated model. *International Family Planning Perspectives, 29*(3), 106–111.

Finkle, J. L., & McIntosh, C. A. (1994). The new politics of population: Conflict and consensus in family planning. In *Supplement to population and development review* (Vol. 20). New York: Population Council.

Guttmacher Institute and UNFPA. (2014). *Adding it up: The costs and benefits of investing in sexual and reproductive health*. New York: Guttmacher Institute.

Handler, A., Kennelly, J., & Peacock, N. (Eds.). (2011). *Reducing racial/ethnic disparities in reproductive and perinatal outcomes*. New York: Springer.

Huber, D., Curtis, C., Irani, L., Pappa, S., & Arrington, L. (2016). Postabortion care: 20 years of strong evidence on emergency treatment, family planning, and other programming components. *Global Health: Science and Practice, 4*(3), 481–494.

International Planned Parenthood Federation (IPPF). (2008). *IPPF charter on sexual and reproductive rights*. Available at: http://www.ippf.org/resource/IPPF-Charter-Sexual-and-Reproductive-Rights. Accessed 2 Oct 2016.

Kantner, A. (2014). The evolution of consensus on population and development: Prospects for resurgent policy and program action. In A. Kulczycki (Ed.), *Critical issues in reproductive health* (pp. 129–251). London/New York/Dordrecht: Springer.

Kassebaum, N. J., Bertozzi-Villa, A., Coggeshall, M. S., et al. (2014). Global, regional, and national levels and causes of maternal mortality during 1990–2013: A systematic analysis for the global burden of disease study 2013. *Lancet, 384*, 980–1004.

Koblinsky, M., Moyer, C. A., & Calvert, C. Campbell, J., Campbell, Oona.M. R., Feigl, A. B., Graham, W. J., Hatt, L., Hodgins, S., Matthews, Z., McDougall, L., Moran, A. C., Nandakumar, A. K., & Langer, A. (2016, September 15) Quality maternity care for every woman, everywhere: A call to action. *Lancet.* Published online. http://dx.doi.org/10.1016/S0140-6736(16)31333-2

Kruk, M.E., Leslie, H. H., Verguet, S., Mbaruku, G. M., Adanu, R. M. K., & Langer, A. (2016). Assessment of quality of basic maternal care functions in health facilities with national health-system surveys of five African countries: A prospective analysis. *Lancet Global Health.* doi: 10.1016/S2214-109X(16)30180-2.

Kulczycki, A. (1999). *The abortion debate in the world Arena*. London/New York: Macmillan/Routledge.

Kulczycki, A. (2007). Ethics, ideology, and reproductive health policy in the United States. *Studies in Family Planning, 38*(4), 333–351.

Kulczycki, A. (2011). Abortion in Latin America: Changes in practice, growing conflict, and recent policy developments. *Studies in Family Planning, 42*(3), 199–220.

Kulczycki, A. (Ed.). (2014). *Critical issues in reproductive health*. London/New York/Dordrecht: Springer.

Kulczycki, A. (2015). Abortion and reproductive health. In D. McFarlane (Ed.), *Global population and reproductive health* (pp. 171–197). Burlington: Jones & Bartlett Learning.

Kulczycki, A., & Windle, S. (2011). Honor killings in the Middle East and North Africa: A systematic review of the literature. *Violence Against Women, 17*(11), 1442–1464.

Kumar, A., Hessini, L., & Mitchell, E. M. (2009). Conceptualising abortion stigma. *Culture, Health & Sexuality, 11*(6), 625–639.

Lee-Rife, S., Malhotra, A., Warner, A., & Glinski, A. M. (2012). What works to prevent child marriage: A review of the evidence. *Studies in Family Planning, 43*(4), 287–303.

Mascarenhas, M. N., Flaxman, S. R., Boerma, T., Vanderpoel, S., & Stevens, G. A. (2011). National, regional and global trends in infertility prevalence since1990: A systematic analysis of 277 health surveys. *PLoS Med, 9*(12), e1001356.

MacDorman, M. F., Declercq, E., Cabral, H., & Morton, C. (2016). Recent increases in the U.S. maternal mortality rate: Disentangling trends from measurement issues. *Obstetrics & Gynecology, 128*(3), 447–455.

May, J. F. (2012). *World population policies: Their origin, evolution, and impact*. New York/London: Springer.

McIntosh, C. A., & Finkle, J. L. (1995). The Cairo conference on population and development: A new paradigm? *Population and Development Review, 21*(2), 223–260.

Miller, S., Lester, F., Webster, M., & Cowan, B. (2005). Obstetric fistula: A preventable tragedy. *Journal of Midwifery & Women's Health, 50*(4), 286–294.

Miller, S., Abalos, E., Chamillard, M., et al. (2016, September 15). Beyond too little, too late and too much, too soon: A pathway towards evidence-based, respectful maternity care worldwide. *Lancet*. Published online. http://dx.doi.org/10.1016/S0140-6736(16)31472-6

Pallitto, C. C., García-Moreno, J. H. A. F. M., Heise, L., Ellsberg, M., Watts, C., et al. (2013). Intimate partner violence, abortion, and unintended pregnancy: Results from the WHO multi-country study on women's health and domestic violence. *International Journal of Gynecology and Obstetrics, 120*(1), 3–9.

Peipert, J. F., Madden, T., Allsworth, J. E., & Secura, G. M. (2012). Preventing unintended pregnancies by providing no-cost contraception. *Obstetrics & Gynecology, 120*(6), 1291–1297.

Pierotti, R. S. (2013). Increasing rejection of intimate partner violence: Evidence of global cultural diffusion. *American Sociological Review, 78*(2), 240–265.

Raj, A., & Boehmer, U. (2013). Girl child marriage and its association with national rates of HIV, maternal health and infant mortality across 97 countries. *Violence Against Women, 19*(4), 536–551.

Robinson, W. C., & Ross, J. A. (Eds.). (2007). *The Global family planning revolution: Three decades of policies and programs*. Washington, DC: World Bank.

Ronsmans, C., Chowdhury, M. E., Dasgupta, S. K., Ahmed, A., & Koblinsky, M. (2010). Effect of parent's death on child survival in rural Bangladesh: A cohort study. *Lancet, 375*(9730), 2024–2031.

Sedgh, G., Singh, S., & Hussain, R. (2014). Intended and unintended pregnancies worldwide in 2012 and recent trends. *Studies in Family Planning, 45*(3), 301–314.

Sedgh, G., Bearak, J., Singh, S., Popinchalk, A., Rossier, C., Gardts, C., et al. (2016). Abortion incidence between 1990 and 2014: Global, regional, and subregional levels and trends. *Lancet, 388*(10041), 258–267.

Singh, S. (2006). Hospital admissions resulting from unsafe abortion: Estimates from 13 developing countries. *Lancet, 368*(9550), 1887–1892.

UN. (2015a). *World population prospects: The 2015 revision*. New York: United Nations.

UN. (2015b). *Trends in contraceptive use worldwide 2015*. New York: United Nations.

UN. (2016). *Global strategy for women's, children's and adolescents' health 2016–2030*. United Nations, New York (2015). http://globalstrategy.everywomaneverychild.org/. Accessed 5 Oct 2016.

UNICEF. (2013a). *Female genital mutilation/cutting: A statistical overview and exploration of the dynamics of change*. New York: United Nations Children's Fund.

UNICEF. (2013b). *State of the world's children 2013: Children with disabilities*. New York: UNICEF.

UNICEF, World Health Organization, The World Bank, & United Nations Population Division. (2015). *Levels and trends in child mortality report 2015: Estimates developed by the UN inter-*

agency group for child mortality estimation. New York: UNICEF. Available at: http://www.childmortality.org/. Accessed 10 Oct 2016.
van Dalen, H. P., & Scharf, M. M. (2014). Reproductive health aid: A delicate balancing act. In A. Kulczycki (Ed.), *Critical issues in reproductive health* (pp. 195–213). London/New York/Dordrecht: Springer.
WHO. (2011). *Unsafe abortion: Global and regional estimates of the incidence of unsafe abortion and associated mortality in 2008* (6th ed.). Geneva: World Health Organization.
WHO. (2012). *Safe abortion: Technical and policy guidance for health systems* (2nd ed.). Geneva: World Health Organization.
WHO. (2013). *Global and regional estimates of violence against women: Prevalence and health effects of intimate partner violence and non-partner sexual violence*. Geneva/London/Tygerberg: World Health Organization, London School of Hygiene & Tropical Medicine and South African Medical Research Council. Available at: http://www.who.int/reproductivehealth/publications/violence/9789241564625/en/. Accessed 27 Sep 2016.
WHO. (2015). *Trends in maternal mortality: 1990 to 2015: Estimates by WHO, UNICEF, UNFPA, World Bank Group and the United Nations Population Division*. Geneva: World Health Organization.
WHO. (2016). *Neonatal mortality; situation and trends*. http://www.who.int/gho/child_health/mortality/neonatal_text/en/. Accessed 12 Aug 2016.
Yoder, P. S., Wang, S., & Johansen, E. (2013). Estimates of female genital mutilation/cutting in 27 African countries and Yemen. *Studies in Family Planning, 44*(2), 189–204.
You, D., Hug, L., Ejdemyr, S., Idele, P., Hogan, D., Malthers, C., Gerland, P., New, J.R., & United Nations Inter-agency Group for Child Mortality Estimation. (2015). Global, regional, and sub-regional levels and trends. *Lancet, 388*(10041), 258–267.

Part IV
Violent Societal Conflict, Human Rights and Justice

Chapter 17
Suffering During the Holocaust and Heroic Rescuers

Samuel P. Oliner

Introduction

What is suffering? The Editor of this volume offers a taxonomy of four forms of suffering: physical suffering, or pain; mental suffering, including distressing thoughts and feelings; interpersonal suffering, trauma caused by interactional problems such as social rejection and isolation; and, finally, social suffering, a loss of a sense of worth and collective value due to social norms that stigmatize and lead to social discrimination of the victims (Anderson 2015, p. 4–5). These varying forms of human suffering are caused and perpetuated by many forces. However, as the primary focus of this volume is the alleviation of human suffering, this chapter explores the forces underlying extraordinary sacrifices made in order to rescue victims from extreme suffering. By examining the nature of suffering, we may envision some novel ways to alleviate human suffering in a variety of contexts.

The purpose of this chapter is threefold. First, after a brief account of the author's survival, suffering and rescue during the Holocaust, we characterize the nature of the Nazi's systematic mass murder of Jews and others, which is considered the most documented genocide in human history. Winston Churchill said of the Holocaust, "This is probably the greatest and most horrific crime ever committed in the whole history of the world" (Weber 2000). Next, is an overview of some heroic rescuers (also called 'righteous gentiles'), who reduced the suffering of thousands of victims by assisting or hiding them and saving their lives. These rescuers chose to act on their principles, risking all to help those in need during the Nazi occupation in Europe. Finally, we highlight several hero-producing projects and point out how altruistic individuals and robust social institutions may evolve to reduce suffering.

S.P. Oliner (✉)
Emeritus Professor of Sociology, Humboldt State University, Arcata, CA 95521, USA
e-mail: spo1@humboldt.edu

R.E. Anderson (ed.), *Alleviating World Suffering*, Social Indicators Research Series 67, DOI 10.1007/978-3-319-51391-1_17

A Holocaust Survivor's Perspective

As a survivor of one of the most extensively documented genocides in human history, the Holocaust, I have been led by my experience to research the various aspects of human nature in order to understand how we may build a brighter future in which another Shoah may never occur. Throughout my career, I have studied altruism, the nature of 'good' and 'evil,' apology and forgiveness, and the motivations of those who give selflessly, such as volunteers, heroes and others who devote themselves to the greater good. Dr. Pearl Oliner and I conducted a major study of rescuers of Jews and others during the Holocaust, *The Altruistic Personality* (1988). Our research team interviewed and taped recorded a number of gentile rescuers in their own language who acted in the interests of those persecuted by the Nazi regime, reducing their suffering and saving their lives. What we found was that although individuals' motives differed, there were consistent characteristics among our rescuers: they were raised by compassionate and non-violent caregivers who encouraged them to think critically and to respect others who were different than themselves (culturally and ethnically); they were instilled with a sense of social responsibility and valued social justice, and they considered themselves responsible for the greater good of their communities, and were willing to act on that sense of responsibility, as opposed to 'bystanders'. Rescuers displayed behavior which can be defined as *heroic altruism*, an altruistic behavior that is voluntary, does not result in personal gain and involves risk of varying degrees to the helper (Oliner 2003, p. 21). Similarly, we interviewed hospice volunteers whom we labeled as *conventional altruists*, those who perform compassionate acts that do not involve risking one's life. Much of the research we have conducted over the years has lent insight into how society may foster and encourage altruistic, caring behavior. While the trauma of my past has partly motivated this research, my focus on the nature of altruistic behavior may be traced in part to a Polish peasant woman named Balwina Piecuch.

I was born in a small village called Zyndranowa, located in southern Poland, on March 10, 1930. I lived with my father Aron, my brother and sister, Moishe and Feigele, and my mother, Jaffa. Sadly, my mother passed away from tuberculosis when I was 7 years of age, but my family lived a relatively happy life on my grandparents' farm until the Nazi occupation of Poland began in 1939. As the occupation progressed, life became worse and worse for Jewish people. Homes and businesses were regularly looted by occupying forces and even some Poles. Food became ever scarcer. Jewish men were forced to shave their beards, and all Jews were forced to wear *opaskas* (stars of David) on the streets. By June of 1942, my family was forced into a hastily constructed ghetto in Bobowa, Southern Poland. Disease and hunger swept through the ghetto, and everywhere people were desperate. I would sneak out of the ghetto, at great risk, to find food for my family by trading thread, needles, and even watches for potatoes and other foods with surrounding Polish peasants. In August 1942, when I was 12 years of age, the fateful call rang through the ghetto—"*Alle Juden—raus!*" (All Jews, out!), shrilly shouted by the *einsatzgruppen*, or mobile killing units. House by house, all occupants of the ghetto were forced to the

Bobowa town square and made to sit on the concrete cobble stones. Loaded onto military trucks, everyone was driven to a pre-dug grave nearby forest of Garbacz, and the *einsatzgruppen* shot them all. I later discovered that my other grandfather and his family had been similarly massacred the day before. There was not enough time to properly bury the victims at the end of the day's massacre, and one victim that I knew crawled out of the grave. Driven insane and wandering aimlessly, he was later caught by the Gestapo and shot.

When the *einsatzgruppen* shouted for all Jews to come out of their homes, my stepmother Ester turned to me. I saw a dreadful look of fear and concern on her face—somehow she knew that our family would not survive this day. Clutching my stepsister Jaffa in her arms, my stepmother said to me, "*Antloif mein kind und do vest bleiben beim leben.*" (Run, my child, run away so that you will save yourself). I asked my stepmother where I should go, and she told me to hide, anywhere. As I contemplated what this warning entailed, what I should do next, I turned to the door and heard my stepmother's last words—"Shmulek, I love you. I know God will protect you."

I hid on the roof, and both heard and saw the horrors taking place below. Eventually I was able to leave the roof, and with great fear and despair made my way out of the ghetto to a nearby village—and to the house of Balwina. She was a Catholic peasant woman who had known my family, and had even traded with them before the war. It was from Balwina that I learned the fate of my family and the others who had been taken from Bobowa. At great risk to herself and her family, Balwina advised me to pose as a Catholic boy. She taught me the catechism, and gave me the name of Jusek Polewski. Balwina's son Staszek posed as my brother, and helped me authenticate my false identity. I was able to get a job as a *pastuch*, or cowhand, on a farm (whose Jewish owners had been killed) that was now rented by a childless Polish couple, the Padworskis. Mr. and Mrs. Padworski hired me to assist on the farm, and in this way I was able to keep up the deception (with the help of Staszek and Balwina) and survive the war.

Why did Balwina help me to reduce my fears and suffering? She was a mother, certainly, and felt great pity for the fate of my family and for all the Jewish people condemned in Nazi-occupied Poland. It was with tears in her eyes and a broken voice that she told me of the liquidation of the Bobowa ghetto. What made Balwina different? The cost of her heroic altruism, had it been discovered, would almost certainly have cost her life, perhaps even the lives of her entire family (Oliner 1979). One way that the Nazis ensured that no help would be offered to Jewish persons during this time was the principle of *collective responsibility*: if anyone was caught giving aid, then there would be consequences not only for the person providing help but also their family and potentially everyone in the community where they lived (Tec 1986, p. 32, 64).

In the Holocaust, as in other genocides, people suffered tremendously. However, the Holocaust is unique in the sense that the Nazis systematically devoted efforts and treasure to murder every Jewish man, woman, and child. The murder took various forms, including mass execution by bullets, gas chambers, starvation, and experimentation. The Holocaust is undoubtedly the most documented genocide;

there are miles of documentary footage, and eyewitnesses, victims and victimizers, many survivors and a number of scholars who have done research on this tragedy. Organizations devoted to Holocaust research include the International Institute for Holocaust Research at Yad Vashem, located in Jerusalem; the Polish Center for Holocaust Research, based in the Polish Academy of Sciences in Warsaw; the Center for Advanced Holocaust Studies, operating from the Holocaust Memorial Museum in Washington, D.C.; the Vienna Weisenthal Institute for Holocaust Studies, and many other academic groups and individuals (Berger 1991; Berger and Berger 2001; United States Holocaust Memorial Museum 2016).

How Was the Holocaust Possible?

It was perpetrated by a "civilized" nation, in collaboration with other nations. In a time marked by the loss of the First World War and the German empire, the punitive Versailles treaty, severe economic depression, a psychological need to blame the 'other', and general social unrest, a charismatic leader named Adolf Hitler was able to come to power. Fascist dictatorship became the political model, resulting in arrest of opposing parties, the establishment of concentration camps such as Dachau, the spread of anti-Semitism, and ultimately *Kristallnacht*—the Night of Broken Glass, during which citizens openly destroyed and looted Jewish homes and businesses, their former occupants dragged away. Nationalist propaganda such as the popularized German phrase "the Jews are our Misfortune" ("*Die Juden sind unser Ungluck*"), hate literature like Hitler's *Mein Kampf, The Protocols of the Elders of Zion* (manufactured by the tsarist secret police), and famous Protestant theologian Martin Luther's book *The Jews and Their Lies* were circulated (Luther 1971; Weber 2000). In a divided nation socially conditioned to punish the 'other,' the tragedy of the Holocaust was possible.

Heroic Rescuers of the Holocaust

After interviewing a number of gentile rescuers, Carnegie Heroes, and Hospice volunteers, we have found common motivating factors of altruistic behavior (Oliner and Oliner 1992). One is *normocentric* motivation; others are *empathic reasoning* and *principled motivation,* all associated with Professor Janusz Reykowski, of the Polish Academy of Sciences (Reykowski 1987a, b).

The normocentrically-oriented respond to an external event that arouses or heightens their empathy. The impact of a direct encounter with a distressed Jewish person was sometimes overpowering. Consider, for example, the following encounter related by a Polish woman, then approximately 35 years of age. In 1942, I was on my way home from town and was almost near home when M. came out of the bushes. I looked at him, in striped cap clothing, his head bare, shod in clogs. He might have been about 30 or 32 years old. And he begged me, his hands joined like for a prayer, that he had escaped from Majdanek and could I help him? He joined his hands in this way, knelt down in front of me, and said: "You are like the Virgin Mary." It still makes me cry. "If I get through and reach Warsaw, I will never forget you." (Oliner 1988, p. 189).

Another rescuer we interviewed, Stanislaus, demonstrated altruism based in normocentric principles as a Holocaust rescuer. During one of our interviews with him, he explained that his reasoning for giving aid to twenty Jewish individuals could be traced back to his mother and grandmother. He stated, "I learned to respect the world from my mother," and learned how to care for others by watching her extend a helping hand to relatives who needed a place to stay until they found work (Oliner 2003, p. 198–199). An interesting factor that contributed to his dedication to helping others were the sacrifices that his maternal grandmother made before he was born. Stanislaus's grandmother was raised Jewish, but decided to leave that part of her life to be with his Polish Catholic grandfather (Oliner 2003, p. 199). Stanislaus's inclination to help stemmed from his mother's teachings and his grandmother's sacrifices, along with the fact that he was raised in a region that had many Jewish people, so he had Jewish friends. In Stanislaus's case, these relationships had a great impact on his appreciation of diversity, which motivated him to provide care for the Jewish people in a time of persecution.

In an interview recounted in *Do Unto Others* (Oliner 2003), Ilsa, another rescuer, initially favored the Nazi view of Jewish people for political reasons. However, she came to disagree with their beliefs because it was affecting her husband negatively. She also believed that the Nazi party was not aligning with the values of her church. Ilsa's actions changed in response to how her most treasured values, such as those of her faith, and her concern for her husband were being affected by the Nazis. Although some people may have initially benefitted from the persecution of the Jewish people, they came to realize that the systematic oppression and the atmosphere of hate and suspicion would affect everyone.

(I suggest dropping the following short section because it does not smoothly fit in with the rest of the chapter.)

The Post-Holocaust Future

Some see the world as having a brighter future. Stephen Pinker, in his book "The Better Angels of Our Nature," argued that violence has been declining and will continue to do so. He wrote: "For all the tribulations in our lives, for all the troubles that remain in the world, the decline of violence is an accomplishment that we can savor—and an impetus to cherish the forces of civilization and enlightenment that made it possible" (Pinker 2011).

Jeremy Rifkin, in his work *The Empathic Civilization* (2009), describes a social world that is evolving to be more altruistic, caring, empathic, and compassionate. I concur with Rifkin, who sees this current century as entering the "Third Revolution," which consists of raising consciousness about the destruction of the biosphere, and the need for economic sustainability. This 'Third Revolution' is associated with what global consciousness, as well as the effects of intergroup apology, forgiveness, and reconciliation.

The Global Consciousness
The emergence of global consciousness, which relates to the digital communication revolution, instantly informs people about events occurring around the world, whether good or ill (Oliner 2003). Remote communication of the hurtful experiences of others arouses an empathic response by many fellow human beings, which we have witnessed time and again during catastrophic events or natural disasters affecting people worldwide.

People's inclinations to help can also be explained by *dual inheritance theory*, which claims that an individual's altruistic and empathic tendencies stem simultaneously from both genetics evolution and cultural evolution. Social groups in which altruism and empathy are exercised tend to live longer and reproduce (Pinker 2011; Rifkin 2009). Neuroscientists and have found convergences between the human brain and social situations. The human brain contains *mirror neurons*, a neurological response to others' actions or emotional displays, allowing people to empathize and experience others' emotions (Winerman 2005).

Our research on rescuers during Nazi occupied Europe, 9/11 first responders, Carnegie heroes, and unpaid volunteers around the world provide examples that many people are innately good. This is due to the influences of important others in an individual's life and the values they internalize. In *Do Unto Others: Extraordinary Acts of Ordinary People* (2003) I found that one of the most common characteristics of empathic people was that they had internalized ethical responsibility for diverse others. The global consciousness now allows people around the world to become aware of the circumstances of others, and thus have more opportunities than ever to take action to alleviate suffering in one's own region or on the other side of the globe.

Intergroup Apology, Forgiveness and Reconciliation

One way of demonstrating social responsibility is to offer apology for wrongdoing and forgiveness to those who seek it. We found positive results from our study on apology, forgiveness, and reconciliation in a number of countries (Oliner and Zylicz 2008). For instance, there are Truth and Reconciliation Commissions around the globe, and many nations, such as Rwanda and South Africa, who have apologized to those that they have harmed in an attempt to heal the hurt and open the path to reconciliation. Another example of apology and reconciliation took place between Poland and Ukraine. Both nations committed tragic massacre of each other's people during World War II, known as the Volhynian Massacres (taking place from approximately 1943 to 1945). Hoping that after the defeat of Hitler, these nations would be free and independent, Ukrainian partisan groups targeted "undesirable" ethnic groups, systematically killing many Polish people. Many Ukrainian citizens heroically aided Polish people, warning them of impending attacks and sometimes hiding them (Zajaczkowski 2013). After World War II, this resulted in the closure of borders and the breaking of economic, cultural, and educational ties, tourism, and other social and political interactions. In 2002, after a historical 2001 visit from Pope John Paul II (the first time a Pope had ever visited Ukraine), the two Presidents, with the approval of their respective Parliaments met on the grounds of the massacre and apologized on the behalf of their people for this tragedy (Zawada 2005). This was a massive step forward in healing for both nations, and resulted in the opening of borders, trade, cultural exchanges, and political cooperation.

Another example of apology is practiced by a group of nuns in Kentucky region who desired to make amends for the exploitation of African Americans. The inherited a group of convents, which were built by slaves in 1800s. In 2001, the Sisters of Charity, Sisters of Loretto, and the Dominicans of Saint Catherine decided to confront the "enduring sin of racism." The nuns publicly apologized to the African American community in Bardstown for historically mistreating them and for not doing more to oppose slavery. As a result of the apology, the three orders helped establish scholarships for African American students in high schools and colleges, and they helped improve diversity in their school boards. While racism has not disappeared, many African American people interviewed in the Kentucky area have reported that race relations have improved in their communities.

There are tangible positive results from both individual and intergroup apology. Forgiveness is a gift and an act of reconciliation that has tangible consequences. Forgiving helps both body and mind to heal. Offering apology and seeking forgiveness has spiritual consequences, and under the right conditions it is able to reestablish a relationship between groups or individuals. "I am sorry" is a difficult phrase in any language. It is particularly crucial that a perpetrator of wrongdoing acknowledges the truth and is willing to apologize when a relationship has been damaged (Oliner and Zylicz 2008). For global harmony, we stress the importance of intergroup apology, forgiveness and reconciliation, a practice that has rendered some of the most positive results in social and political reparation throughout the twenty-first century.

Humanitarian Projects Facilitating Heroic Rescue

Suffering occurs when people hurt because they are deprived of their basic needs, both physiological and social. Social connections and physical safety are endangered by violence, conflict and instability in the social environment. Suffering, then, can be reduced through efforts to provide safety and stability for all people. What follows are examples of organizations and projects where aid workers and others function as heroic rescuers and thus reduce suffering. We begin with an overview of the exemplary non-government organization Doctors Without Borders.

During the time of the Holocaust, where hate, racial discrimination and genocide abounded, many compassionate individuals risked their lives to help and protect. On a macro level, it can be observed that different organizations have grown in order to address economic and social inequalities that have contributed to human suffering. One global humanitarian effort that was born from the tremendous need of medical care in war-torn countries is called *Doctors Without Borders*, also known as *Medecins Sans Frontieres (MSF)*, the title chosen by the French doctors who founded the organization. A quote from the Doctors Without Borders website (http://www.msf.org) sums up its purpose: "MSF was created on the belief that all people have the right to medical care regardless of gender, race, religion, creed, or political affiliation and that the needs of these people outweigh respect for national boundaries."

According to psychologist Maslow's "hierarchy of needs," in order for a person to achieve higher levels of well-being (love, self-esteem, and self-actualization), their basic needs must be met, and for most people, having basic safety and security means having access to shelter or housing (McLeod 2014). *Habitat for Humanity*, a non-profit organization created in 1976 addresses poverty and lack of housing (Habitat for Humanity, 2016). This organization has been able to gather resources in order to build homes with families under certain requirements, and has successfully been able to address these issues not on in the United States of American but also in over 70 countries worldwide. Every year the Habitat for Humanity attracts over one million volunteers, who make it possible to place 310,000 families per year into housing units. In their 40 years of operation they placed three million people into safe housing solutions worldwide.

The *Danish Refugee Council* (DRC) is a humanitarian, non-profit, nongovernmental organization (NGO) that works in more than 30 countries throughout the world. Its mandate is to develop durable solutions among conflict-ridden populations, particularly those with refugees and displaced persons. Denmark itself has integrated many of these refugees helped elsewhere. Established in 1956 they have aided over one million people in their history. Established in 1956 they have aided over one million people in their history. In recent years it has ranked among the top ten of the Global Journal's ranking of the top 100 NGOs.

Mercy Corps is a small NGO with a budget well under a half million dollars. Yet they have a major presence in several countries achieving demonstrable impact. Mercy Corps started out as an organization to help the Cambodian refugee crisis, but evolved into a much broader role of a combination of disaster relief and development. From their beginning, their primary mission was to "alleviate suffering." That is still their primary goal but their focus is to eliminate oppression and to help build productive and just communities. Unlike most NGOs, they explicitly define their stakeholders as the people and communities their serve. And their explicit value premises are the dignity of human life; the stewardship of the earth's health; and their stakeholders participate in all decisions. Mercy Corps was ranked in the top 10 NGOs in 2013.

Bringing in the Bystander is an unusually robust violence prevention program, of which there are hundreds of programs. Rather than focusing strictly on the roles of perpetrator and victim, this highly interactive, researched and evaluated program offers a curriculum and evaluation tools using a community of responsibility approach. It teaches bystanders how to safely intervene in instances where an incident may be occurring or where there may be risk of violence. The program, which was developed and evaluated by University researchers and program practitioners, is customizable to reflect the locations, colloquialisms and cultures of diverse campuses. The program was developed and currently managed at the Prevention Innovations Research Center (http://cola.unh.edu/prevention-innovations-research-center) at the University of New Hampshire (UNH), Durham NH USA. The Center designed several Bystander Program Evaluation Tools. The program is working in colleges and other organizations all over the world. Research such as that of Moynihan et al. (2015) demonstrates significant impact in training young adults in intervening or rescuing victims of sexual violence.

An organization called Humanitarian Outcomes maintains the international Aid Worker Security Database available at (https://aidworkersecurity.org/about). In their 2015 report, there were an estimated 450,000 aid workers worldwide and over the past decade, an estimated 3000 workers encountered extreme violence. About a third of these workers were killed, a third wounded, and a third kidnapped. These estimates do not include the local or national aid workers. Often these violent victimizations of international aid workers are widely publicized in the media. Therefore, the aid workers are truly heroic rescuers, knowing that they are risking their lives by the decisions they make in the field.

This risk applies to workers for all of the organizations above except the Bystander project. In Bystander projects, ordinary students and adults are trained to take risks in order to reduce the likelihood of violent relationship, usually sexual violence. Undoubtedly, on occasions the bystander person engaged in intervention encounters physical harm, however, these project organizations do not report statistics on such instances. Those engaged in (or considering) intervention are called *bystanders* because this label has emerged from the enormous number of academic research projects that have examined the factors that predict whether or not an individual will intervene if s/he observes a violent or morally reprehensible action taking place. The most persistent finding is that the larger the group of observers of a situation or crisis, the less likely someone is to help, which is called the *bystander effect.* The Bystander projects are designed to counteract the bystander effect.

Conclusions

The pursuit of education and the process of personal and social growth are deeply connected. From research on the nature of people's moral and altruistic motivations we can conclude that building upon the altruistic impulse from early life into the adult years is crucial to cultivating a caring society (Oliner and Oliner 1995). In the classroom environment, where young people spend so much of their formative years, there is unlimited opportunity to teach and reward compassionate, socially responsible behavior. One model, called the "jigsaw classroom," places students in ethnically diverse groups and requires them to work together to complete a task. Students who experience diversity and learn cooperation in the classroom tend to be less prejudiced, more cooperative and more empathic than students who are not required to work with others of different cultural backgrounds and cognitive abilities. The students are intrinsically rewarded for working together, and tend to internalize and retain the values of cooperation and empathy (Clay 2006).

Reduction of suffering is possible by encouraging and empowering the altruistic potential within each individual. Any contribution to others, whether volunteer work, donation or random acts of kindness offers the potential, if not the reality, of the reduction of suffering. The key to promoting this type of behavior is to teach children and youth the importance of caring and social responsibility. It is encouraging to see that education in caring and empathy in the classroom can be effective (Clay 2006). Empathy in classrooms builds positive classroom culture, strengthens community and reduces suffering. Empathy training prepares students to be responsible leaders in the community. Teaching tolerance can build a positive classroom culture and results in reduced bullying. By instilling the values of caring and social responsibility in our young people, and rewarding those behaviors and practices that empower and assist, the future of our world can look much brighter.

Because of the risk involved in aid work or bystander intervention, ordinary persons are not likely to take on these challenging roles unless they are altruistic and have a moral sense of social responsibility. Such an inclination may be inculcated within the family, the school, communities, or other social institutions where training is offered. Fortunately, there seems to be a growing trend in North America to incorporate empathy and social responsibility in elementary and secondary schools.

The Holocaust has become a metaphor in Western societies for both the evil and good hidden in the human spirit. It is comforting that contemporary societies continue the heroic rescuing that emerged from the *righteous gentiles* of the Holocaust. In continues in the form of select altruistic individuals and specific social institutions that maintain the recruitment and training of professionals and ordinary people to engage in heroic rescuing when violence comes to our attention.

Acknowledgement The author thanks Nichole Wagner for extensive and very helpful assistance in completing this chapter.

References

Anderson, R. (Ed.). (2015). *World suffering and quality of life*. Dordrecht: Springer.

Berger, A. (Ed.). (1991). *Bearing witness to the Holocaust, 1939–1989*. Lewiston: E. Mellen Press.

Berger, A., & Berger, N. (Eds.). (2001). *Second generation voices: Reflections by children of Holocaust survivors and perpetrators*. Syracuse: Syracuse University Press.

Clay, R. (2006). Helping kids care. *Monitor On Psychology*, *37*(11), 42. American Psychological Association. Retrieved from http://www.apa.org/monitor/dec06/kids.aspx

Luther, M. (1971). The jews and their lies. In *The christian society.* Vol. 4, of Luther's Works. F. Sherman (Ed.). Philadelphia: Fortress Press.
McLeod, S. (2014). Maslow's Hierarchy of Needs. *Simply Psychology*. Retrieved from http://www.simplypsychology.org/maslow.html
Moynihan, M. M., Banyard, V. L., Cares, A. C., Potter, S. J., Williams, L. M., & Stapleton, J. G. (2015). Encouraging responses in sexual and relationship violence prevention: What program effects remain one year later? *Journal of Interpersonal Violence, 30*, 110–132.
Oliner, S. P. (1979). *Restless memories: Recollections of the Holocaust years. St.* Paul: Paragon House.
Oliner, S. P. (2003). *Do unto others: Extraordinary acts of ordinary people*. Boulder: Westview Press.
Oliner, S. P., & Oliner, P. (1988). *The altruistic personality: Rescuers of Jews in Nazi Europe*. New York: The Free Press.
Oliner, S. P., & Oliner, P. (1992). *Embracing the other: Philosophical, psychological, and historical perspectives on altruism*. New York: New York University Press.
Oliner, S. P., & Oliner, P. (1995). *Toward a caring society: Ideas into action*. Westport: Praeger.
Oliner, S. P., & Zylicz, P. (2008). *Altruism, intergroup apology, forgiveness and reconciliation*. St. Paul: Paragon House.
Pinker, S. (2011). *The better angels of our nature: Why violence has declined*. Penguin Books.
Reykowski, J. (1987a). *Activation of helping motivation: The role of extensivity*. Unpublished paper.
Reykowski, J. (1987b). Dimensions of development in moral value: Two approaches to the development of morality. In N. Eisenberg, J. Reykowski, & E. Staub (Eds.), *Social and moral values: Individual and societal perspectives*. Hillsdale: Lawrence Erlbaum.
Rifkin, J. (2009). *The empathic civilization: The race to global consciousness in a world in crisis*. New York: Penguin Books.
Tec, N. (1986). *When light pierced the darkness*. New York: Oxford University Press.
United States Holocaust Memorial Museum. (2016). *Research in collections*. Retrieved from https://www.ushmm.org/research/research-in-collections
Weber, L. (2000). Winston Churchill. In*The holocaust chronicle*. Lincolnwood: Publications International.
Winerman, L. (2005, October). The mind's mirror. *Monitor on Psychology*. American Psychological Association.
Zajaczkowski, M. (2013). *Polish-Ukrainian historical disputes over the Volhynian massacres*. Institute of National Remembrance. Retrieved from http://www.volhyniamassacre.eu/spory-o-wolyn/polish-ukrainian-historical-disputes-over-the-volhynian-massacres
Zawada, Z. (2005, April 10). Ukraine mourns Pope John Paul II, recalls 2001 visit. *Ukrainian Weekly*, Vol. LXXIII, No. 15. Retrieved from http://www.ukrweekly.com/old/archive/2005/150504.shtml

Chapter 18
Digitized Suffering, Actual Healing: Empathy, Reconciliation, and Redress Through a Virtual Indian Residential School

Adam Muller, Struan Sinclair, and Andrew Woolford

Introduction

Before it can be adequately alleviated, suffering must be acknowledged and its causes and consequences properly understood. Not all forms of distress are visible, either to the sufferer (who may exist in a state of denial) or to secondary witnesses (who may lack the information necessary to make sense of suffering's symptoms). Absent this visibility, it is difficult, if not impossible, to care about another's enduring pain and misery, and so be motivated to try to put things right. It can be even more difficult to care, or even to comprehend, collective experiences of suffering resulting from the imposition of negative quality of life upon a targeted group, not to mention the attempted negation of the group itself. If visible but improperly understood, suffering may end up misrecognized or unacknowledged and thereby prolonged or made worse. If we really want to reduce others' suffering, and redress past and/or ongoing wrongs, we must first recognize suffering for what it is, have some idea where it comes from, and imagine what experiencing it must be like.

Our chapter begins with an overview and comparison of the collective experience of the many different kinds of suffering found in both Canadian and American Indigenous boarding schools. We pay particular attention to how this suffering negated important forms of social and cultural capital within Indigenous communities in a manner that we argue is consistent with Raphael Lemkin's conceptualization of genocide (Lemkin 1944, 2013). Next we examine the ways in which Canadians have been working to acknowledge Indian Residential School (IRS) harms, most

A. Muller (✉) • S. Sinclair
Department of English, Film, and Theatre, University of Manitoba,
Winnipeg, MB R3T 2N2, Canada
e-mail: Adam.Muller@umanitoba.ca; Struan.Sinclair@umanitoba.ca

A. Woolford
Department of Sociology, University of Manitoba, Winnipeg, MB R3T 2N2, Canada
e-mail: Andrew.Woolford@umanitoba.ca

R.E. Anderson (ed.), *Alleviating World Suffering*, Social Indicators Research Series 67, DOI 10.1007/978-3-319-51391-1_18

conspicuously through a public apology and the Indian Residential School Settlement Agreement, including the activities of the Truth and Reconciliation Commission of Canada (TRC). We will draw upon testimony given by residential school Survivors to the TRC on the topic of reconciliation to illustrate some of the complications associated with attempts to alleviate suffering in this context. Amongst other things this testimony expresses concerns about the limited potential of prescribed reconciliatory mechanisms to redress the losses of social and cultural capital imposed on Indigenous peoples through their experience of residential schools. Indeed, a prominent theme in Survivor reflections on reconciliation is their sense that settler colonial wrongs have been made visible in the IRSSA through a performance of alleviation that is superficial and delimited in such a manner that it will not adequately address the full brunt of settler colonialism's destructive assault on Indigenous nations and identities.

We will conclude by reflecting on strategies for deepening and enriching Canadians' understanding of what reconciliation with Indigenous people needs to become. Our remarks will primarily concern the possibilities for advancing reconciliation afforded by *Embodying Empathy*, a critical and creative collaboration between scholars, IRS Survivors, and technologists who are working to construct a virtually immersive IRS "storyworld." We will discuss relevant aspects of *Embodying Empathy*'s attempt to alleviate suffering and further reconciliation – not just between Indigenous and non-Indigenous Canadians but between IRS Survivors, their families, and their communities – through the cultivation of a morally and politically salient form of empathy.

Indigenous Boarding Schools in Canada and the United States

Providing a general history of assimilative education through Indigenous boarding schools in Canada and the United States is difficult. First, it is hard to speak of a distinct experience of assimilative schooling in either country.[1] Although each country sought to develop policy around the use of schools, in practice these schools took specific shape depending on a variety of factors, including the power of local Indigenous communities and the attitudes of principals, superintendents and other staff. Assimilative education was an uneven experience with the brunt of suffering felt more strongly in some regions and periods than others. Second, Indigenous boarding schools were parts of complex settler colonial networks. These networks included other educational institutions, such as day and public schools, as well as diverse agents from the fields of religion, health, justice, and politics who were enlisted in the project of Indigenous assimilation. In addition, the assimilative

[1] It is also hard to quantify the number of students physically or sexually harmed through these schools. For example, 150,000 students are said to have passed through Canadian residential schools, and at least 6000 to have perished therein or soon after their departure, but the extent of abuse within the schools, which is known to be widespread, as not yet been accurately calculated.

schools were deployed alongside other techniques of forced collective identity transformation, for example laws against Indigenous spiritual practices, efforts to impose individualized property ownership, and interventions to erase Indigenous modes of governance. For these reasons, one risks over-simplifying the impact of settler colonialism on Indigenous lives by focusing solely on boarding schools. Finally, Canada and the United States did not operate in isolation from one another in developing Indigenous boarding school policy. Cross-border conversations and borrowing were not uncommon (Woolford 2015).

With these caveats in mind, it is possible to make a few generalizations about Indigenous boarding schools in the U.S. and Canada. In both countries, the turn toward concerted use of assimilative schooling occurred in the late nineteenth century (Reyhner and Eder 2004). At this time, discussion of the so-called "Indian problem," a notion of the Indigenous group as an obstacle to land acquisition and settlement, turned toward the ideas of "assimilation" and "civilization" as solutions. Education – a technique long used by missionaries in efforts to proselytize and convert Indigenous young people – came to be viewed as a primary vehicle for addressing the Indian problem. Lieutenant Richard Henry Pratt's experiment with "industrial" education was particularly influential.

Pratt's model involved removing Indigenous children from their home communities and placing them in schools closer to "civilization." Such propinquity to European settlers was seen as a necessary means to distance Indigenous children from the ways of their parents and attach them instead to European life. To facilitate this transformation, Pratt sought to discipline children through a combination of military regimentation, work training, and basic education. Students would spend each day of the school year rising early to assemble on the grounds for marching and inspection before splitting the remainder of their day between work and school (Fear-Segal 2007).

Pratt's ideas travelled across the border to influence Canada's initial effort to systematize assimilative education. Canada had not engaged in warfare to the extent experienced in the U.S., and had long sought a more assimilative path for dealing with its "Indian problem." However, after Nicholas Flood Davin was dispatched by John A. MacDonald's Conservative government in 1879 to study Indian education in the U.S., a clearer embrace of an industrial style education was promoted with one exception – Davin felt that a state run system was impractical and that Canada should build its Indigenous boarding school system through the missions that were already established near Indigenous communities (Davin 1879). Indeed, though Canada would initially seek to establish an industrial school system comprised of large schools equipped to prepare male students for menial labour in agriculture and the trades, and females for caring for the household, the costs of such a system would eventually lead Canada to opt for a residential school system featuring many smaller schools located closer to Indigenous communities.

The role of the churches represents an important difference between Indigenous boarding schools in the U.S. and Canada. In the U.S., religious involvement through "contract schools" began to fade in the late nineteenth century as the government stopped funding such schools – in part because there was concern among Protestant advocates of assimilative education about the degree of influence Catholics maintained through contract schools (Keller 1983). In contrast, the Canadian government depended on Protestant (Methodist, Presbyterian, and Anglican) and Catholic missionaries to operate their schools. This resulted in a symbiotic relationship that had negative quality of life consequences for the children attending these schools. First, the churches maintained a great deal of influence over educational policy given the government's dependence on their services. This resulted in less change in policy over the history of residential schools in Canada than was true in the U.S. The U.S. Bureau of Indian Affairs shifted its policies alongside trends in the logic of governance, for example moving from a more militaristic model of schooling to one more defined by a managerial ethos directed towards encouraging the students to become responsible for governing themselves. Meanwhile, Canada's schools were consistently defined by a regime of monastic discipline oriented first and foremost toward shaping the souls of the students (Woolford 2015). Second, the relationship between government and churches in Canada was an unhealthy one, and the government sought to provide the minimum funding possible to operate the schools, which were often deliberately crowded in hopes of accessing more funds. U.S. schools were in general better funded than Canadian schools, though one should not make the mistake of thinking of them as adequately resourced. At both schools, children often suffered from overcrowding, poor nutrition, inadequate clothing, a lack of health care, and other problems associated with underfunding (Woolford 2015).

U.S. boarding schools also operated in a more systematic fashion than those in Canada. According to the American model, though this policy was not always followed in practice, young children would typically begin their education at reserve-based day schools before graduating to a reserve-based boarding school and then enrolling at a non-reservation boarding school for the final few years of education. Therefore most students were in their teens at the latter institutions, though this was not always the case. In Canada, the policy that determined who would and would not be sent to a day or boarding school was more haphazard. After 1920, when the Indian Act clarified that Indigenous children belonged to the Christian denomination assigned to their community, children were sent to a school run by that denomination whether it was a day or boarding institution. For this reason, children were often sent to boarding schools at ages as young as five or six (Reyhner and Eder 2004).

Finally, the temporal shifts in Indigenous boarding school policy were less dramatic in Canada than the U.S. In Canada, there was very little turnover among the bureaucrats running the residential school system. Deputy Superintendent of Indian Affairs Duncan Campbell Scott, in particular, kept a close eye on residential schools (and their costs to government) for almost 20 years between 1913 and 1932, and did so in a manner quite consistent with those who came before and after him. In contrast, the U.S. Bureau of Indian Affairs experienced multiple and sometimes radical leadership changes, conspicuously when John Collier, a former Indian rights advocate, became Commissioner from 1933 to 1945. It was under Collier that the BIA sought to address concerns raised in the 1928 Meriam Report, which lambasted the many failings of the schools even if it did not challenge the practice of assimilative education itself (Szasz 1999; Woolford 2015).

Indigenous Boarding Schools, Genocide, and the Loss of Social and Cultural Capital

Several scholars, activists, and Survivors have described the suffering experienced by children at Indigenous boarding schools as genocide (e.g., Chrisjohn and Young 1997; Macdonald 2014; Starblanket 2015; Woolford 2015). It is worthwhile to take a moment to reflect on this assertion.

Raphael Lemkin (1900–1959), a Polish-Jewish jurist, coined the term genocide to address his concern that no law existed to protect the life of groups. For Lemkin (1944: 79), genocide represents a purposeful effort to destroy the "essential foundations of the group." This effort might occur through the physical murder of group members, but it could also take place through the destruction of the various cultural institutions (e.g. family, politics, art, religion) that make group life possible. Lemkin was a tireless advocate for his genocide concept, and after escaping the Holocaust he fled to the United States where he helped draft the 1948 *United Nations Convention on the Prevention and Punishment of the Crime of Genocide* (UNGC). It was during the United Nations General Assembly debates on early drafts of the UNGC that Lemkin saw his genocide concept receive legal recognition. But it was also here that his notion of cultural genocide was largely excised from the Convention (Abtahi and Webb 2008). Lemkin felt this to be an unfortunate but necessary compromise. For him, culture was that which defined the "groupness" of a group, binding members to one another through the sharing of traditions, practices, languages, and other resources of group life. He hoped that later revisions to the UNGC would include the destruction of culture in the crime of genocide (Lemkin 2013).

Article III of the UNGC, which covered the topic of cultural genocide, was opposed by several General Assembly members on the grounds that it was too vague to be justiciable and that its protections were already covered under various other minority protection laws. Some members also noted that it would be ridiculous to protect the cultures of those groups perceived to be backward and primitive. Canada and the U.S. were among these members opposed to Article III. The Canadian delegation, for example, was advised by Ottawa: "You should support or initiate any move for the deletion of Article III on 'Cultural' Genocide. If this move is not successful, you should vote against Article III and if necessary, against the Convention." (quoted in Brean 2015, n.p.). They were also instructed to look toward the U.S. for support on this issue. In the end, 26 nations voted in favour of excluding cultural genocide from UNGC versus 16 against and 4 abstentions.

These complexities of the formation of genocide law lend some insight into why genocide remains an "essentially contested concept" (Powell 2011). The political self-interest that was often transparent in the creation of genocide law leaves social scientists, historians, lawyers, philosophers, and others engaged in the study of genocide in conflict over what exactly the term seeks to protect. Does it merely protect individuals in the aggregate? Or is it the group? And if the latter, what is a group? How does one protect something that is dynamic and itself subject to change?

Rather than limit ourselves to the narrowing and politicized concepts of genocide law, we understand genocide sociologically (and more in keeping with Lemkin's broader understanding of the concept). Drawing from a Bourdieuian framework (e.g., Bourdieu 1990; Bourdieu and Wacquant 1992), genocide's target, the group, can be understood as a network of social relations that is also the site of multiple fields of practice (e.g., art, education, language, law, politics, etc.). Each of these fields is defined by a valuational structure that privileges certain arrangements of power or capital. To appear competent within the field and abide by its rules, individuals muster their dispositions gained through experience (their *habitus*, which is their store of various forms of capital). These are the tools that allow them to feel at home within the various institutions of group life. In this fashion, participants in the group's activities use their capital to navigate the conditions of the group's fields, both contributing to the dynamism of the group through everyday negotiations and innovations in its constitutive fields and its persistence by reaffirming the logic of practice within these fields. When these forms of capital are damaged through genocidal actions, the individual is left disconnected and rootless and experiences layers of suffering from this loss of sociality.

Returning to our example of Indigenous boarding schools, we can now look more closely at how these institutions targeted the fields and forms of capital inherent in Indigenous group life. First, however, we must note that there exist a multiplicity of Indigenous groups in what is now North America, and we are thus not speaking of a homogenized "Indian" or "Native American." Second, we must be clear that boarding schools were just one strand in U.S. and Canadian efforts to address the so-called Indian problem. For more than a century multiple strategic interventions were launched in an effort to transform Indigenous *persons* and divorce them from Indigenous *peoples*.

For the sake of brevity, we will focus here on only two ways in which boarding schools disrupted important forms of capital transmission thereby working to negate group life. Let's begin with social capital, which refers to the power accessible through one's social networks. Indigenous boarding schools in both the U.S. and Canada sought to sever ties between the student and his or her community and family. Soon after their arrival at boarding schools, children were stripped of the Indigenous names that connected them to community and territory. The clothes they wore, which may have been constructed from local materials, were taken away and destroyed. Siblings of the opposite sex were housed in separate wings of schools, and little to no contact between brothers and sisters was permitted. Some Survivors recount that they were told to no longer refer to their parents as "mom" and "dad," while teachers, matrons, and other supervising staff were directed to act as their surrogate family (Woolford 2015). Additionally, the physical distance between the school and the community, as well as the school's fence, kept children in and visiting relatives out. Together interventions such as these destroyed Indigenous networks. Children were deprived of a sense of collective identity, but also a sense of being grounded within a family, community, and territory. New networks of social capital arose that connected students to staff, school, work, and the settler nation, but all those anchoring them to their home communities were severely weakened if not destroyed. Indeed, former students often experienced great difficulty returning to their communities in summers and at the conclusion of their schooling. They no longer felt at home in the fields of traditional group life, in part because they no longer possessed the right sort of social capital – the power of strong and deep relations with kin, neighbours, animals and territory.

Similarly, Lemkin's emphasis on cultural genocide can be better understood when we examine how cultural capital was attacked through residential and boarding schools. A primary attack was linked to the prohibition against speaking Indigenous languages. These verb-based languages, uniquely suited to opening one's thinking to the processual and dynamic nature of Indigenous collective life, were replaced with noun-based languages that sought to fix and delimit the world. This effort at linguistic destruction overlapped with efforts to alter Indigenous cultural practices related to land. The assimilative education that students received taught that land was not something alive and related to the student; instead it was to be surveyed, marked, farmed, landscaped, and individually owned. Students were taught that land was a resource rather than a relation. Likewise, animal life was instrumentalized through instruction in husbandry, altering the traditional sense that animals were to be lived with in harmony. Children also lost out on much of their cultural learning, as entire story cycles were missed while students boarded at school over the winter. Songs, practices, traditions, games, jokes, ceremonies, and other aspects of Indigenous cultural learning were not transmitted. Upon leaving school, students often lacked the cultural resources required to maintain a feel for Indigenous group life.

These experiences were in addition to the physical and sexual violence that was often present at boarding and residential schools, and the combined suffering from these experiences had the potential to upset all forms of capital group members possessed, preventing them from connecting meaningfully with others. Survivors have spoken at great length about how these forms of intimate physical violence compromised their efforts to form relationships. The following testimony from a Canadian IRS Survivor captures well the many ways in which physical, cultural, and sexual violence affected group relations[2]:

> I called those people who ran the boarding school, 'stone people.' What did I learn from those stone people? I learned how to suppress my natural feelings, my feelings of love, compassion, natural sharing and gentleness. I learned to replace my feelings with a heart of stone. I became a non-human, non-person, with no language, no love, no home, no people, and a person without an identity. (Quoted in Dalseg 2003, pp. 76-7)

[2] Pseudonyms have been used for all Survivor testimony.

Redressing Boarding Schools in Canada and the U.S.

Conceptualizing the forms of capital that help maintain the network of social relations comprising the group allows for a more careful examination of the forms of redress heretofore made available to deal with the suffering connected to Indigenous boarding schools. The following Survivor's description of her aftermath of residential school education is not atypical:

> I found alcohol when I arrived in the city. I just became alcoholic. I didn't drink to enjoy it; I didn't even like the taste of it. I like what it did to make me forget. … I became suicidal, slashed my wrists because I was so embarrassed what I did to my kids. Same thing happened [inaudible] that's exactly what my mom did to us. What I was doing (Jane 2010).

In 2007, the Supreme Court of Canada approved the Indian Residential Schools Settlement Agreement (IRSSA). This agreement ended years of lawsuits and failed resolution processes that had presented Canada with the risk of huge liabilities, and residential school Survivors with the threat of remaining trapped in retraumatizing and lengthy struggles for redress. Final agreement on the IRSSA was made possible through the federal government's acceptance of the need to provide a public apology in the House of Commons, which was delivered by then Prime Minister Stephen Harper on June 11, 2008.

The IRSSA itself has several components. First, the settlement provided "at least" $1.9 billion dollars for Common Experience Payments (CEP) allotted to any individual having attended a residential school, regardless of his or her experience. This included a base amount of $10,000 for the first year of schooling and $3000 for every year thereafter. Second, the settlement created an Independent Assessment Process (IAP) for those who had suffered sexual or substantial physical abuses, or other abuses that caused severe psychological trauma. Compensation awarded through this process can range between $5000 and $275,000, or more if a loss of income can be demonstrated. IAP amounts were determined through a point system, which involved itemizing the types of harm suffered by students while in attendance at a residential school. Finally, $125 million was provided to the Aboriginal Healing Foundation and $60 million set aside to create the Truth and Reconciliation Commission (TRC), with a further $20 million earmarked for community commemorative projects (Indian Residential Schools Settlement Agreement 2006). The TRC conducted seven national events at which Survivors and others connected to the schools delivered either public or private statements about their residential schooling experiences and feelings about reconciliation, supplemented by community-based events that were more numerous than the national events and less rigidly structured, allowing communities to adapt these hearings to local practices and traditions (Truth and Reconciliation Commission of Canada 2010).

In comparison, in the U.S. movement to redress the harms of Indigenous boarding schools has been very slow. The Canadian example may therefore seem especially praiseworthy. However, Canada's has been an uneven process. On the plus side, for the duration of its 2008–2015 mandate the TRC worked hard to ensure that Canadians would not view its efforts as the "end" but rather as the beginning of reconciliation. It also sought to educate Canadians and show them that residential schools were part of a broader set of colonial harms that are multilayered and ongoing (Truth and Reconciliation Commission 2015). However, other aspects of the IRSSA were panned for narrowing the TRC's historical focus to exclude suffering beyond the residential schools.

On the federal government's apology, one Survivor noted the ongoing nature of her suffering: "as if some words are going to make up for all the lives that are, have been ruined. Yet really, it's not just my life, my other son's life has been ruined, my granddaughter's life has been ruined. …. The trauma just goes on and on and on" (Ellen 2011). In another instance, a Survivor pointed to inconsistencies between the language of reconciliation and its actual practice: "What did Harper do since the apology? Well, now, he's starting to implement a system where they do [mandatory minimum] punishment, where he's gonna punish people. And who are the people that he's punishing? It's our people!" (Sandra 2011) Likewise, the compensation programs were condemned for their failure to address ongoing feelings of trauma: "no … amount of money …is gonna release what's inside that I have. I'm going to do that in my own time, in my own way" (Mike 2012). Furthermore, compensation was deemed inadequate to deal with the complexity of the suffering that had been endured: "The IAP (Independent Assessment Process) is asking me … to measure the amount of hurt and pain I have experienced in the residential school. What I find most difficult is trying to separate my whole life experience from what happened to me in the school and the events before and after the residential school" (Annette 2012).

These are but a few examples intended to foreground the voices of Survivors as they struggled (and still struggle) to come to terms with their traumatic pasts. They are, however, emblematic of what we have heard from Survivors more generally (see also Woolford 2015). We make no claim that the digital IRS storyworld we discuss in the next section can overcome all of these shortcomings. We have, though, become increasingly optimistic that our project can deepen diverse audiences' empathy for Survivors and Indigenous groups generally by immersing them in the everyday losses of social and cultural capital – in the persistent acts and threats of physical, sexual, symbolic, and cultural violence – that pervaded these schools.

Embodying Empathy, Unsettling Reconciliation

How can empathy be "designed into" a virtual environment? How long will the empathetic connections arising within virtual worlds last? Should psychological and affective contiguity between virtual and actual be expected, or even contemplated? The *Embodying Empathy* (EE) project (*EE*) is an interdisciplinary collaboration linking researchers and IRS Survivors in order to create and evaluate the reconciliatory potential of a virtual Indian Residential School. Essentially a museum-quality dynamic and immersive exhibition, EE is being created both as a standalone installation (it will debut publicly at Winnipeg's Indigenous-run Urban Shaman Gallery early in 2018) and as a mobile non-immersive app suitable for use on tablets and cell phones. The project has three core aims. It seeks: 1) to make knowledge about IRS experiences widely accessible; 2) to promote reconciliation between IRS Survivors, their families, and their communities, as well as between Indigenous and non-Indigenous Canadians, by cultivating empathetic connections; and 3) to test the hypothesis that immersive media can enhance the representation of complex experiences, including traumatic ones held to be "difficult," to use Deborah Britzman's influential term designating representational resistance (Britzman 1998). More broadly, the *EE* storyworld can contribute to larger discussions about the composition and function of empathy in virtual environments, how such empathy might be coded and evaluated, and the relation of virtual environments (VEs) to real ones.

In recent years, scholarly interest in the potential of VEs to facilitate affective engagement has seen researchers from across the disciplines increasingly making use of "virtual laboratories" to conduct a wide range of experimental inquiries, in the process helping to overcome a prevailing cynicism about the capacity of virtual environments to model and sustain real emotions. Sun Joo Ahn et al. (2013), for example, make the case that digitally recreating and extending human sensory capabilities exploits our readiness to temporarily accept the illusion of sufficiently realistic experiences. On their view, "the realism of virtual experiences is likely to produce mental schema about the simulated event as if he or she had firsthand experience of it, to be recalled later when necessary" (Ahn et al. 2013, p. 9). Likewise, Garry Young (2010) offers a detailed analysis of experiments that demonstrate the efficacy of virtual environments in fostering emotional connections. His view is shared by Andreas Mühlberger and his colleagues (2007, p. 340), who claim that working exclusively within VEs can yield a "valid and reliable assessment of phobic fear" and induce "true emotional responses."

In 2006, Mel Slater and his team replicated the Milgram obedience experiments in a VE using a virtual learner in order to gauge how participants respond to "interactions with a virtual character in the type of extreme social situations exemplified by the conflict created within the Milgram paradigm" (Slater et al. 2006). Slater's results include his conclusion that "humans tend to respond realistically at subjective, physiological, and behavioral levels in interactions with virtual characters," despite their "cognitive certainty" that the virtual character positioned as the "learner" was not real (Slater et al. 2006). The potential advantages of virtual spaces as sites of social inquiry thus now include spatial, sensory, behavioral, and *affective* verisimilitude.

Insofar as the *EE* storyworld is concerned, the promise of immersive VEs includes the idea that they may exceed standard fictional worlds in terms of the range and availability of emotions they are able to provide. Grant Tavinor (2005, pp. 24-25) observes of video game play that it is possible "to feel guilty or ashamed for what one does in the fictional world," since one is an actor rather than observer within the fiction:

> Contrast this with the fictive engagement one has with a film or novel; there the epistemic access the audience has to a fictional world is constrained by the narration. With most traditional fictions, the rule is that audiences are passive observers of a predetermined fiction

> unfolding before them.... [immersive VEs] however, seem to be active pursuits in a more robust sense. (Tavinor 2005, p. 26)

Immersive interactivity potentially allows for those immersed in a virtual environment to become personally involved with characters at a level impossible with traditional fictions, while the requirement of personal (agential) intervention and narrative construction permits a whole host of previously unavailable emotional states to be directed toward characters and/or events in the VE (Young 2010). The balance of evidence therefore currently suggests that VEs represent an appropriate framework for studying the formation and persistence of empathy responses, even though they exist at one remove from actual experience.

Embodying Empathy follows established "participatory design" (PD) protocols, which have been modified to conform to principles for working with and disseminating Indigenous knowledge developed by the Assembly of First Nations known as OCAP (Ownership, Control, Access, and Possession). Our approach has been designed to reflect the variety and particularity of Survivor experiences of collective suffering, and it makes a great deal of room available for taking seriously Survivors' desires and concerns, even as they change over time. In nearly every respect *Embodying Empathy* is a Survivor-led undertaking, and Survivors will have the final word on what the storyworld looks like, where it is installed, and how it is used. In conjunction with our refusal to profit from any of the technology created through our efforts (we have ceded our intellectual property rights), *Embodying Empathy*'s consultative and fully participatory approach is intended to model a certain kind of reconciliatory praxis, one that takes Indigenous perspectives seriously. The project has been guided by an advisory council of IRS Survivors. In our consultations to date we have focused on the range of experiences to represent within the storyworld, and explored a variety of ways of interacting in the world with an emphasis on ease of access and in-world navigation, modularity and scalability, and the possibility of using the world to inculcate long-term behavioural change conducive to reconciliation (Greitemeyer and Osswald 2010); in particular, behavioural change that recognizes and redresses the continuing impact of settler colonialism on Indigenous social and cultural capital.

Such a possibility is anything but remote. Ahn et al. (2013, p. 8) explain that the kind of technology we are using "allows for a literal demonstration of climbing into another person's skin to embody his or her experiences first hand. Vivid, multilayer perceptual information simulated by digital devices enables individuals to see, hear, and feel as if they were undergoing the sensory experiences in the physical world—what we call 'embodied experiences' [that] allow the user to experience the closest realization of the portal to enter another person's mind and body." The combination of this kind of embodiment, and the presence in the storyworld of IRS-related documents and photographs, replica furniture, and Survivor testimony, some available through links we'll be providing to the TRC's (Truth and Reconciliation Commission's) testimonial archive, will deepen the immersivity of the *EE* user's experience. Together with the complex topography and elaborate matrix of possible social interactions available in the virtual IRS, this immersivity should facilitate critical reflection on the reality of residential schools' harms and their aftermaths, contributing to an increase in "unsettling" behaviour, in Paulette Regan's (2010) sense of the term, whereby Canadians may confront the ways in which settler colonialism has shaped their ways of seeing and knowing the world.

The persistence or contiguity of behavioural change between virtual and actual worlds has been extensively documented. According to Ahn et al. (2013, p. 31), the capacity of the kinds of technologies *Embodying Empathy* is using to facilitate the merging of self and other within virtual environments "transfers to the physical world and translates into actual helping behavior, even when the other person is a complete stranger." And these affective connections can endure. In his work on long-term interactions with relational virtual agents, Timothy Bickmore (2010, p. 661) notes that "the use of social and relational behaviors [such as] empathy and social chat, can serve to establish a social bond with users that in turn serves to maintain engagement over time and keep users returning again and again." That the empathetic connections forged during a visit to the *Embodying Empathy* storyworld may contribute to the goals of reconciliation that are central to this and other attempts to reckon with the traumatic history of the IRS has proven to be a powerful motivator for the project's advisors and extended network of partners and collaborators, including archives, community groups, commemorative agencies, Indigenous rights advocates, and scholars.

The storyworld we are creating requires users to experience it actively. It is through such activity that empathetic bonds will be forged, and the outlooks of IRS Survivors and secondary witnesses will (ideally) become aligned. We understand empathy to be a practice rather than simply a feeling. As a practice it is something we can improve at. According to Dan Zahavi (2008, p. 522), empathy "simply refers to our ability to access the life of the mind of others in their bodily and behavioural expressions; an ability that moreover can improve with familiarity, learning, and salience." Empathy arises from constant assessments we make within and between various contexts, including virtual ones. Users operating as virtual agents within the *EE* storyworld should be capable of empathizing with the virtual children they meet and interact with there. This empathy will tend to be either be "parallel" or "reactive," a significant distinction since, as Scott McQuiggan et al. (2008) explains, "parallel empathy refers to mere replication of another's affective state, whereas reactive empathy exhibits greater cognitive awareness." The opportunities to experience reactive empathy modelled within and primed by Embodying Empathy (*EE)* are intended to reach the "stone hearts" not just of secondary witnesses to IRS trauma but of the Survivors themselves, hopefully thereby contributing to a richer awareness of our shared humanity, vulnerability, and moral and political agency.

Conclusion: Prospects and Challenges

Notwithstanding the arguments above, empathy's power to spur and sustain subsequent "unsettling" behavioural change is far from assured. Walter Stephan and Krystina Finlay, for example, have shown that people direct comparatively little empathy towards members of groups against which they are already prejudiced (Stephan and Finlay 1999). The *EE* interface as well as its content will be crucial to overcoming such prejudice. Entry points into the storyworld, along with the array of perspectives open to users, and the mechanisms by which each may be primed to respond affectively are all design considerations that will impinge on the power of the virtual IRS to dislocate users from their extant beliefs, desire, and habits. Doing so will be vital to the storyworld's success, for as Jonathan Belman and Mary Flanagan (2010, p. 9) argue, those immersed in virtual environments "are likely to empathize only when they make an intentional effort to do so [...]. [W]ithout some kind of effective empathy induction at the outset, most people will play 'unempathetically.'"

Can a well-designed virtual IRS foster reconciliation by helping to initiate and also sustain empathetic connections and encourage unsettling behaviour? The balance of the research available to date suggests that, properly integrated into virtual environments and suitably "embodied," empathy will impact learning and may aid in realizing long-term goals of reconciliation and the ongoing alleviation of the negative effects of a genocidal assault on Indigenous social and cultural capital. How successfully *Embodying Empathy*'s immersive storyworld achieves this integration and embodiment, along with its specific short- and long-term effects, remains to be precisely determined. As of this writing, the project is completing its second year of concentrated work and entering its design phase. After more than a year and a half of consultations with IRS Survivors, we have begun discussing with intergenerational Survivors their hopes for and concerns about an immersive representation of their relatives' experiences of residential school life, experiences that often went unmentioned even though their effects were cruelly felt. We and our research partners and collaborators remain optimistic about *Embodying Empathy*'s prospects, and deeply committed to the twin tasks assigned to all Canadians by Murray Sinclair (2015), the Truth and Reconciliation Commission's chair, following the 2015 release of the summary of the commission's final report: "The Survivors have entrusted us, and by extension, all the people in Canada, with two priorities. First, the Survivors need to know before they leave this earth that people understand what happened and what the schools did to them. Second, the Survivors need to know that, having been heard and understood, that we will act to ensure the repair of damages done." Through *Embodying Empathy* we hope to enhance awareness of the damage done by Canada's IRS system to Indigenous students and their cultures, while in the process exploring new means for beginning to successfully acknowledge and redress the suffering arising in its wake.

References

Abtahi, H., & Webb, P. (2008). The genocide convention: The travaux preparatoires (2 vols.). Leiden: Brill Academic Publishing.

Ahn, S. J. (Grace), Le, A. M. T., & Bailenson, J. (2013). The effect of embodied experiences on self-other merging, attitude, and helping behavior. *Media Psychology, 16*, 7–38.

Annette. (2012, April 13). *Statement to the Truth and Reconciliation Commission of Canada; 2011–3967*. Winnipeg: National Centre for Truth and Reconciliation Archives.

Belman, J., & Flanagan, M. (2010). Designing games to foster empathy. *Cognitive Technology, 14*(2), 5–15.

Bickmore, T., Schulman, D., & Yin, L. (2010). Maintaining engagement in long-term interventions with relational agents. *Applied Artificial Intelligence, 24*(6), 648–666.

Bourdieu, P. (1990). *The logic of practice*. Stanford: Stanford University Press.

Bourdieu, P., & Wacquant, L. (1992). *An invitation to reflexive sociology*. Chicago: University of Chicago Press.

Brean, J. (2015, June 8). Canada opposed concept of 'cultural genocide' in 1948 accord. *The National Post*.

Britzman, D. P. (1998). *Lost subjects, contest objects: Toward a psychoanalytic inquiry of learning*. Albany: State University of New York Press.

Chrisjohn, R., & Young, S. (1997). *The circle game: Shadows and substance in the Indian residential school experience*. Penticton: Theytus Books.

Dalseg, B. A. (2003). *In their own words: Manitoba's native residential schools remembered*. MA thesis, Winnipeg: University of Manitoba.

Davin, N. F. (1879, March 14). *Report on industrial schools for Indians and Half Breeds*. Ottawa: Government of Canada.

Ellen. (2011, October 13). *Statement to the Truth and Reconciliation Commission of Canada; 2011–3291*. Winnipeg: National Centre for Truth and Reconciliation Archives.

Fear-Segal, J. (2007). *White man's club: schools, race, and the struggle of Indian acculturation*. Lincoln: University of Nebraska Press.

Greitemeyer, T., & Osswald, S. (2010). Playing prosocial video games increases empathy and decreases schadenfreude. *Emotion, 10*(6), 796–802.

Herman, D. (2002). *Story logic: Problems and possibilities of narrative*. Lincoln: University of Nebraska Press.

Indian Residential Schools Settlement Agreement. (2006). *Detailed notice for the Indian residential school settlement*. Ottawa: Government of Canada. Retrieved from: http://www.residentialschoolsettlement.ca/detailed_notice.pdf

Jane. (2010, June 18). *Statement to the Truth and Reconciliation Commission of Canada; 02-MB-18JU10–057*. Winnipeg: National Centre for Truth and Reconciliation Archives.

Keller Jr., R. H. (1983). *American protestantism and the United States Indian policy, 1869–82*. Lincoln: University of Nebraska Press.

Lemkin, R. (1944). *Axis rule in occupied Europe: Laws of occupation, analysis of government, proposals for redress*. Washington, DC: Carnegie Endowment for International Peace.

Lemkin, R. (2013). *Totally unofficial: The autobiography of Raphael Lemkin* (D. L. Frieze, Ed.). New Haven: Yale University Press.

Macdonald, D. B. (2014). Genocide in the Indian residential schools: Canadian history through the lens of the UN genocide convention. In A. Woolford, J. Benvenuto, & A. Hinton (Eds.), *Colonial genocide in Indigenous North America* (pp. 306–324). Durham: Duke University Press.

McQuiggan, S.W. Robison, J. L., Phillips, R. & Lester, J. C. (2008). Modeling parallel and reactive empathy in virtual agents: an inductive approach. In L. Padgham, D. Parkes, J. Mueller, and S. Parsons (Eds.), *Proceedings of AAMAS*. Estoril: Portugal, 2008. Retrieved from https://www.intellimedia.ncsu.edu/wp-content/uploads/empathy-aamas-2008.pdf

Mike. (2012, June 24). *Statement to the Truth and Reconciliation Commission of Canada; 2011–1776*. Winnipeg: National Centre for Truth and Reconciliation Archives.

Mühlberger, A., Bülthoff, H., Wiedemann, G., & Pauli, P. (2007). Virtual reality for the psycho-physiological assessment of phobic fear: Responses during virtual tunnel driving. *Psychological Assessment, 19*, 340–346.

Powell, C. (2011). *Barbaric civilization: A critical sociology of genocide*. Montreal/Kingston: McGill-Queen's University Press.

Regan, P. (2010). *Unsettling the settler within: Indian residential schools, truth telling, and reconciliation in Canada*. Vancouver: University of British Columbia Press.

Reyhner, J., & Eder, J. (2004). *American Indian education: A history*. Norman: University of Oklahoma Press.

Sandra. (2011, February 5). *Statement to the Truth and Reconciliation Commission of Canada; 01-ON-28 05FE11–009*. Winnipeg: National Centre for Truth and Reconciliation Archives.

Sinclair, M. (2015, June 15). For the record: Justice Murray Sinclair on residential schools. *Macleans Magazine*. Retrieved from: http://www.macleans.ca/politics/for-the-record-justice-murray-sinclair-on-residential-schools/

Slater, M. et al. (2006). A virtual reprise of the stanley milgram obedience experiments. *PLoS One, 1*(1), e39. Web.

Starblanket, T. (2015). *Suffer the little children: Genocide, Indigenous nations, and the Canadian state*. Atlanta: Clarity Press.

Stephan, W. G., & Finlay, K. (1999). The role of empathy in improving intergroup relations. *Journal of Social Issues, 55*(4), 729–743.

Szasz, M. C. (1999). *Education and the American Indian: The road to self-determination since 1928*. Albuquerque: University of New Mexico Press.

Tavinor, G. (2005). Videogames and interactive fiction. *Philosophy and Literature, 29*(1), 24–40.

Truth and Reconciliation Commission of Canada. (2010). *Mandate for the Truth and Reconciliation Commission of Canada*. Ottawa: Government of Canada, Retrieved from: http://www.trc-cvr.ca/pdfs/SCHEDULE_N_EN.pdf

Truth and Reconciliation Commission of Canada (TRC). (2015). *Honouring the truth, reconciling for the future: Summary of the final report of the Truth and Reconciliation Commission of Canada*. Ottawa: Truth and Reconciliation Commission of Canada.

Woolford, A. (2015). *This benevolent experiment: Indigenous boarding schools, genocide and redress in Canada and the United States*. Lincoln/Winnipeg: University of Nebraska Press and the University of Manitoba Press.

Young, G. (2010). Virtually real emotions and the paradox of fiction: Implications for the use of virtual environments in psychological research. *Philosophical Psychology, 23*(1), 1–21.

Zahavi, D. (2008). Simulation, projection and empathy. *Consciousness and Cognition, 17*, 514–522.

Chapter 19
Women and Genocide: Ending Impunity for Sexual Violence

Ellen J. Kennedy

Introduction

Women and girls are targeted and victimized during genocides and mass atrocities. To strike at them is to strike at the heart of a culture and a society. Such strikes provoke fear and intimidation; prevent the possibility of retaliation; break up families; destroy communities; and change the ethnic identity of subsequent generations. This chapter explores epidemics of violence against women during some of the major genocides of the twentieth century, including the kidnapping and sexual slavery of Armenian women during World War I; the medical cruelty and forced prostitution perpetrated in the Ravensbruck women's concentration camp during the Holocaust; the use of 'rape camps' in Bosnia in the 1990s war; the rape and intentional transmission of HIV/AIDS to more than 500,000 Rwandan women during the 1994 genocide; and sexual slavery of Yazidi women and girls in Syria and Iraq perpetrated by the terrorist organization ISIS. Significant advances in human rights in the past several decades have classified rape and other forms of sexual and gender violence as crimes against humanity, genocide, and war crimes, not as unavoidable collateral damages of war. This chapter examines prosecutions for these crimes as part of a profound legal shift towards ending impunity for perpetrators of violence against women and girls. This change is influenced, in part, by the increased numbers of women prosecutors and judges in national and international tribunals and an increased attention to 'gender justice' on a global scale. The impact of this profound shift is to communicate clearly the penalties of such crimes, provide deterrence for future sexual violence against women, and promote some measure of justice and the alleviation of suffering.

E.J. Kennedy (✉)
World Without Genocide, Mitchell Hamline School of Law, St Paul, MN 55105, USA
e-mail: kennedy@worldwithoutgenocide.org

R.E. Anderson (ed.), *Alleviating World Suffering*, Social Indicators Research Series 67, DOI 10.1007/978-3-319-51391-1_19

Gender and Genocide

"The women are those who hold their families and communities together. Their physical and emotional destruction aims at destroying social and cultural stability. In many cultures, the female body embodies a nation as a whole. The rape of women of a community, culture, or nation can be regarded as symbolic rape of the body of a community" (MacKinnon 2006).

In recent years, prosecutors of genocide and crimes against humanity have sought successfully to include rape as a crime of genocide. This 'gendering' of genocide and mass atrocities represents a relatively recent phenomenon in both legal scholarship and in efforts to prosecute perpetrators who target women and girls. Females are victimized during genocides and mass atrocities because to strike at them is to strike at the heart of a culture and a society. These strikes also provoke fear and intimidation and prevent the possibility of retaliation; break up families and destroy communities; and the offspring born of rapes change the ethnic identity of subsequent generations. Sexual torture of women is used to cause terror sufficient to drive whole populations out of an area or to deter males from revolutionary activity.

Men and boys are targeted as well, as perpetrators attempt to eliminate retaliation from battle-age males. However, the nature of the targeting by sex is vastly different: males are typically killed, whereas women are violated – and then killed. Although sexual violence is also perpetrated against men (Féron 2014) and those who identify as LGBTQ (Flaherty et al. 2014), their rates of victimization are much lower. This discussion focuses only on crimes of sexual violence perpetrated by men against women, which not only constitute the preponderance of sexual violence crimes but also the greatest range of crimes within that category.

Margot Walstrom, Special Representative of the UN Secretary-General on Sexual Violence in Conflict, has said, "[Sexual violence] is a way of demonstrating power and control. It inflicts fear on the whole community. And it is unfortunately a very effective, cheap, and silent weapon with a long-lasting effect on every society" (Walstrom 2011). Sexual violence against women during armed conflict takes many forms: rape, forced sexual intercourse or other sexual acts with family members, forced pregnancy, sexual mutilation, sexual humiliation, medical experimentation on women's sexual and reproductive organs, forced abortion, forced sterilization, forced prostitution, being compelled to exchange sexual favors for essential items or services or for the return of children, forced sexual slavery, being the subject of pornography, and forced cohabitation. In recent years, women and girls have been raped with burning wood, knives and other objects. They have been sexually assaulted and raped by government forces and non-state actors, friendly forces, police responsible for their protection, checkpoint guards, prison guards, administrators and staff of refugee camps, fellow refugees, looters, lawless gangs, local politicians, neighbors, and family members under threat of death. They have been maimed or sexually mutilated and later killed or left to die (Schneider 2006).

Rape and sexual violence are crimes of opportunity – and crimes of impunity, with deeply-rooted precedent in the historical license to 'rape and pillage' in the context of war, and indeed, with raping and pillaging often used as incentives and rewards for other acts of atrocity. These crimes of sexual and gender-based violence are often unpunishable because the victims remain silent, unable or afraid to accuse their violators. The women bear great shame and stigma in cultures that value their 'purity' and they become pariahs and outcasts, rejected from their own communities and from their own families. In some societies, women also have few legal rights to bring charges against their perpetrators or they face life-threatening reprisals for taking action. Women and girls have too little chance for justice – or for healing.

The twentieth century is replete with sexual violence against women perpetrated in the context of genocide. Although most of the stories remain unheard, the wall of silence is slowly crumbling. For example, in 2013, during the prosecution of former Guatemalan dictator Jose Efrain Rios Montt, the first former head of state to stand trial in his own country and by his own courts for crimes against humanity, ten rape victims came forward to break the taboo surrounding their own experiences.

"This is the first time in a national court that the issue of sexual violence has been aired more than fifteen years after the war ended," said Alejandra Castillo, assistant director of Guatemala's Human Rights Legal Action Centre. "It's an issue that has until now remained invisible. It's very important because it's a recognition that sexual violence of this nature happened" (Moloney 2013). Under conditions of utmost security, brave women testified about their own rapes and one woman spoke about being forced to witness the rape of her 12-year-old daughter by four soldiers.

These stories are coming to light from conflicts that stretch across the globe and span a century. The next few sections of this chapter describe five major genocides spread across the twentieth century and ways in which women and girls were sexually victimized in each case. (NB: Many other tragic examples from the last century are not included because of space limitations, e.g. the abductions of babies and children from women in Argentina; brutal victimization of women and girls in the Democratic Republic of the Congo, referred to as 'the rape capital of the world' (Brown 2012); torture and violence against women in East Timor; and more). In each example, progress in prosecuting these crimes of sexual violence is summarized. Impunity for these crimes is slowly receding as the truth is brought forward.

Genocide of the Armenians

Sexual Violence and Tattoos

From 1915 to 1923, an estimated 1.5 million Armenians living in the Ottoman Empire perished in a genocide led by Turkish armed forces, militias, and ordinary members of the public. This death toll constituted three-fourths of the total Armenian population. The systematic use of rape during this genocide was verified by Turkish, American, Austrian, and German witnesses and officials (Dadrian 2008).

Young girls were assaulted in their homes before forced relocation or on forced marches into the Syrian desert. Deported women were subjected to murder, rape, mutilation, and abduction. Those who were abducted were eventually forced into slavery and marriage. The abducted women were tattooed on the cheek, forehead, below the lip, and on the neck and chest with tattoos that indicated the name of the owner. Each time a slave girl changed owners, additional tattoos were placed on her (Sanasarian 1989).

An eyewitness testified, "It was a very common thing for them to rape our girls in our presence. Very often they violated eight- or ten-year-old girls, and as a consequence many would be unable to walk, and they were shot." Another testified that every girl in her village aged over twelve, and some even younger, had been raped (Smith 2013).

Once the men had been separated from the women, the women were systematically raped and then killed, along with any children. According to eyewitness accounts, the practice of rape was "more or less universal" (Theriault 2007).

Prosecutions

At the urging of the British government, military trials were held in Turkey after World War I for those accused of crimes against humanity. More than one hundred Turkish officials were arrested by April 1919.

A police chief testified that he had given young girls as a gift from the governor-general to the members of the central committee. A merchant testified that not only were children being killed at the Red Crescent Hospital, but young girls were also being raped and the governor-general himself kept fifteen girls there for his own sexual gratification. A military officer testified to the British that "government officials at Trebizond picked out some of the prettiest Armenian women of the best families. After committing the worst outrages on them, they had them killed" (Dadrian 2008). The court found Lieutenant-Governor Kemal Bey guilty of murder and forced relocation; he was given the death penalty. Major Tevfik Bey, a police commander, was also found guilty and received a 16-year prison sentence (DeLaet 2005). While the number of prosecutions was trivial, at least small steps were taken to address some of the crimes of sexual violence.

The Holocaust – Ravensbruck Concentration Camp for Women

Forced Sterilization and Forced Prostitution

Although there were approximately 42,500 concentration camps in the Nazi network throughout occupied Europe (Lichtblau 2013), only one main camp was built exclusively to house women prisoners. Ravensbruck concentration camp, about 50 miles north of Berlin, began operating in 1939 and housed women from more than 30 countries, Jews and non-Jews. Over the 6 years of the camp's operations, an estimated 132,000 women were imprisoned there. Fully 90% perished from various causes: starvation, disease, torture, and extermination, either after transport to Auschwitz or other extermination centers, or through killing practices instituted at Ravensbruck itself, including poisonings and death in a gas chamber built on the premises near the end of the war.

Because Ravensbruck's population was almost exclusively women, including the guards, the practices related to sexual violence that were often carried out by the female guards are particularly heinous to me. Two practices in particular are noteworthy: medical experiments to determine the 'best' methods of forced sterilization, and the use of Ravensbruck's women prisoners as prostitutes in brothels that Heinrich Himmler established in many of the concentration camps.

In 1933, the Nazis passed the Law for the Prevention of Genetically Defective Progeny. This legalized the involuntary sterilization of people with various characteristics and encouraged the growth of the Aryan race. The Nazis sterilized about 400,000 German women (United States Holocaust Memorial Museum 2016), using techniques that were developed at Ravensbruck and other concentration camps.

Ravensbruck women were sterilized through multiple means including surgery, drugs, or severe radiation under the direction of Dr. Carl Clauberg. Clauberg's earlier experiments at Auschwitz had failed and he experimented again at Ravensbruck in the final months of the war. In particularly horrific tests, sterilization started at Ravensbruck on Roma and Sinti (also known as Gypsy) girls aged eight to ten. "Clauberg sprayed a substance into the womb under pressure and watched the effect on the fallopian tube through an X-ray screen" (Helm 2014). According to figures discovered in German records after the war, "between Christmas 1944 and February 1945, 500 Gypsies [sic] were sterilized at Ravensbruck, including 200 young girls" (Helm 2014).

In 1942 the SS began opening brothels in some of the concentration camps. Camp authorities used the women who were forced to work in these brothels as a reward to male prisoners for meeting production quotas. Most of the women were prisoners from Ravensbrück; their numbers are estimated to be at least 100. Ravensbruck doctor Gerhard Schiedlausky selected women to be prostituted at Mauthausen, Dachau, Buchenwald, and Flossenburg concentration camps. The women often were forced to service at least ten men each night (Helm 2014).

Ravensbruck Prosecutions

Following the war, national trials were held in Germany (most notably the Hamburg Ravensbruck Trials from 1946 to 1948), Poland, and the United States to prosecute the SS leadership and the female guards from Ravensbruck, many of whom were sentenced to death or to various terms of imprisonment. Ravensbruck commandant Fritz Suhren was captured and tried by a French military court in 1949 and was sentenced to death and hanged in 1950 (Cook 2006). These trials did not focus specifically on crimes of sexual violence but served to punish perpetrators for a wide range of heinous crimes against the women.

Rape Camps in Bosnia

Fifty years after the Holocaust, war broke out again in Europe in the former Yugoslavia. This conflict was marked by intense sexualized violence, most notably the creation of "rape camps" in which women were tortured and repeatedly violated.

Although violence was perpetrated by all sides in this conflict, Bosnian Serbs were responsible for most of the sexualized attacks, which were directed against Bosnian Muslim women. Estimates of the number of women raped range from 20,000 to 60,000 (Hirsch 2012).

Rape and sexualized violence were used as several different types of weapon in this war (Hirsch 2012). *For ethnic cleansing,*[1] women testified that soldiers told them, during rape, that they wanted to get the women pregnant or force them to have children who would look ethnically different from their mother (Cohen 2011). *To humiliate*, women were raped in front of their husbands and children, who were held at gunpoint; even elderly women were raped, clearly not to impregnate them but to demean them and their families. *To instill fear*, women were raped in public, which caused the flight of entire Muslim communities. Rapes were even committed outdoors, in broad daylight. *To coerce information*, women were raped to force them to divulge the whereabouts of men who were hiding in the forests. *As spoils of war*, women were raped alongside the looting and theft of private property (Hirsch 2012).

One of the most notorious sites of gang rape during the beginning of the war, April to July 1992, was in Foča, a town in southeastern Bosnia. Rape camps were

---

[1] The United Nations Commission of Experts defined "ethnic cleansing" as "rendering an area ethnically homogenous..." Ethnic cleansing was carried out in the former Yugoslavia through murder, torture, arbitrary arrest and detention, extrajudicial executions, rape and sexual assault, confinement of the civilian population, deliberate military attacks or threats of attacks on civilians and civilian areas, and wanton destruction of property. http://www.crimesofwar.org/a-z-guide/ethnic-cleansing/#sthash.Bilw6RGn.dpuf

set up in restaurants, motels, schools, and other large buildings. In one single location in Foča, more than 70 women were held captive and tortured for months.

Prosecution

In 2001, the International Criminal Tribunal for former Yugoslavia, a United Nations ad hoc tribunal established solely to adjudicate crimes that occurred during the Yugoslav war, pronounced 'guilty' verdicts for three Foča defendants accused of rape and sexual enslavement as a crime against humanity. This was the first time in history that rape had been labeled a crime against humanity (International Criminal Tribunal for the Former Yugoslavia 2001), and it represents a landmark shift in human rights law. It is not coincidental that lead prosecutors and judges in the case were women (Women, War, and Peace 2011).

Rape and AIDS in Rwanda

In 1994, during the hundred-day genocide in Rwanda, an estimated 500,000 women were raped (Aginam 2012), and thousands were intentionally infected with HIV/AIDS. Hundreds of male patients who were suffering from AIDS had been released from hospitals and formed into "rape squads" by Hutu perpetrators, with the deliberate intent to infect Tutsi and moderate Hutu women with the disease and to cause a "slow, inexorable death" (Drumbl 2012). Some observers believe that almost every woman and adolescent girl who survived the genocide was raped. Although the exact number of women raped will never be known, testimonies from survivors confirm that thousands of women were individually raped, gang-raped, raped with objects such as sharpened sticks, machetes, knives, or gun barrels, held in sexual slavery (either collectively or through forced "marriage"), or sexually mutilated (Human Rights Watch 1996).

In Rwanda, as elsewhere in the world, rape and other gender-based violations carry a severe social stigma. The physical and psychological injuries suffered by Rwandan rape survivors were aggravated by a sense of isolation and ostracism. Rwandan women who have been raped or who suffered sexual abuse generally do not dare reveal their experiences publicly, fearing that they will be rejected by their family and wider community and that they will never be able to reintegrate or to marry. Others fear retribution from their attackers if they speak out. Often, rape survivors suffer extreme guilt for having survived and having been held for rape, rather than having been executed (Human Rights Watch 1996).

Many of the rapes during the genocide resulted in what were called "pregnancies of war." According to estimates of the National Population Office, survivors of rape have given birth to between 2000 and 5000 children who are known as "enfants non-desirés" (unwanted children), "enfants de mauvais souvenir" (children of bad memories), or "children of hate" (Human Rights Watch 1996).

Prosecution of Rape

The International Criminal Tribunal for Rwanda (ICTR), a United Nations ad hoc tribunal established in the aftermath of that genocide to prosecute the perpetrators, handed down the first conviction for the use of rape as a weapon of war. It was the first time that mass rape during wartime was found to be an act of genocide (Office of the UN Special Adviser on the Prevention of Genocide 2016; Russell-Brown 2003).

Jean-Paul Akayesu of Rwanda is the first person to have been convicted for using rape as genocide. While the Yugoslav tribunal, ICTY, had classified rape under the category of a 'crime against humanity,' the Akayesu case was the first instance in which rape also became part of the definition of 'genocide.' Initially gender- based violence had not been included in the indictment against Akayesu. However, after pressure was brought to bear by non-governmental organizationsan amendment was made to the indictment. During Akayesu's trial, the ICTR affirmed that sexual violence, including rape, fell under paragraph B of the Convention on the Prevention and Punishment of the Crime of Genocide, as the rapes had been carried out with the sole intent to destroy, in whole or in part, a specific group. The ICTR also ruled that the sexual violence against the Tutsi women was a systematic part of the genocide, which was carried out against all Tutsi women. To this extent the finding against Akayesu, that rape can be an act of genocide, is a major step forward in international jurisprudence for prosecutions on charges of genocide. On September 2, 1998, Akayesu was sentenced to life imprisonment after being found guilty of genocide and crimes against humanity, which included rape. Like the result from the ICTR 'rape camp' trial, this was a major achievement in promoting justice for victims of sexual violence.

ISIS and Sexual Slavery

Sexual Violence Against Yazidis

The extremist group ISIS (aka Islamic State, ISIL, or Daesh) has perpetrated rape, sexual slavery, forced marriage, and other forms of sexual and gender violence against the Yazidis, a Kurdish ethnic group who follow an old religion that teaches a single God created seven archangels to help rule the world. The Yazidis are located primarily in the Nineveh province of northern Iraq (Joshua Project 2016).

According to a 2014 Human Rights Watch report, ISIS forces took several thousand Yazidis into custody in 2014 (Muscati 2015). Men and women were separated; the men were killed and several thousand women and girls were sold into sexual slavery and repeatedly bought and sold.

The trade in Yazidi women and girls created an ISIS infrastructure that includes a network of warehouses where victims are held, viewing rooms where they are inspected and marketed, and a fleet of buses used to transport them from one area to another.

A total of 5270 Yazidis were abducted in 2015, and at least 3144 are still being held as of this writing, according to community leaders. To handle them, the Islamic State has developed a detailed bureaucracy of sex slavery, including sales contracts notarized by the ISIS-run Islamic courts. And the practice has become an established recruiting tool to lure men from deeply-conservative Muslim societies where casual sex is taboo and dating is forbidden (Callimachi 2015).

But unlike the situation for women in Rwanda, Bosnia, and other cases examined in this chapter, Yazidi women who have been sexually violated by ISIS are promised to be welcomed back into the Yazidi community. Baba Sheikh, a Yazidi religious leader, issued a statement on September 6, 2014 welcoming escaped women to return and stating that no one should harm them. Six months later he re-issued the appeal, saying, "These survivors remain pure Yazidis and no one may injure their Yazidi faith because they were subjected to a matter outside their control.... We therefore call on everyone to cooperate with and support these victims so that they may again live their normal lives and integrate into society" (Musicati 2015). The Yazidi community in this way demonstrates that the alleviation of all suffering from mass sexualized violence includes strategies to eliminate social suffering through community acceptance of victims.

Prosecutions

A report released in 2015 by the U.N. Assistance Mission in Iraq and the U.N. High Commissioner for Human Rights concluded that actions by ISIS "may amount to war crimes, crimes against humanity, and possibly genocide" (Keating 2015). There have been an increasing number of calls for ISIS leaders to be prosecuted by the International Criminal Court (ICC, or Court) at The Hague. The ICC's chief prosecutor, Ms. Fatou Bensouda, addressed the issue, saying that while ISIS has committed "crimes of unspeakable cruelty," her jurisdiction is too narrow to launch a prosecution (ICC Office of the Prosecutor 2015). Neither Iraq nor Syria, where the crimes in question have taken place, is a party to the Rome Statute, which in 1998 established the ICC, the world's only permanent court to prosecute genocide, war crimes, and crimes against humanity. Since most of the crimes in question took place in these two countries and most known ISIS leaders are thought to be citizens of one of them, the crimes and the perpetrators fall outside the Court's jurisdiction. However, foreign fighters from ICC member countries could theoretically be tried by the ICC. The Court *can* start an investigation of crimes by outside member states if the situation is referred to the ICC by the U.N. Security Council.

Prosecutor Bensouda has said, "I remain profoundly concerned by this situation and I emphasise our collective duty to respond to the plight of victims whose rights and dignity have been violated. The international community pledged that appalling crimes that deeply shock the conscience of humanity must not go unpunished" (ICC Office of the Prosecutor 2015).

Conclusion – Gendering Justice and Alleviating Suffering

Customary international law refers to international obligations that arise from established practices and custom, as opposed to formal laws, treaties, or other related documents. Earlier sections of this chapter illustrate that customary international law is moving in the direction of prosecuting crimes of sexual violence. There are important reasons to applaud this shift. One is, without doubt, that our collective moral imperative is charged with eliminating these brutal crimes. Second is that, although nothing can ever provide closure to the survivors or their communities, prosecution establishes confidence in the rule of law and develops a social and legal infrastructure that promotes long-term peace and stability. Finally, sexual violence is a known component in enabling genocides, crimes against humanity, and war crimes to occur. The reduction or elimination of sexual and gender violence would herald an important step towards genocide prevention.

The International Criminal Court

The various cases examined in this chapter illustrate that significant efforts occurred during the twentieth century to reduce impunity for sexual violence. The most significant commitment to date has been undertaken by the International Criminal Court, the permanent tribunal in operation in The Hague, Netherlands since 2002. Most nations in the world have ratified the Rome Statute, the 1998 treaty that formed the basis for this Court. Although the United States has not yet ratified the Rome Statute, the US supports many of the Court's activities, and the challenges to address both gender justice and 'gendered justice' are central to the mission and vision of this Court.

The Rome Statute explicitly codifies crimes of sexual and gender violence as war crimes and crimes against humanity. These crimes include rape, sexual slavery, enforced prostitution, forced pregnancy, enforced sterilization, and sexual violence. In addition to the legal codification of these human rights violations that overwhelmingly apply to women and girls, the Rome Statute also requires that the Court must have an adequate representation of women judges as well as experts on gender and violence against women who are required to serve on the Court (Spees 2003).

At the International Criminal Court today, six of the 18 judges are women, which reflects women's increasing rise in the field of international criminal law as well as the achievements of the Court in enhancing 'gendered justice.' This female representation at such high levels is notable in a field where male judges typically outnumber female judges by a significant number.

In 2014, Chief Prosecutor Ms. Fatou Bensouda's office published A Policy Paper on Sexual and Gender-Based Crimes to guide the Office of the Prosecutor in combating impunity for sexual and gender-based crimes (International Criminal Court Office of the Prosecutor 2014). The policy was designed to insure not only the effective investigation and prosecution of these crimes, but to enhance access to justice for victims of these crimes through the Court. The Court's public statement accompanying release of the policy adds, "Sexual and gender-based crimes are among the gravest under the Rome Statute, and investigating and prosecuting such crimes is a key priority for the Office" (International Criminal Court Office of the Prosecutor 2014).

The Court also has a mandate to address victims' concerns, including providing safety, reparations, support services, access to the Victims' Trust Fund, and other programs that serve to alleviate, in at least a small measure, some of the harm and suffering that was experienced (Human Rights Center, UC Berkeley School of Law 2015).

United Nations

The United Nations Security Council (SC) has also taken many steps to address this historical, systemic, global problem at a world-wide level and to promote action against sexual violence in conflict. There have been seven Security Council Resolutions on this topic since 2000 (United Nations, Outreach Program on the Rwanda Genocide and the United Nations 2013):

- SC Resolution 1325 (2000) calls for increased participation of women in the prevention and resolution of conflicts, the maintenance and promotion of peace and security, and the incorporation of policies and procedures to protect women from gender-based crimes such as rape and sexual assault.
- SC Resolution 1820 (2008) calls for an end to acts of sexual violence against women and girls as a war tactic, an end to perpetrators' impunity, and protection in UN-led security endeavors including refugee camps.
- SC Resolution 1888 (2009) calls for a special UN representative to lead the UN work on this issue, to send experts to situations of particular concern, and to mandate peacekeepers to protect women and children.
- SC Resolution 1889 (2009) reaffirms Resolution 1325 and calls for greater empowerment of women and girls in post-conflict programming.
- SC Resolution 1960 (2010) asks the Secretary-General to establish monitoring, analysis, and reporting specific to conflict-related sexual violence.

- SC Resolution 2106 and 2122 (2013) calls for stronger monitoring and prevention of sexual violence in conflict and reiterates the importance of women's roles in conflict prevention, resolution, and peace-building.

In 2007, the work of thirteen separate UN agencies that all address the elimination of sexual violence was put under one umbrella: UN Action Against Sexual Violence in Conflict. The goal was to improve coordination, accountability, and to support national efforts at violence prevention and to respond to survivors' needs (Stop Rape Now: UN Action 2014)

At present, despite UN resolutions and actions, best efforts of the International Criminal Court, and changes in the definitions of genocide and crimes against humanity to include sexual violence, women and girls continue to constitute 90% of casualties of war and 80% of those who are displaced by violence. Despite their overwhelming victimization and vulnerability during times of conflict, women still comprise only 8% of participants in peace negotiations and fewer than 3% of signatories in peace negotiations (United Nations Entity for Gender Equality and the Empowerment of Women 2012).

The Legal Profession

A critical step in advancing justice for women and insuring their representation in peace processes is to increase women's presence in the highest reaches of the law and in equal proportion to their male counterparts. Equal representation of men and women in the criminal law process enhances normative legitimacy and frees decisions from gender biases, while also including the unique perspectives of both men and women in the courtroom. Although empirical studies of women judges and international courts have been quite rare, one study of ICTY sentencing practices showed that ICTY panels with female judges imposed more severe sanctions on defendants who assaulted women than did their male counterparts (Grossman 2011).

Former Inter-American Court of Human Rights Judge Cecilia Medina Quiroga has recounted how her woman's perspective affected the elicitation of facts relevant to reparations in a Guatemalan massacre and rape case (Grossman 2011). Further, women judges have, in fact, had an impact on the actual development of law and facts on international criminal courts. Judge Navi Pillay, the only woman judge on the ICTR panel trying Jean-Paul Akayesu, is widely credited with taking the initiative to question witnesses about evidence of sexual violence. Her insistence, combined with the efforts of non-governmental organizations, resulted in amending Akayesu's indictment to include charges of sexual violence (Grossman 2011).

Alleviating Suffering

The sexualized atrocities in large-scale violent conflict produce intense suffering among girls and women. This genocidal aggression results in deep mental suffering, severe physical injury and pain, and often a lifetime of humiliation and stigma. This social suffering accompanies hopelessness and despair, the essence of existential suffering. The cases of genocide examined in this chapter illustrate that the situation of civilians in armed conflict zones, especially women, remained "grim and bleak" throughout the twentieth century.

"Even war has rules," stressed Jan Eliasson, United Nations Deputy Secretary-General, as he addressed the Security Council. While progress had been made over the past 40 years in establishing international norms to enhance the protection of civilians, large numbers of civilians today are still deliberately or recklessly killed, maimed, tortured or abducted. The United Nations has announced that 2016 must be a time to turn rhetoric into concrete action to mitigate civilian suffering (Eliasson 2016). This focus is embodied at the United Nations Security Council, in countless resolutions, in programs at the International Criminal Court, and as the mission of thousands of governmental and nongovernmental organizations around the world.

The genocides profiled in this chapter together reveal that gender-based victimization and suffering continue to occur over and over again. The progress made by the International Criminal Court, other tribunals, and related initiatives of the UN give hope for the future. While these changes at the international level have been ground-breaking, sexualized violence will continue until the spirit of the international steps filters down to the national, city, community and family levels.

At a domestic level, the levels of sexual assault and violence in the United States are shocking. According to the National Sexual Violence Resource Center, one in five women will be raped at some point in their lifetimes. Annually, rape costs the U.S. more than any other crime ($127 billion). Nearly 20,000 women in the U.S. military report sexual assaults (Military Times). The Centers for Disease Control reports that one in five undergraduate women on college campuses will experience an attempted or completed sexual assault. The CDC also reports that for more than half of all women rape victims, the perpetrator was their intimate partner.

We will never end all sexual violence, and we will certainly never prosecute all cases of rape. But as this chapter demonstrates, the changes in both customary and official laws are sending a message that gender-based violence will not to be tolerated. Prevention is a more effective strategy than prosecution, and protection begins with educating young girls and boys about respectful relationships and gender equality (UN Women). The alleviation of sexualized suffering depends upon replacing gender-based aggression with gender-based justice from the couple upward to the whole of society.

"If we can travel to the moon and back—then of course we can end sexual violence." - Charlotte Isaksson, Senior Gender Advisor, Swedish Armed Forces, Sweden.

References

Aginam, O. (2012). *Rape and HIV as weapons of war*. United Nations University. http://unu.edu/publications/articles/rape-and-hiv-as-weapons-of-war.html. Accessed 27 May 2016.

Brown, C. (2012). Rape as a weapon of war in the democratic republic of the Congo. *Torture, 22*(1), 24.

Callimachi, R. (2015). ISIS enshrines a theology of rape. *New York Times*. http://www.nytimes.com/2015/08/14/world/middleeast/isis-enshrines-a-theology-of-rape.html?_r=0. Accessed 27 May 2016.

Center for Disease Control. (2016). *Sexual violence: Facts at a glance*. https://www.cdc.gov/violenceprevention/pdf/sv-datasheet-a.pdf. Accessed 7 Oct 2016.

Cohen, R. (2011). *Ethnic cleansing*. Crimes of War. http://www.crimesofwar.org/a-z-guide/ethnic-cleansing/#sthash.Bilw6RGn.dpuf. Accessed 7 Sept 2016.

Cook, B. (2006). *Women and war: A historical encyclopedia from antiquity to the present*. Santa Barbara: ABC-CLIO.

Dadrian, V. (2008). The Armenian genocide: An interpretation. In J. Winter (Ed.), *America and the Armenian genocide of 1915* (p. 3). New York: Cambridge University Press.

DeLaet, D. (2005). *The global struggle for human rights* (pp. 162–163). Belmont: Wadsworth Publishing.

Drumbl, M. (2012). 'She makes me ashamed to be a woman': The Genocide Conviction of Pauline Nyiramasuhuko, 2011. *Michigan Journal of International Law*, 2013.

Eliasson, J. (2016). *Concrete action critical to alleviating human suffering, speakers say, at security council debate on protection of civilians*. http://www.un.org/press/en/2016/sc12210.doc.htm. Accessed 28 May 2016.

Féron, É. (2014). Suffering in silence? The silencing of sexual violence against men in war torn countries. In R. Anderson (Ed.), *World suffering and quality of life* (pp. 31–44). Dordrecht: Springer.

Flaherty, M. P., Byrne, S., Tuso, H., & Matyok, T. (2014). *Gender and peacebuilding: All hands required*. Lanham: Rowman & Littlefield.

Grossman, N. (2011). Sex representation on the bench and the legitimacy of International Criminal Courts. *International Criminal Law Review*. http://www.law.qmul.ac.uk/eji/docs/73685.pdf. Accessed 28 May 2016.

Helm, S. (2014). *Ravensbruck: Life and death in Hitler's concentration camp for women* (p. 480). New York: Nan A. Talese/ Doubleday.

Hirsch, M. (2012). *Conflict profiles: Bosnia*. Women Under Siege. Women's Media Center. http://www.womenundersiegeproject.org/conflicts/profile/bosnia. Accessed 28 May 2016.

Human Right Watch. (1996). *Shattered lives: Sexual violence during the Rwandan Genocide and its Aftermath*. Human Rights Watch Women's Rights Project. https://www.hrw.org/reports/1996/Rwanda.htm. Accessed 28 May 2016.

Human Rights Center, UC Berkeley School of Law. (2015). *The victims' court? A study of 622 victim participants at the International Criminal Court*. https://www.law.berkeley.edu/wp-content/uploads/2015/04/VP_report_2015_final_exe-sum.pdf. Accessed 28 May 2016.

International Criminal Court, Office of the Prosecutor. (2014). *Policy paper on sexual and gender-based crimes*. https://www.icc-cpi.int/iccdocs/otp/OTP-Policy-Paper-on-Sexual-and-Gender-Based-Crimes--June-2014.pdf. Accessed 28 May 2016.

International Criminal Court, Office of the Prosecutor. (2015). *Statement of the Prosecutor of the International Criminal Court*. Fatou Bensouda, on the alleged crimes committed by ISIS. https://www.icc-cpi.int/Pages/item.aspx?name=otp-stat-08-04-2015-1. Accessed 28 May 2016.

International Criminal Tribunal for the Former Yugoslavia (ICTY). (2001). *Facts about Foča*. http://www.icty.org/x/file/Outreach/view_from_hague/jit_foca_en.pdf. Accessed 28 May 2016.

Joshua Project. (2016). *Yazidi in Iraq*. https://joshuaproject.net/people_groups/20455/IZ. Accessed 25 May 2016.

Keating J. (2015). *Why its' so hard to prosecute ISIS for war crimes*. Slate. http://www.slate.com/blogs/the_slatest/2015/04/08/isis_and_the_icc_why_it_s_will_be_tough_to_prosecute_the_islamic_state_for.html. Accessed 28 May 2016.

Lichtblau, E. (2013). The holocaust just got more shocking. *New York Times*. http://www.nytimes.com/2013/03/03/sunday-review/the-holocaust-just-got-more-shocking.html?_r=1. Accessed 28 May 2016.

MacKinnon, C. (2006). *Genocide's sexuality: Are women human?* (pp. 209–233). Cambridge, MA: The Belknap Press of Harvard University Press.

Military Times. (2016). *Incidents of rape in military much higher than previously reported*. http://www.militarytimes.com/story/military/pentagon/2014/12/04/pentagon-rand-sexual-assault-reports/19883155/. Accessed 7 Oct 2016.

Moloney, A. (2013). *Guatemalan war rape victims break silence in genocide trial*. http://news.trust.org//item/20130510144558-362tb?view=print. Accessed 28 May 2016.

Muscati, S. (2015). *Iraq: ISIS escapees describe systematic rape*. Human Rights Watch. https://www.hrw.org/news/2015/04/14/iraq-isis-escapees-describe-systematic-rape Accessed 28 May 2016.

National Sexual Violence Resource Center. (2016). *Statistics about sexual violence*. http://www.nsvrc.org/sites/default/files/publications_nsvrc_factsheet_media-packet_statistics-about-sexual-violence_0.pdf. Accessed 7 Oct 2016.

Office of the UN Special Adviser on the Prevention of Genocide. (2016). *Analysis framework*. http://www.un.org/en/preventgenocide/adviser/pdf/osapg_analysis_framework.pdf. Accessed 28 May 2016.

Russell-Brown, S. (2003). Rape as an act of genocide. Berkeley *Journal of International Law*, 21:2. Article 5, p. 352.

Sanasarian, E. (1989). Gender distinction in the genocidal process: A preliminary study of the Armenian Case. *Holocaust and Genocide Studies, 4*(4), 449–461.

Schnall, M. (2016). Feminist.com. "Quotes from participants at the women forging a new security: Ending sexual violence in conflict conference. http://www.feminist.com/conferencequotes.html. Accessed 28 May 2016.

Schneider, M. (2006). Women, war and darfur: Implementing and expanding gender violence justice. REVUE Asylon(s), N°1, http://www.reseau-terra.eu/article497.html. Accessed 28 May 2016.

Smith, R. (2013). Genocide and the politics of rape. In J. Apsel & E. Verdeja (Eds.), *Genocide matters: Ongoing issues and emerging perspectives* (p. 94). London/New York: Routledge.

Spees, P. (2003). Women's advocacy in the creation of the International Criminal Court: Changing the landscapes of justice and power. *Signs: Journal of Women in Culture and Society, 2*, 1233–1254.

Stop Rape Now: UN Action. (2014). http://www.stoprapenow.org/about/. Accessed 7 Sept 2016.

Theriault, H. (2007). Rethinking dehumanization in genocide. In R. G. Hovannisian (Ed.), *The Armenian genocide: Cultural and ethical legacies* (p. 30). New Brunswick: Transaction Publishers.

UN Women. (2016). *Focusing on prevention to stop the violence*. http://www.unwomen.org/en/what-we-do/ending-violence-against-women/prevention

United Nations Entity for Gender Equality and the Empowerment of Women. (2012). *Women's participation in peace negotiations: Connections between presence and influence*. http://www.unwomen.org/~/media/headquarters/attachments/sections/library/publications/2012/10/wpssourcebook-03a-womenpeacenegotiations-en.pdf. Accessed 28 May 2016.

United Nations, Outreach Programme on the Rwanda Genocide and the United Nations. (2013). *Background information on sexual violence used as a tool of war*. http://www.un.org/en/preventgenocide/rwanda/about/bgsexualviolence.shtml. Accessed 28 May 2016.

United States Holocaust Memorial Museum. (2016). The biological state: Nazi Racial Hygiene, 1933–1939. Holocaust Encyclopedia. https://www.ushmm.org/wlc/en/article.php?ModuleId=10007057. Accessed 28 May 2016.

Walstrom, M. (2011). In Schnall, M. Peace laureates take on the war on women. http://www.huffingtonpost.com/marianne-schnall/peace-laureates-take-on-t_b_876348.html. Accessed 7 Sept 2016.

Women, War, and Peace. (2011). I came to testify. PBS. http://www.pbs.org/wnet/women-war-and-peace/full-episodes/i-came-to-testify/. Accessed 7 Sept 2016.

Chapter 20
Support Programs for Male Survivors of Conflict-Related Sexual Violence

Élise Féron

Introduction

Instances of sexual violence against men have been documented in a great number of conflicts and wars, both ancient and contemporary. A study conducted by Johnson et al. (2010) has, for example, established that 23.6% of men and boys living in Eastern DRC (39.7% of women and girls) have experienced some form of conflict-related sexual violence. In Bosnia, a survey of 6000 concentration-camp inmates in Sarajevo found that 80% of men reported having been raped during the war (Stemple 2009: 613). In Liberia, Johnson, et al. (2008) have shown that approximately one-third of adult male ex-combatants in their sample had experienced sexual violence. Numerous cases have also been reported in Colombia where 15% of victims of conflict-related sexual violence are male (Quijano and Kelly 2012: 490), in Chile (Oosterhoff et al. 2004: 68), in El Salvador (Leiby 2012), in Afghanistan and Syria (UN 2015), in Kashmir (Sengupta 2011); also in Sri Lanka (Sooka 2014), in Sudan and South Sudan (UN 2015), and in the Central African Republic (UN 2015), among many others cases.

The extent of suffering generated by sexual violence against men in conflict zones is increasingly recognized by the international community and especially by the UNHCR, which has issued guidelines in July 2012 on how to identify and support male victims of rape and other forms of sexual violence in conflict settings and displacement situations (UNHCR 2012). The challenges in dealing with that suffering are significant and varied, and pertain mostly to the medical, psychosocial, legal and social consequences for the survivors. But because the suffering induced by wartime sexual violence against men has long been ignored and silenced at the international and national levels, its alleviation has up to very recently not even been an issue considered worth addressing.

É. Féron (✉)
Tampere Peace Research Institute, University of Tampere, Tampere, Finland
e-mail: Elise.Feron@uta.fi

R.E. Anderson (ed.), *Alleviating World Suffering*, Social Indicators Research Series 67, DOI 10.1007/978-3-319-51391-1_20

As awareness grows, voices in the academia, the NGO and the policy fields have started to point at shortcomings and limits in existing programs dealing with wartime sexual violence, and to ask for responses targeting the specific needs of male survivors to be conceptualized and implemented (see for instance Carpenter 2006, Gorris 2015, Sivakumaran 2010). So far however, responses are very limited, and specific support mechanisms for male survivors are almost nonexistent in conflict zones, where most humanitarian organizations focus on female survivors of sexual violence. Only a few survivors groups have spearheaded programs directly and specifically addressing the suffering induced by sexual violence against men. But funding is hard to come by, and numerous social, cultural and technical obstacles hamper these initiatives.

After briefly presenting the general characteristics and specificities of suffering induced by wartime sexual violence against men, this contribution will review existing local and international programs and initiatives for the relief of male survivors, and will highlight the important role played by organizations and groups led by survivors themselves. What are the strengths, promises, shortcomings and limits of these programs and organizations? By putting the stress on the challenges faced by relief programs, this contribution intends to underscore the necessity for a long-term prevention approach, as well as the importance of a combined study and strategy for alleviating the suffering of both male and female survivors of wartime sexual violence.

Wartime Sexual Violence Against Men

Wartime sexual violence, including rape, sexual torture, sexual mutilation, sexual humiliation and sexual slavery, is an important feature of most contemporary conflicts. While most policies as well as much of the existing literature have shown a tendency to treat sexual violence as a women's issue, recent research and empirical evidence have drawn attention to the significant proportion of males among survivors of wartime sexual violence and sexual torture (Carpenter 2006, Sivakumaran 2007, Johnson et al. 2010, Mervyn et al. 2011). Admittedly, there are many similarities between the needs of male and female victims of conflict-related sexual violence, but the alleviation of the suffering of male survivors faces specific challenges, mostly related to underreporting, stigma and shame in contexts where conceptions of masculinity render the sexual brutalization of men unthinkable.

Suffering is not just physical; it often co-occurs with mental and social suffering (Anderson 2014: 8–27). In the case of wartime sexual violence, the physical (e.g. fistula, HIV infection), mental (e.g. anxiety, humiliation) and social (e.g. social rejection, distrust) consequences for female victims are already well documented (see for instance Okot et al. 2005). Male survivors suffer from various types of physical pain too, related to castration, genital infections, ruptures of the rectum, physical impotence, etc., but also from sexually transmitted diseases and HIV. Physical injuries are often the main reason why survivors decide to overcome their shame and to seek support, but because of the lack of medical knowledge and training on wartime sexual violence on men, many male survivors' physical symptoms are not addressed in time (Féron 2015). The suffering created by sexual violence on men is also mental, emotional, and psychological, and pertains to the trauma, shame, guilt, and confusion that survivors experience. Alleviating that type of psychological suffering requires a good knowledge and understanding not only of post traumatic disorder symptoms, but also of the relevant gender roles and representations that male survivors feel they are not able to uphold anymore. They often blame themselves for what happened, and fear that they will no longer be able to behave as a man "should." In addition, many male survivors find it difficult to open up and to express their emotions, especially in societies where this is seen as a feminine trait. Psychological pain is accompanied, and reinforced, by the suffering that they also experience at the societal level. When they speak out about what happened to them, they are often discriminated against, accused of being homosexual, they face marital problems and might even lose their job. This in turn can lead to further destructive behavior like antisocial behavior, alcohol and drug abuse and, in the most extreme cases, suicide.

Because of the interrelated nature of these different aspects of suffering caused by wartime sexual violence against men, support for survivors has to be conceived in a holistic way and not merely focus on the alleviation of physical pain. The UNHCR guidelines on "Working with men and boys survivors of sexual and gender-based violence in forced displacement" (2012: 10) for instance, lists beyond medical treatment, mental and social health issues, livelihood support, and legal protection as survivors' major needs. Similarly, Chris Dolan, the director of the Refugee Law Project that has spearheaded several support initiatives in this field, underscores the importance of a series of key challenges such as "medical and psychosocial service provision, legal redress (both immediate, and in terms of transitional justice measures after a conflict is over), survivor organization (particularly to recover lost voice, lost livelihoods and lost respect in their communities), and dealing with community shaming so that the community can once again become a source of support to survivors rather than the driver of stigmatization" (Refugee Law Project 2013: 10–11).

As we will see, offering such support to male survivors in conflict zones is particularly challenging, not least because in such contexts sexual violence is perpetrated alongside other types of violence, which leads to the prioritization of the alleviation of physical pain over other dimensions of suffering.

International Programs and Measures for the Relief of Male Survivors

Over the past few years the international community's awareness of the existence, and extent of conflict-related sexual violence against men has been steadily growing. A series of important international reports have shed light on this phenomenon, for example the Final Report of the UN Commission of Experts on the war in former Yugoslavia (UN 1994), which recognized the existence and extent of sexual violence and torture against men, or more recently the UN Security Council Report published in 2015 on "Conflict-related sexual violence" (UN 2015), which explicitly recognizes the existence of sexual and gender-based violence against men and boys, especially in detention settings (§6, p. 2). The report documents specific cases of sexual violence against men that occurred in 2014 in Afghanistan, the Central African Republic, the Democratic Republic of the Congo, South Sudan, Sudan and Syria, among others. Similar cases had been documented in previous UN yearly reports on conflict-related sexual violence.

However, most measures proposed at the international level do not target male survivors specifically and seem geared toward the prosecution of acts of sexual violence rather than toward the provision of support for survivors, such as the recently published "Guidelines for Investigating Conflict-Related Sexual and Gender-Based Violence Against Men and Boys," compiled by the Institute for Criminal Investigations (2016). The objective is to help criminal justice and human rights investigators to monitor, document, and investigate wartime sexual and gender-based violence against men and boys. Similarly, regarding the UN yearly reports on conflict-related sexual violence for instance, measures range from training for UN peacekeepers to the deployment of Women's Protection Advisers in Democratic Republic of the Congo and Côte d'Ivoire, and to the setting up of early warning indicators of conflict-related sexual violence to be used by UN forces in countries like South Sudan. The UN has also been providing technical support to relevant countries through the training of envoys, mediators, and mediation experts whose main task is to ensure that provisions on sexual violence are included in peace and ceasefire agreements (§89, p. 26). The Secretary General Report includes only one paragraph addressing the issue of support to survivors, stating the importance of ensuring "differentiated and appropriate services" for male survivors, but it remains very vague, stating responsibilities without guidelines for practical implementation: "I encourage Member States, donors and regional organizations: (a) To support the delivery of multisectoral assistance for survivors of sexual violence, including the full range of sexual and reproductive health services; HIV awareness and response measures; and psychosocial, legal and livelihood support, ensuring differentiated and appropriate responses for children and male survivors" (§100, p. 29).

The aforementioned UNHCR report (UNHCR 2012), which directly focuses on the alleviation of the suffering of male survivors of conflict-related sexual violence, stands out as an exception among these documents primarily interested in prosecution and in raising awareness on wartime sexual violence in general. This report, published in 2012, provides guidelines for staff and other aid workers on how to identify and support male victims of rape and of other types of sexual violence in conflict and displacement situations. The report underscores the reasons for the vulnerability of refugee men and boys, and "provides guidance on how to access survivors, facilitate reporting, provide protection and deliver essential medical, legal and social services" (p. 2). It also advocates for the setting up of inclusive programs for both male and female survivors of sexual violence (p. 8), and for the creation of peer support groups (p. 13) which, as we will see, have so far constituted one of the most effective, though scattered, sources of support for survivors.

Though it undoubtedly represents great progress toward the alleviation of male survivors' suffering, one of the main limits of this report, however, is that it does not develop proactive strategies to prevent sexual violence against men from occurring. This is representative of the generally reactive rather than proactive attitude of the international community on conflict-related sexual violence against both women and men. In this perspective, it is quite complicated to assess the real impact that this report has on practices. It seems that most health-care professionals working on the ground are not aware of the existence of the UNHCR Guidelines, or find them too vague to really help, be it in refugee camps located in conflict areas, or in Western countries' structures providing healthcare services for refugees fleeing war.

Other available guidelines or toolkits for providing medical, mental health and psychosocial support to survivors of wartime sexual violence, like those published by the World Health Organization in 2012, or by the Australian Civil-Military Centre in 2014, only mention male victims of sexual violence in passing. Similarly, the UN-led campaign "Stop Rape Now" (UN action against sexual violence in conflict) does not seem interested in male survivors and is rather structured as a campaign against conflict-related sexual violence against women (Grey and Shepherd 2012).

Fortunately, over the past few years, major international nongovernmental organizations like Physicians for Human Rights or Médecins Sans Frontières (MSF) have started to open up their programs and awareness campaigns to the plight of male survivors. For instance in 2015 MSF launched its first comprehensive program dedicated to survivors of sexual violence in Port Harcourt in Nigeria, which includes among other initiatives an awareness campaign targeting different facilities including universities, schools, and health clinics, and which organizes discussions around male sexual abuse. In July 2014 MSF also opened in Bangui (Central African Republic) a medical and psychological care service for victims of sexual violence, where male survivors are also cared for. Similar initiatives have been implemented by the International Rescue Committee and other international NGOs like Care, which has developed a Training Manual on "Gender Peace and Conflict," acknowledging male victimhood in situations of conflict-related gender-based violence. Resistance to this inclusion is, however, still strong among regional organizations. In its Wababa project on gender and masculinity,[1] Heal Africa for instance only refers to men as either indirect victims (men witnessing female relatives being sexually abused) or perpetrators of sexual violence.

In parallel to these initiatives directly implemented in conflict areas, the alleviation of the suffering generated by sexual violence and sexual torture is an important issue for refugees fleeing war zones toward Western countries, too. In receiving Western countries however, the level of awareness on these issues is still very low, and when the non-physical consequences of sexual violence are addressed, it is in

[1] Wababa Project (accessed 25 February 2016): http://www.healafrica.org/wababa

centers specialized in support for torture victims in general, and not for survivors of sexual violence specifically, such as the Centre for Torture Survivors in Finland. Major institutions such as the International Rehabilitation Council for Torture Victims, located in Denmark, have also developed training programs such as the project PROTECT-ABLE,[2] which aims at improving the access to psychological and medical care for asylum seekers and refugees who have been victims of torture.

The Major Role Played by Local and Survivors' Organizations

On the ground, too, most support programs remain entirely focused on female survivors, and very few local organizations have developed specific programs or premises dedicated to the alleviation of the suffering of male survivors. According to a study conducted by Del Zotto and Jones at the beginning of the 2000-decade, out of more than 4000 non-governmental groups tackling conflict-related sexual violence, "only 3% mention the experiences of males at all in their programs and informational literature. About one quarter of the groups explicitly deny that male-on-male violence is a serious problem" (Del Zotto and Jones 2002). If things seem to have evolved slightly over the past decade, it remains that most of the grassroots organizations still provide services to women and girls only. In Burundi, for instance, where numerous cases of sexual torture against men have been documented since 2015 (see Amnesty International 2015), organizations like Nturengaho still focus exclusively and explicitly on girls and women. Sometimes this reluctance to offer support to male survivors can be explained by the agenda of donors who usually prioritize support to women, or by the religious background of these organizations.

In such a context, the emergence over the past 5 years of structured groups of male survivors seeking to organize themselves and to provide support to other survivors constitutes a major development. In many ways, survivors' organizations are well ahead of any public initiative or program in this field. Most of these groups are located in Uganda and in the broader Great Lakes Region of Africa, though there are a few in Asia as well, such as First Step Cambodia. The Makerere University-based Refugee Law Project supports several of these survivors groups, like Men of Hope and Men of Courage, both founded in 2011, and Men of Peace, founded in 2013. Their membership varies from a few dozen to several hundreds, almost all recruited in the refugee camps scattered throughout Uganda. These survivors-led organizations share similar goals, like raising awareness on wartime sexual violence and on its consequences, protecting male survivors, advocating for them, and providing medical and psychosocial support. In addition, most of them have set up educational programs for male survivors to help them become more autonomous and self-

[2] PROTECT-ABLE Project (accessed 25 February 2016): http://protect-able.eu/

confident. These organizations also liaise with donors, and some also support projects for survivors with disabilities, by building houses, for example.

The Men of Peace and Men of Hope associations provide good illustrations of the support that can be offered to male survivors of wartime sexual violence. Their members (around 200 registered members each), are refugees settled in camps in Uganda who have experienced conflict-related sexual abuse and/or have been forced to participate in such acts. Membership is of course voluntary, and those who wish to join usually have to write a letter to the association before being interviewed. Though these groups do not provide direct medical treatment such as surgery, they support their members at the material and psychological levels, and also organize visits for those who are hospitalized (Men of Peace Association 2014). Beyond support to survivors, their main activities center on raising awareness or advocacy work conducted among refugee-hosting communities in Uganda. Their members also receive training in various relevant areas such as human rights, trauma counselling, issues related to forced migration, sexual and gender-based violence, post-traumatic stress disorder, and so on (Men of Hope Refugee Association Uganda 2015). As such, they can be considered as a form of "therapeutic activism" (Edström et al. 2016), and they provide invaluable support to male victims of sexual violence, especially in a context where many male survivors face significant challenges, particularly at the legal level. In countries like Uganda, where an Anti-Homosexuality Bill was passed by Parliament in December 2013, and where some judges refuse to distinguish between consensual and nonconsensual same-sex relationships, male survivors are often assumed to be homosexual, which threatens their security. Organizing collectively can help improve survivors' psychological and material security, even though heightened security threats have sometimes been reported (see for instance Men of Peace Association 2014).

But the impact of these survivors-led organizations is often geographically limited, notably for financial reasons. The general lack of public awareness on wartime sexual violence against men impedes fund raising, and the low socioeconomic status of their members prevents them from relying on members' financial contributions. Their capacity for reaching out to other male survivors is also often very limited, and many operate only within the limits of a single refugee camp. In this perspective, the support offered by larger organizations like the Refugee Law Project or the African Centre for the Treatment and Rehabilitation of Torture Victims, also located in Uganda, is paramount. In addition to providing direct support to male survivors, these organizations cover the expenses related to many reconstructive surgery operations, and to related medical treatments. They also contribute to raising awareness on conflict-related sexual violence against men by organizing training programs targeted toward health services or policy makers, and they have participated in the launch of several research initiatives, such as the "South-South Institute on Sexual Violence against Men and Boys in Conflict and Displacement" which was launched in April 2013 in Kampala. However, neither of these organizations can afford to cover the other related costs for the survivors, such as compensation for job loss, provision of food, or housing costs, which therefore constitute areas where major progress is needed.

Main Challenges and Obstacles to Alleviation

Recent changes in the international narratives on wartime sexual violence have shed light on the plight of male survivors, though they still largely remain under the shadow of female survivors. But as we have seen, it seems that these changes in international discourses have largely failed to translate at the policy and programming level, where support for survivors remains overwhelmingly concerned with female survivors only. While some support is offered to male victims of rape in many Western countries, they are hardly transferrable to conflict settings, where sexual and gender-based violence displays specific characteristics, is arguably more frequent, and where survivors face different challenges following their ordeal. By contrast, support facilities for male survivors in conflict zones are lacking (with the above-mentioned exception of survivors-led groups), and most relief programs focusing on sexual violence against women, including the most important ones like the previously mentioned "Stop Rape Now" UN campaign, still ignore the plight of male survivors.

One of the reasons for this obliviousness lies in the role played by stereotypes, according to which men cannot be victims of sexual and gender-based violence. When they are not trapped in the perpetrator role, men are seen as strong and able to defend themselves. And even when the possibility of sexual violence against men is acknowledged, female survivors are always presented as making up the "vast majority" of victims (a highly credible assumption, but based on reported cases and not on "actual" figures, which are in any case almost impossible to gather), thus *de facto* dismissing the importance of the suffering of male survivors. This dismissal in turn hampers the setting up of dedicated prevention and support programs: "The absent presence of masculinity and the silencing effects of the logic of 'the vast majority' in scholarly literature on war-time rape denies the materiality of the violated male body. For us, this is problematic, as without envisioning the violated male body we can neither hope to prevent its violation nor seek redress for violence committed against it." (Grey and Shepherd 2012: 122).

Another reason explaining the lack of support for male survivors pertains to the lack of data and of information available on prevalence rates, mostly due to underreporting. Programming is indeed often based on statistical reports, and in the case of wartime sexual violence against men, reports are rare and scattered. In addition, the number of male victims who report sexual assault depends greatly on whether the clinic or hospital has the reputation to treat those issues, which feeds a kind of vicious circle—male victims being more likely to avoid places that have a reputation of treating women only, thus reinforcing existing patterns. What is more, male survivors are ashamed and sometimes feel responsible for what happened to them, and thus only come forward when their injuries are life threatening. Most other cases seem to be left unreported, and the level of reporting for wartime sexual violence against men is generally thought to be significantly lower than for women and girls (Sivakumaran 2007). Rather than seeking help, most male survivors isolate themselves, and, because they fear being rejected by their own communities and families, and possibly also being targeted for retaliation by perpetrators, try to hide what happened to them. This reluctance to speak about what happened is not only maintaining the level of reporting, and therefore of awareness, at very low levels, but it is also impeding the provision of proper support and care: "Some male survivors do not want the person they have confided in to share the information further, making referrals for additional service provisions problematic" (Refugee Law Project 2013: 26).

One of the most immediate consequences of this low level of reporting and general lack of awareness is an un-preparedness of medical facilities and staff for dealing with cases of sexual violence against men. Medical staff and health care professionals lack training with regard to detecting, identifying, and tackling the injuries related to this type of violence, and many doctors even seem to ignore that such cases exist (Féron 2015: 37). Because most services for survivors of sexual and gender-based violence are located in gynecology departments, many male survivors are referred to them, but medical staff in these departments is not trained and prepared to take care of psychological and physical suffering induced by sexual violence on males. The knowledge and training about how to deal with survivors of violence and torture is very low, and most of the time limited to general guidelines like the 2004 Istanbul Protocol (UNHCR 2004). Male survivors of sexual violence often have very different needs—different kinds of physical injuries—from female survivors, for whom existing programs and facilities have been designed. Some male survivors also find it difficult to talk to female service providers, who often are the majority in departments offering support to sexual violence survivors. All of this is further complicated by the fact that most health systems in conflict-affected countries are underfunded and understaffed. When they are still operating, hospitals and clinics struggle to cope with the number of patients and often prioritize those who present the most serious diseases and injuries, and also those whom they think they can really help.

Because of the lack of awareness and training in how to deal with sexual violence against men, and because humanitarian assistance also tends to prioritize female survivors, male survivors are often left in limbo. And even in the few instances when their physical injuries are taken care of, the widespread understanding of health as absence of disease, overlooking the psychosocial aspects of relief, prevents the other dimensions of their suffering from being addressed and alleviated. If, as we have seen, survivors-led organizations existing in some countries like Uganda provide psychological support, the deep social impact that sexual violence can have on male survivors seems much more complicated to tackle, especially in terms of lost livelihoods and work incapacity. Alleviating that type of suffering lies well beyond the competences and expertise of medical services, but it does not seem to be tackled by any other public or private institution or initiative either.

The great majority of male survivors of wartime sexual violence thus have access to scattered and limited support, if at all. But if the few NGO-led programs specifically targeting wartime sexual violence—be it against men or women—admittedly offer much better support, they also display a potentially major flaw, which is to focus exclusively on that type of violence and hence neglect other forms of violence that are perpetrated during conflict times, and to which sexual violence is tightly connected. This type of approach might lead to a situation where sexual violence is treated as disconnected from the other experiences of war that the person has had, and which are paramount for making sense of sexual violence itself. Taking the broader context of conflict and violence into account seems essential for helping survivors overcome their trauma. As with every person who has been victim of any form of torture or violence, male survivors of wartime sexual violence strive to understand why this has happened to them (McCLure 2015). Whether these acts are committed in a random fashion, or can be explained by the specific religious, political, or ethnic belonging of the victim, they ultimately only make sense in the broader context of the war situation and the spread of uncontrolled violence. Wartime sexual and gender-based violence is tightly connected to other forms of violence, and is a highly multicausal phenomenon linked, among other factors, to specific gender roles and images in the relevant society, but also to impunity, poverty, and so on. Furthermore, the other experiences of violence that survivors have faced often make it more difficult for them to recover from the physical and psychological trauma entailed by sexual violence. Having been forced to leave their country or region of origin, having lost several or all members of their family, having witnessed atrocities—all dramatically hamper their capacity to deal with, and recover from, the suffering induced by sexual violence.

Conclusion: The Need for Longer-Term Prevention Strategies

What current support programs at local, national, and international levels obviously lack is an emphasis on longer-term prevention. Admittedly, programs addressing conflict-related sexual violence against women have just started developing prevention strategies, focusing on education, awareness-raising activities and on associating men "as central agents of change."[3] It is therefore no surprise that support programs for male survivors, which are still in their infancy, have not yet worked much on the issue of prevention. But since wartime sexual violence against women and against men are both tightly related to how masculinities are built in times of war, and in particular to models of militarized and dominant masculinities, it would be worth considering the implementation of prevention programs addressing all types of wartime sexual violence in a holistic way. This would necessitate acknowledging and better understanding the core relationship between conceptions of masculinity and the conduct of war, while taking into account the fact that male and female survivors have specific needs in terms of support.

[3] Wababa Project developed by Heal Africa (checked on 25 February 2016): http://www.healafrica.org/wababa

Several obstacles stand in the way of such an approach, though. One is that when it comes to conflict-related sexual violence, programming is still too often done in terms of either/or, as if including male survivors in the overall picture would somehow undermine the hard-won advances in the fight against sexual and gender-based violence against women. This is particularly true of prevention activities, as explained by Sivakumaran (2010: 268): "When it is at the level of heightening awareness and responsiveness, the language is inclusive—all civilians, including women and children. However, as the provision goes on, and when the matter shifts to the more onerous prevention of sexual violence, the objects of protection are exclusively women and girls." Another obstacle lies in the fact that the phenomenon of wartime sexual violence is not well understood, and too often boiled down to "rape as a weapon of war" explanations, which overlook its relation with the wider structures of power in society, between but also within groups. More generally, preventive policies are notoriously difficult to implement in conflict settings, where they are seen as too complicated to design and set up, expensive, and where their efficiency is difficult to demonstrate (Ackermann 2003). Harnessing support for prevention on the part of the policy-making community, and also of donors, is, however, imperative if we want to significantly reduce the suffering induced by wartime sexual violence against both men and women.

References

Ackermann, A. (2003). The idea and practice of conflict prevention. *Journal of Peace Research, 40*(3), 339–347.

Amnesty International. (2015, August). *Just tell me what to confess to, torture and other ill-treatment by Burundi's police and intelligence service since April 2015*, Amnesty International. http://www.amnestyusa.org/sites/default/files/burundi_torture_report.pdf. Accessed 03 Mar 2016.

Anderson, R. E. (2014). *Human suffering and quality of life, conceptualizing stories and statistics*. New York: Springer.

Carpenter, R. C. (2006). Recognizing gender-based violence against civilian men and boys in conflict situations. *Security Dialogue, 37*(1), 83–103.

Del Zotto, A. & Adam, J. (2002). *Male-on-Male sexual violence in wartime: Human Rights' Last Taboo?* Paper presented to the Annual Convention of the International Studies Association (ISA), New Orleans, LA, 23–27 March. http://adamjones.freeservers.com/malerape.htm. Accessed 29 Feb 2016.

Edström, J., Dolan, C., Shahrokh, T., & Onen, D. (2016). Therapeutic activism: Men of Hope Refugee Association Uganda. Breaking the silence over male rape in conflict-related sexual violence. *Institute of Development Studies*, Evidence Report no 182.

Féron, É. (2015). Suffering in silence? The silencing of sexual violence against men in war torn Countries. In R. Anderson (Ed.), *World suffering and quality of life* (pp. 31–44). New York: Springer.

Gorris, E. A. P. (2015). Invisible victims? Where are male victims of conflict-related sexual violence in international law and policy? *European Journal of Women's Studies, 22*(4), 412–427.

Grey, R., & Shepherd, L. J. (2012). Stop rape now?: Masculinity, responsibility, and conflict-related sexual violence. *Men and Masculinities, 16*(1), 115–135.

Institute for Criminal Investigations. (2016). *Guidelines for investigating conflict-related sexual and gender-based violence against men and boys*. http://refugeelawproject.org/files/others/IICI_Guidelines_for_Investigating_Conflict_Related_SGBV_against_Men_and_Boys.pdf. Accessed 29 Feb 2016.

Johnson, K., Asher, J., Rosborough, S., et al. (2008). Association of combatant status and sexual violence with health and mental health outcomes in post-conflict Liberia. *JAMA, 300*(6), 676–690.

Johnson, K., et al. (2010). Association of sexual violence and human rights violations with physical and mental health in territories of the Eastern Democratic Republic of the Congo. *JAMA, 304*(5), 553–562.

Leiby, M. (2012). The promise and peril of primary documents: Documenting wartime sexual violence in El Salvador and Peru. In M. Bergsmo, A. Butenschø Skre, & E. J. Wood (Eds.), *Understanding and proving international sex crimes* (pp. 315–366). Beijing: Torkel Opsahl Academic EPublisher.

McClure, N. R. (2015). Injured bodies, silenced voices: Reclaiming personal Trauma and the narration of pain in Northern Ireland. *Peace and Change, a Journal of Peace Research, 40*(4), 497–516.

Men of Hope Refugee Association Uganda. (2015). *We believe in the future*. http://www.refugeelawproject.org/files/others/men_of_hope_magazine_may_2015.pdf. Accessed 22 June 2016.

Men of Peace Association. (2014). *Together we can, 2014 activity report*. http://www.refugeelawproject.org/files/others/Men_of_Peace_2014_report.pdf. Accessed 29 Feb 2016.

Mervyn, C., et al. (2011). Sexual and gender based violence against men in the Democratic Republic of Congo: Effects on survivors, their families and the community. *Medicine, Conflict and Survival, 27*(4), 227–246.

Okot, A. C., Amony, I., & Otim, G. (2005). *Suffering in silence: A study of Sexual and Gender Based Violence (SGBV) In Pabbo Camp, Gulu District, Northern Uganda*. UNICEF, District Sub-Working Group on SGBV. http://reliefweb.int/sites/reliefweb.int/files/resources/BEFB77D29CC17FE74925702200095601-unicef-uga-15jun.pdf. Accessed 3 Mar 2016.

Oosterhoff, P., Zwanikken, P., & Ketting, E. (2004). Sexual torture of men in croatia and other conflict situations: An open secret. *Reproductive Health Matters, 12*(23), 68–77.

Quijano, A. A., & Kelly, J. (2012). A tale of two conflicts: An unexpected reading of sexual violence in conflict through the cases of Colombia and Democratic Republic of the Congo. In M. Bergsmo, A. Butenschø Skre, & E. J. Wood (Eds.), *Understanding and proving international sex crimes* (pp. 437–493). Beijing: Torkel Opsahl Academic EPublisher.

Refugee Law Project. (2013). *Report on the 1st South-south institute on sexual violence against men and boys in conflict and displacement*. Kampala, refugee law project, 8–12 April, 10–11. http://refugeelawproject.org/files/others/SSI_2013_report.pdf. Accessed 29 February 2016.

Sengupta, S. (2011). Kashmir's Abu Ghraib. In S. Kak (Ed.), *Until my freedom has come: The New Intifada in Kashmir* (pp. 71–85). New Delhi: Penguin Books.

Sivakumaran, S. (2007). Sexual violence against men in armed conflict. *The European Journal of International Law, 18*(2), 253–276.

Sivakumaran, S. (2010). Lost in translation: UN responses to sexual violence against men and boys in situations of armed conflict. *International Review of the Red Cross, 92*(877), 259–277.

Sooka, Y. (2014). *An unfinished war: Torture and sexual violence in Sri Lanka 2009–2014*. The Bar Human Rights Committee of England and Wales (BHRC) and The International Truth & Justice Project, Sri Lanka.

Stemple, L. (2009). Male rape and human rights. *Hastings Law Journal, 60*, 605–645.

UN. (1994). *Final report of the commission of experts established pursuant to Security Council Resolution 780 (1992)*. http://www.icty.org/x/file/About/OTP/un_commission_of_experts_report1994_en.pdf. Accessed 29 Feb 2016.

UN. (2015). *Conflict-related sexual violence*. http://www.securitycouncilreport.org/atf/cf/%7B65BFCF9B-6D27-4E9C-8CD3-CF6E4FF96FF9%7D/s_2015_203.pdf. Accessed 29 Feb 2016.

UNHCR. (2004). *Istanbul protocol. Manual on the effective investigation and documentation of torture and other cruel, inhuman or degrading treatment or punishment*. http://www.ohchr.org/Documents/Publications/training8Rev1en.pdf. Accessed 29 Feb 2016.

UNHCR. (2012). *Working with men and boy survivors of sexual and gender-based violence in forced displacement*. http://www.refworld.org/cgi-bin/texis/vtx/rwmain?docid=5006aa262. Accessed 29 Feb 2016.

Chapter 21
Success in Reducing Female Genital Cutting: A Multilevel Framework of Social Change

Elizabeth Heger Boyle and Joseph Svec

FGC as a Form of Suffering

The World Health Organization (World Health Organization 2016) recognizes four types of FGC. Type 1, known as clitoridectomy, is the partial or total removal of the clitoris or, in rarer cases, the hood of the clitoris. Type 2, known as excision, is the partial or total removal of the clitoris, the labia minora, and sometimes the labia majora. Type 3 is infibulation, the most serious form of FGC, which involves the narrowing of the vaginal opening by cutting and repositioning the labia to create a covering seal of skin. This type may or may not involve the removal of the clitoris. The WHO also recognizes a fourth category that includes other procedures imposed on female genitalia for non-medical purposes, such as pricking, piercing, scraping or cauterizing.

FGC has been documented in parts of Indonesia, Malaysia, among the Bedouin of Israel, and in several other countries, but the practice occurs primarily in 29 African countries and in migrant communities from those countries (UNICEF 2013). Within Africa, FGC prevalence and types vary by regional concentrations (Yoder et al. 2013). For example, in the Horn of Africa, including Djibouti, Egypt, Eritrea, Somalia, and Sudan, the prevalence of FGC, and Type 3 in particular, are very high. Fifty-nine percent of all African women who have experienced FGC live in this region of the continent. Another concentration occurs in western Africa, with rates ranging from 72 to 96% across Burkina Faso, the Gambia, Guinea, and Mali (a set of culturally-similar countries), and Liberia and Sierra Leone. FGC

E.H. Boyle (✉)
Faculty of Sociology, University of Minnesota, Minneapolis, MN 55455, USA
e-mail: Boyle014@umn.edu

J. Svec
Department of Sociology, University of Minnesota, Minneapolis, MN 55455, USA
e-mail: Svecx006@umn.edu

R.E. Anderson (ed.), *Alleviating World Suffering*, Social Indicators Research Series 67, DOI 10.1007/978-3-319-51391-1_21

occurs across other sub-Saharan African countries but rates are often much lower there—below 50% of women. In these countries, FGC is typically performed within particular religious or ethnic groups.

When girls are cut, they will experience severe pain if the procedure is completed without anesthesia, and they will experience pain and discomfort during the healing process. Immediate health risks are hemorrhaging, infection, and shock (World Health Organization 2016). Later in life, women who have been cut are more likely to experience urinary tract and other types of infections (WHO 2016). The intended health effect of most forms of FGC is to reduce or eliminate female orgasm. FGC also negatively affects some obstetric outcomes, increasing the chances of prolonged labor, obstetric tears, post-partum hemorrhaging, and difficult deliveries (Berg and Underland 2013).

Importantly, the nature and seriousness of FGC's physical consequences depend greatly on the type of cutting. The side effects of infibulation (Type 3) are much more serious than the health consequences of Type 1. Yount and Carrera (2006) found, for example, that Type 3 FGC increased primary infertility among women, while Type 1 and Type 2 FGC had no effect on fertility. A multi-country study run by the World Health Organization also found that Type 3 FGC increased the chances, during deliveries, of an infant having to be resuscitated and of infant death immediately after birth. While eliminating FGC altogether would be the most effective approach to alleviate suffering, transitions from Type 3 to Type 1 FGC also represents progress.

Given the physical suffering involved, a common question is why girls are subject to such procedures. In communities where FGC occurs, FGC plays an important social role for women's future well-being. Often framed as a religious requirement, FGC functions as a physical marker that enhances marriage prospects for girls. FGC as a physical alteration constitutes an important social marking which makes girls more hygienic and attractive (UNFPA-UNICEF 2014). Moreover, reducing women's sexual pleasure through the procedure also acts to eliminate women's promiscuity, enhancing girls' marriageability by marking one's femininity and purity. Given the context of many resource poor communities, as well as women's often economically dependent roles as domestic caretakers, marriageability can be essential for their survival. From the perspective of the communities where FGC occurs, FGC is physical suffering designed to offset social suffering. Until recently, FGC was a deeply entrenched social institution in many places where it occurred. Consider the field notes of American ethnographers Lane and Rubenstein (1996: 35) in Egypt in the 1990s:

> In the rural Egyptian hamlet where we have conducted fieldwork some women were not familiar with groups that did not circumcise their girls. When they learned that the female researcher was not circumcised, their response was disgust mixed with joking laughter. They wondered how she could have thus gotten married and questioned how her mother could have neglected such an important part of her preparation for womanhood. It was clearly unthinkable to them for a woman not to be circumcised.

The notes indicate that, in this community, a *failure* to arrange for FGC is viewed as a form of child neglect or abuse.

Despite the physical consequences of FGC, the underlying socio-cultural logic rationalizes girls' physical suffering as a method to avoid social suffering. In many communities, the importance of marriage and social identity is perceived to offset the physical pain that is endured. In some communities, FGC and male circumcision happen to many young people at once in a collective celebration. These communities view FGC as an important coming-of-age marker and abstaining from the practice can have tremendous social ramifications. The practice of FGC exists at the nexus of different forms of suffering which, as we show, are interrelated with broader social issues.

Social Change

In the last quarter century, there has been a sea change in attitudes toward FGC and notable reductions in the occurrence of the practices (UNICEF 2013). The Demographic and Health Surveys began measuring levels of FGC in the 1990s, providing a valuable resource for assessing change (ICF International, various years; see also IPUMS-DHS, 2016). As of 2013, 15 out of the 20 countries with at least two surveys saw a significant decrease in support for the practices. For example, in Egypt in 1995, 82% of women (15–49 year olds who were currently or previously married) thought FGC should continue, but that number had dropped to 62% for a similar sample of women by 2008. Out of 20, only one country—Guinea-Bissau—has seen a small increase in support for FGC over time.

Changing attitudes are having an effect as rates of FGC are decreasing in most places. Comparing rates of FGC in 29 countries with DHS data reveals lower rates of FGC among 15–19 year olds than among 45–49 year olds, indicating that the practices are becoming less common over time. For example, in Burkina Faso, a recent DHS survey showed that 89% of 45–49 year old women had been cut, but only 58% of 15–19 year old girls had been. All 29 countries saw a decrease in FGC; for over half, the difference was statistically significant (UNICEF 2013). In addition, families in regions where Type 3 infibulation has been common are beginning to turn to less invasive forms of FGC, meaning less harmful health consequences for girls (Yoder and Wang 2013). Overall, the relatively rapid abandonment of FGC makes the practices an important case for understanding effective reforms to reduce suffering.

What Made Revolutionary Change Possible in the Case of FGC?

The case of FGC reveals that alleviating suffering is a complex multi-level, multi-stage process. Change required institutional transformations first in international law and then in national and local community contexts. Importantly, the keys to effective change were very different, sometimes even contradictory, across the different spheres. As with many other sources of suffering, this meant that cultural translation was essential for social change. While garnering support from the international community was an important step toward change, it was not in itself sufficient. National governments had to endorse change, and mothers ultimately had to be convinced to stop having their daughters cut.

Change at the Macro Level At the international level, the greatest barrier to action against FGC was the institution of sovereign autonomy. The UN Charter of 1948 protects the domestic jurisdiction of states from international encroachment. For decades, "cultural" matters, such as FGC, were deemed outside the scope of the UN's authority based on this doctrine. For example, in 1961, when African women attending a UN seminar in Addis Ababa asked the WHO to study FGC, the organization refused, stating that it had no jurisdiction (Boulware-Miller 1985). It was essential to narrow the scope of the sovereign autonomy doctrine, which was justifying a lack of compassion (Boyle 2002).

Social mobilization affected the necessary change toward the doctrine of sovereign autonomy by drawing attention to the problem of FGC. Radical feminists used incendiary rhetoric and sympathetic (but exaggerated) stories to challenge international organizations to be more responsive to women's suffering. For example, Daly (1978:154) called it a "sado-ritual" done in the interest of "planetary patriarchy"; Hosken (1979) described it as castration derived from a worldwide fear by men of female sexuality. Their claims eventually became part of the Western public consciousness. In the US, novelist Alice Walker wrote *Possessing the Secret of Joy*, a story about the travails of a circumcised woman. Abe Rosenthal began to write reports on FGC for *The New York Times*, and in 1994 CNN broadcast live the circumcision of a 12-year-old Egyptian girl. American women began to clamor for action against the practice.

Thus, collective action forced international actors to take moral responsibility for the relief of suffering from FGC. Under pressure, they found a way to challenge FGC without explicitly rejecting the principle of sovereign autonomy. Their solution was to redefine FGC as a health issue rather than a cultural issue (Boyle 2002). The WHO was already intervening in national arenas to provide family planning programs and vaccinations. By placing FGC within the health framework, international actors were not singling out African nations—health problems were a universal concern, affecting every nation. This framing thus preserved the idea of sovereign autonomy, even as the WHO began to take action to reduce FGC.

Pressure on national governments to condemn FGC accompanied international interventions in the name of health. The US passed a law in 1996 that made aid contingent on taking action against FGC. At the same time, the US State Department began to feature actions against FGC in its annual Human Rights Country Reports. Because of these and other actions, nearly every country where FGC occurs had a law against the practices by the end of the millennium (Boyle and Preves 2000).

Research suggests that global norms, and by extension national laws, are important components to the elimination of FGC. Yet, legal mechanisms on their own have been insufficient to create change. In response to international pressure, countries may adopt laws, but merely as window dressing without any real intention of implementing them. After a 2012 UN General Assembly resolution to abandon FGC, 25 countries enacted *new* laws to curtail FGC prevalence (PRB and Feldman Jacobs 2013). This suggests that, in the FGC context, laws are primarily symbolic since new laws would be unnecessary if old laws were effective.

A lack of enforcement is an obvious problem (Muthumbi et al. 2015), but even when anti-FGC laws are enforced, the results are mixed. For example, Eritrea's legal prohibition, accompanied by arrests and prosecutions, is estimated to have decreased rates of FGC by 13% for girls under 5 and 33% for girls under 15 (UNFPA-UNICEF 2012). However, Rasheed et al. (2011) observe that although FGC prevalence in Upper Egypt declined following the 2007 criminalization of the procedure, that decline was slower than the years preceding criminalization. Rahman and Toubia (2000: 13) argue laws are most effective in providing leverage for other agents of change. In short, legal prohibitions can be useful compliments to other activities that raise awareness of the health consequences of FGC in villages, recruit local allies against FGC, and connect FGC elimination with broader development goals.

Change at the Micro Level Certain local accompaniments to legal prohibitions are more effective than others. Feminist rhetoric did not easily translate to the community level. The Western message that parents were mutilating their children (calling FGC "female genital mutilation") was offensive, and exaggerated claims concerning health consequences marked activists as uninformed. Different approaches were necessary—approaches that understood community contexts and the local impetus for FGC. Change in local communities has rested on (1) education about the negative health consequences of FGC, especially relating to reproduction, (2) community-wide declarations that parents will not cut their daughters and men will marry women who have not been cut, and (3) connecting FGC with broader development agendas that incorporate enhanced socioeconomic status for women.

Health education and awareness programs are a common strategy to promote FGC abandonment. The assumption is that once mothers know the harmful effects, the practice of FGC will end (Shell-Duncan 2008). Orubuloye et al. (2000) observe that only 8% of rural women in Nigeria knew that FGC was associated with child-bearing complications and infertility. Other studies also observe that FGC has been supported by conventional beliefs that the practice benefits women's reproductive health (van der Kwaak 1992). Such studies contend that a lack of information on the health consequences of FGC contributes to the perpetuation of the practice. Thus, publicizing medical knowledge to communities is an important step toward FGC abandonment. In an evaluation of health education programs in Nigeria, Ekwueme et al. (2010) found that the percentages of those in favor of FGC continuation in participating villages declined from 70% to 11%. However, scholars (Orubuloye et al. 2000; Sedgh et al. 2005; Mackie 2000) note that a health education emphasis that focuses on the physical consequences of FGC (bleeding, infection) can promote the medicalization of the practice rather than its elimination. Thus, education campaigns can promote harm reduction while allowing the practice to continue (McChesney 2015).

Another shortcoming of health education is that it does not address the religious beliefs that support the practice in some locations. Women will continue to circumcise their daughters regardless of the health consequences if they believe that FGC is a religious requirement (Johnson 2000). FGC predates Islam, it not practiced in most Islamic countries, and is not required by the Koran. Nevertheless, in some parts of Africa, such as Egypt, Mali, and Nigeria, the practice is associated with the Islamic faith. For FGC-practicing communities in these countries, religious education from respected Islamic leaders is as important as health education. One example of effective education is when, in 2006, the Grand Mufti of Al-Azhar University issued a religious edict condemning FGC, and the Al-Azhar Supreme Council for Islamic Research issued a statement explaining that FGC has no basis in Islamic law (UNICEF 2013). This type of education can be an important compliment to health-based education.

In addition to education, almost all elimination programs now include community dialogue leading to community-wide agreements to abandon FGC. Mackie's (1996) notion of "social conventions" explains that practices continue when communities require them and rejection of conventions lead to social sanctions. Parental decisions to circumcise their daughters operate within familial preference and community normativity. Norm violation can be the basis of social sanctions, such as unmarriageability and ostracism (Shell-Duncan et al. 2013).

The most successful programs tend to be community driven, recruiting trusted local members to advocate abandonment. Mackie (2000) describes Tostan, a non-governmental organization, in Senegal as an effective program due to its inclusiveness. A key factor in Tostan's approach is the effort to recruit local village members, approved by the community, to enroll in a basic education program. The knowledge and skills they acquired in the program, including FGC information, was then shared with the rest of the community. Local recruits lend credibility to Tostan's FGC message, which is highly important as "rural Africans regularly encounter novel factual claims" and "must evaluate the credibility of information coming from clearly interested or unknown outside sources" (Mackie 2000: 259). Over the past decade in Senegal, nearly 6000 villages publicly declared an intention to abandon FGC. In Egypt, education programs and community member recruitment operate within a holistic approach to encourage critical dialogue about FGC practices and the norms surrounding it. Medical professionals were specifically targeted (as well as religious leaders, media, and village members) due to the rise of medicalization in FGC procedures. From 2003 to 2009, approximately 50 Egyptian villages publicly declared to end FGC in their communities (UNICEF 2013).

Not all public declarations are the same. Some fail while other succeed. The difference is the level and nature of community involvement. Examples from Ethiopia demonstrate this clearly. NGO interventions in Yilmandensa District and Wolayta Zone of Ethiopia conducted outreach activities that resulted in broader agreements to abandon FGC. The intervention in Yilmandensa District, supported by the Amhara HIV/AIDS Prevention and Control Office selected village representatives to attend education sessions and return to the village to facilitate dialogue on harmful practices. In the Wolayta Zone, the Women's Affairs Office funded a program that successfully culminated in a public declaration to abandon FGC and establish a monitoring system to expose violators. However, only 10% of people in Yilmandensa District participated in the discussions and participants in Wolayta Zone consisted of NGO employees rather than villagers. In both cases, uncut girls were still subject to ridicule and stigma while facilitators for abandonment faced intimidation by those who supported FGC continuation. Evaluators later found that FGC had simply continued underground despite public declarations of abandonment because villagers did not consider abandonment as a collective decision. Rather, the decision was viewed as a governmental directive because the interventions only engaged village members through trained facilitators, many of whom were from other areas.

Unlike Yilmandensa and Wolayta interventions, NGO interventions in Gewane District and Kembatta Tembaro Zone of Ethiopia relied on local participation. Gewane and Kembatta Tembaro NGOs worked directly within village community structures, recruiting local elites (traditional and religious leaders) and conducted FGC discussions in the villages. In Gewane and Kembatta, the public declaration to abandon FGC came from months of direct conversations with village members and elites. Over the course of both interventions, 75% of villagers in Gewane and 85% of villagers in Kembatta rejected FGC while indicating that uncut girls were no longer "despised" (UNICEF 2013). In short, changing a long standing practice depends heavily on the credibility of the message and messenger. Gerry Mackie (2000) argues that the most successful programs to end FGC are "nondirective" interventions which avoid telling people what should or should not be done. Unlike early international campaigns which portrayed the practice as a malicious act against women and daughters, cultural sensitivity and awareness of the local realities enables social change rather than heavy-handed directives from outsiders.

Finally, as a parallel aspect of local participation, successful anti-FGC interventions were often embedded within general economic development programs. The Kembatta interventions mentioned above integrated FGC discourses into other projects and services such as HIV/AIDS prevention, community schools, livelihood projects for women and other income-generating activities (UNICEF 2013). As concrete results emerged, new information (including FGC abandonment) was received as useful or at least well-intentioned.

Likewise in Egypt, successful reductions in FGC prevalence relied on achieving development goals that directly benefited women (Hadi 2006). Through the development initiatives of the Coptic Evangelical Organization for Social Services (CEOSS), the Upper Egyptian village of Deir El Barsha experienced a rapid decline in FGC that was connected to women's increasing participation in income earning activities, higher levels of literacy, and women's increasing control over household earnings and decisions. By contrast, FGC rates remained high in the neighboring El Barsha where women were far less likely to engage in development activities. Scholars such as Hadi and Mackie argue that community development that challenges women's subservient roles is central to eliminating FGC, a practice rooted in patriarchal ideologies.

Ultimately, FGC reduction largely depends on undermining the social roots that necessitate the procedure. While laws (and enforcement) can deter the practice, individual decisions are informed by real or perceived social expectations. As successful programs highlight, communities must perceive the information provided through education as credible and well-intentioned. Trusted local leaders, including religious leaders and community elders, can legitimize new information on conventional practices. Moreover, consensus building through local participation in FGC dialogues tends to generate meaningful declarations of abandonment. Health education that encourages FGC abandonment is especially effective when coupled with development priorities in the villages. Not only do tangible development benefits lend credibility to FGC discussions, but such interventions can also alter the underlying gender systems that justify FGC.

A Model Case

The approaches to FGC abandonment provide a useful model for alleviating suffering in many other contexts. Similar to other forms of suffering, FGC is an institutionalized practice, rooted in sexist and patriarchal structures that have no functional justification. Moreover, FGC occurs in the global south which brings about unique challenges to programs that aim to eliminate the practice. FGC is rooted within a gendered logic that privileges men's position at the cost of women's subjected state and challenging those foundations is a paramount, albeit tricky, undertaking. The most successful programs are keenly aware of social control factors and surrounding institutions that maintained the importance of FGC in people's lives. Education and development programs that are sensitive to local needs are effective foundations for social change. Even in cases where education programs drove the practice toward medicalization, subsequent harm reduction strategies are arguably successful in reducing suffering if not entirely eliminating it. Ultimately, knowledge of the physical consequences of FGC are effective instruments of change when interventions are built on mutual trust and respect.

Various forms of suffering arise from deeply held belief systems, such as sexism, that subjugate one group over another. In the particular case of FGC, women are the primary perpetuators of the practice. A key factor in the persistence of FGC is the context of women's economic dependence of men. In communities where women do not inherit property and are discouraged from or sanctioned for participating in the labor market, marriage is essential for survival. The successes of Tostan in Senegal and the Coptic Evangelical Organization for Social Services (CEOSS) in Egypt highlight the socially transformative power of economic development. Such NGOs engaged local development priorities, producing tangible gains to education and incomes for men and women. Women's increased economic status translated to improved social statuses as well, triggering grass-roots challenges to FGC and underlying rationales for the practice. In short, development projects eroded the economic basis (i.e. marriageability for survival) of FGC.

Education and economic development can also redefine the gender roles that subjugate women. Women's denial of access to incomes not only deprives them economically but also imposes normative constraints on their public and relational roles. Take for instance, the practice of foot-binding in China. Like FGC, foot-binding was a physical marking of women's femininity and marriageability, based on the importance of women's dependence and fidelity to their husband (Mackie 2000). In terms of FGC and foot-binding, expectations of women as wife and domestic caretaker is a normative foundation for both practices and deviation from those expectations result in physical and social sanctions. Sociologists such as Greenhalgh (1977) linked the demise of foot-binding with employment and educational expansion which weakened patriarchal control over women in China. Similarly, Hadi (2006) notes, women's economic autonomy in Deir El Barsha triggered their willingness to openly challenge FGC privately and publicly.

As successful FGC interventions show, the institutional foundations (i.e. sexism, normative femininity) for FGC are responsive to education and development. However, development planners should also be mindful of the global south contexts in which FGC occurs. Although there have always been opponents of the practice in the practicing countries, international action was prompted primarily by feminists in the global north. As with many other sources of suffering, this meant that cultural translation was essential for social change. For example, the depiction of FGC as child abuse did little to generate local support for abandonment. Rather, promoting FGC abandonment indirectly, coupled with other local priorities, enabled a sincere dialogue between NGOs and communities. Resulting consensuses were far more effective when they were homegrown agreements and not external directives from what locals viewed as self-interested others.

Numerous other efforts to alleviate suffering would benefit from adopting similar anti-FGC strategies. Like FGC, global and international efforts can trigger action to alleviate suffering by drawing attention to critical problems such as natural disasters and sexual violence in conflict. As Western feminists were instrumental in raising global consciousness of suffering from FGC, global advocacy groups can coalesce wider efforts to alleviate physical, economic and social hardships. Generating widespread recognition of a problem unites people and facilitates new and innovative solutions to circumvent barriers to action such as national sovereignty and culturally translating values and practices. However, many other forms of suffering that are entrenched in social systems require more than education and discourse. Consequential outcomes such as child battering and racial, gender and age discrimination are all founded on social systems that normalize and even legitimize such behaviors. As successful anti-FGC interventions worked within the layers of social, economic and political realities of communities, addressing multifaceted types of suffering would also be most effective when utilizing existing community support systems and institutions. The global advocacy against intimate partner violence (IPV), particularly domestic violence against women, is instructive to contextual awareness in suffering alleviation. Like FGC, policy and academic research attributes women's high risk of domestic violence to their subjected status. Women's economic empowerment is touted as a solution to IPV; however, many women's development projects were ineffective or even exacerbated partner violence as women's economic gain was perceived as a threat to men's dominant status. These acts of violence share with FGC an exaggerated concern that individuals will become threats to a community unless they are physically altered or managed.

Importantly, some of the weaknesses in anti-IPV projects highlight why some anti-FGC projects worked and some did not. Engaging the local community and facilitating active participation, beyond development interventions, was critical to FGC abandonment. In short, if change is directly expected among individuals in a community, then the impetus of change should not fall on individuals alone. In the case of IPV, women risk physical "corrections" when their economic independence deviates from the norm. In the case of FGC, if one family abandons FGC while the rest of the community continues to support it, the daughters in that one family will suffer serious social consequences.

Gerry Mackie (1996: 1009) posits that social conventions are maintained through a "belief trap." Entrenched beliefs about a practice despite contrary information are often difficult to change because the cost of dissent is too high. Successfully challenging a deeply embedded practice thus depends on a broad community consensus. In such global south contexts, NGOs have been the most effective when engaging community members and leaders, the latter of whom must take action on behalf of those who are victims of the practice. Given the outsider status of many organizations, gaining the mutual trust and respect of communities is vital. Development planners could learn a lot from the failures of the "stop FGC" movement in these cases as well. Rather than directly contest a practice from an outside perspective, successful approaches recruited and leveraged high status individuals who legitimized the abandonment of a long-standing practice. Logics of social control can erode in a longer discourse between global movements and local contexts. However, effective strategies to eliminate FGC also operated within the institutional realities of the places. The information and even the sentiments behind FGC abandonment are often the same, but it was when villagers felt that the decision to abandon came from within the community, rather than externally derived, that declarations to abandon FGC coincided with actual abandonment.

Conclusion

By contrasting the successful and unsuccessful interventions to eliminate FGC, we emphasize key approaches that facilitate suffering alleviation in general. Medical experts consistently show that FGC is a physically harmful procedure that results in long-term pain and reproductive health consequences. Educational programs that inform parents of health effects are an important step toward elimination. Yet, social conventions that maintain gender inequality can perpetuate the practice regardless of the information. Thus, health programs that simultaneously alter the social and institutional environments of a community are the most effective interventions. Leveraging local elites, engaging village members, and addressing broader development priorities lends credibility to the education programs. Furthermore, generating educational and economic opportunities for women can change the normative logic that FGC is important for a girls' future survival. FGC elimination highlights the utility of a multi-pronged approach to suffering alleviation. Trust, credibility and goodwill are underused concepts in development interventions (Mackie 2000). As the successes of numerous NGOs (such as Tostan and CEOSS) show, mutual respect can be a vital platform for change and enhances the effectiveness of education and development agendas.

References

Berg, R. C., & Underland, V. (2013). Obstetric consequences of female genital mutilation/cutting (FGM/C). *Obstetrics and Gynecology International, 2013*, 1–15.

Boulware-Miller, K. (1985). Female circumcision: Challenges to the practice as a human rights violation. *Harvard Women's Law Journal, 8*, 155–179.

Boyle, E. H. (2002). *Female genital cutting: Cultural conflict in the global community*. Baltimore: Johns Hopkins.

Boyle, E. H., & Preves, S. E. (2000). National politics as international process: The case of anti-female genital cutting laws. *Law and Society Review, 34*, 703–737.

Daly, M. (1978). *Gyn/Ecology: The metaethics of radical feminism*. Boston: Beacon.

Ekwueme, O. C., Ezegwui, H. U., & Ezeoke, U. (2010). Dispelling the myths and beliefs toward female genital cutting of woman: Assessing general outpatient services at a tertiary health institution in Enugu State, Nigeria. *East African Journal of Public Health, 7*(1), 66–69.

Greenhalgh, S. (1977). Bound feet, hobbled lives: Women in old China. *Frontiers, 2*, 7–21.

Hadi, A. A. (2006). A community of women empowered: The story of Deir El Barsha. In R. M. Abusharaf (Ed.), *Female circumcision: Multicultural perspectives* (pp. 104–124). Philadelphia: University of Pennsylvania Press.

Hosken, F. P. (1979). *The Hosken report: Genital and sexual mutilation of females*. Lexington: Women's International Network News.

ICF International. (1989–2014). Demographic and Health Surveys (various) [Datasets]. Calverton, Maryland: ICF International [Distributor], 2016. http://dhsprogram.com/data/

Johnson, M. (2000). Becoming a Muslim, becoming a person: Female 'circumcision,' religious identity, and personhood in Guineau-Bissau. In B. Shell-Duncan & Y. Hernlund (Eds.), *Female "Circumcision" in Africa: Culture, controversy, and change* (pp. 215–233). Boulder: Lynne Reiner Publishers.

Lane, S. D., & Rubinstein, R. A. (1996). Judging the other: Responding to traditional female genital surgeries. *Hastings Center Report, 26*(3), 31–40.

Mackie, G. (1996). Ending footbinding and infibulation: A convention account. *American Sociological Review, 61*(6), 999–1017.

Mackie, G. (2000). Female genital cutting: The beginning of the end. In B. Shell-Duncan & Y. Hernlund (Eds.), *Female "Circumcision" in Africa: Culture, controversy, and change* (pp. 253–282). Boulder: Lynne Reiner Publishers.

McChesney, K. Y. (2015). Successful approaches to ending female genital cutting. *Journal of Sociology and Social Welfare, 42*(1), 3–24.

Muthumbi, J., Svanemyr, J., Scolaro, E., Temmerman, M., & Say, L. (2015). Female genital mutilation: A literature review of the current status of legislation and policies in 27 African countries and Yemen. *African Journal of Reproductive Health, 19*(3), 32–40.

Orubuloye, I. O., Caldwell, P., & Caldwell, J. (2000). Female circumcision among the Yoruba of southwestern Nigeria: The beginning of change. In B. Shell-Duncan & Y. Hernlund (Eds.),

Female "Circumcision" in Africa: Culture, controversy, and change (pp. 73–94). Boulder: Lynne Reiner Publishers.
PRB, & Feldman-Jacobs, C. (2013). Ending female genital mutilation/cutting: Lessons from a decade of progress.
Rahman, A., & Toubia, N. (2000). *Female genital mutilation: A practical guide to worldwide laws & policies*. London/New York: Zed Books.
Rasheed, S. M., Abd-Ellah, A. H., & Yousef, F. M. (2011). Female genital mutilation in Upper Egypt in the new millennium. *International Journal of Gynecology & Obstetrics, 114*(1), 47–50.
Sedgh, G., Jackson, E., & Ibrahim, B. (2005). Toward the abandonment of female genital cutting: Advancing research, communication and collaboration. *Culture, Health & Sexuality, 7*(5), 425–427.
Shell-Duncan, B. (2008). From health to human rights: Female genital cutting and the politics of intervention. *American Anthropologist, 110*(2), 225–236.
Shell-Duncan, B., Wander, K., Hernlund, Y., & Moreau, A. (2013). Legislating change? Responses to criminalizing female genital cutting in Senegal. *Law and Society Review, 47*(4), 803–835.
UNFPA-UNICEF. (2012). Joint Programme on Female Genital Mutilation/Cutting: Accelerating Change. UNFPA-UNICEF: Retrieved May 31, 2016. http://www.unfpa.org/sites/default/files/pub-pdf/UNICEF-UNFPA%20Joint%20Programme%20AR_final_v14.pdf
UNFPA-UNICEF. (2014). 2014 Annual Report of the UNFPA-UNICEF Joint Programme on Female Genital Mutilation/Cutting: Accelerating Change. UNFPA-UNICEF: Retrieved May 31, 2016. http://www.unfpa.org/sites/default/files/pub-pdf/UNFPA_UNICEF_FGM_14_Report_PDA_WEB.pdf
UNICEF. (2010). The Dynamics of Social Change: Towards the Abandonment of Female Genital Mutilation/Cutting in Five African Countries. *Innocenti Insight*: Retrieved May 31, 2016. http://www.unicef.org/chinese/videoaudio/PDFs/fgm_insight_eng(1).pdf
UNICEF. (2013). Female Genital Mutilation/Cutting: A Statistical Overview and Exploration of the Dynamics of Change. UNICEF: Retrieved May 31, 2016. http://www.unicef.org/media/files/UNICEF_FGM_report_July_2013_Hi_res.pdf
Van der Kwaak, A. (1992). Female circumcision and gender identity: A questionable alliance? *Social Science & Medicine, 35*(6), 777–787.
World Health Organization. (2016). Female Genital Mutilation. Retrieved May 31, 2016. http://www.who.int/mediacentre/factsheets/fs241/en/
Yoder, P. S., & Wang, S. (2013). *Female genital cutting: The interpretation of recent DHS Data*. Calverton: ICF International.
Yoder, P. S., Wang, S., & Johansen, E. (2013). Estimates of female genital mutilation/cutting in 27 African countries and Yemen. *Studies in Family Planning, 44*(2), 189–204.
Yount, K. M., & Carrera, J. S. (2006). Female genital cutting and reproductive experience in Minya, Egypt. *Medical Anthropology Quarterly, 20*(2), 182–211.

Chapter 22
International Criminal Law as One Response to World Suffering: General Observations and the Case of Darfur

Joachim J. Savelsberg

Introduction: Human-Induced World Suffering

Human suffering in the world can result from natural disasters, earthquakes, floods, or epidemics. The biblical book of Exodus lists many plagues, and more can be added, some appearing only millennia later (no Ebola then, no HIV, and no Zika Virus). Other episodes of suffering are indirect consequences of human action. They include the ongoing desertification of many arid areas around the globe, resulting from, at least partly human-made, climate change. Consequences are competition for resources, hunger, and intensified conflict between social groups. And such conflicts are one of the conditions of suffering that can be directly attributed to human action: mass violence, much of which is today categorized as human rights crimes. In this chapter I (1) briefly sketch the dimension of mass violence in recent history; (2) describe efforts to reduce such episodes by way of a diversity of historically new institutions (focusing on criminal law, including international criminal law); and (3) juxtapose the promise of such efforts with some cautionary notes.

Suffering from Human Rights Crime

In 1994, near the end of a murderous century, political scientist R.J. Rummel assembled one of the most comprehensive accounts of government-induced democides committed during the twentieth century through 1987. By democide, Rummel (1994:31) means "the murder of any person or people by a government, including genocide, politicide [the murder of groups because of their politics or for political

J.J. Savelsberg (✉)
Department of Sociology, University of Minnesota, Minneapolis, MN 55455, USA
e-mail: savel001@umn.edu

R.E. Anderson (ed.), *Alleviating World Suffering*, Social Indicators Research Series 67, DOI 10.1007/978-3-319-51391-1_22

purposes], and mass murder [indiscriminate killing]" (Rummel 1994:31–43 for terminological specifics).

The numbers are staggering. Rummel (1994:4) lists "Dekamegamurderers," those who killed in the tens of millions (e.g., USSR from 1917–1987; PRC 1949–1987; Germany 1933–1945; nationalist China [KMT] 1928–1949). The death toll adds up to more than 128 million people. Lesser "Megamurderers" took the lives of another more than 19 million humans (e.g., Japan from 1936–1945; Mao's Soviets in China 1923–1949; Cambodia 1975–1979; Turkey 1909–1918; Vietnam 1945–1987; Poland 1945–1948; Pakistan 1958–1987; and Yugoslavia under Tito 1944–1987). Adding other suspected Megamurderes and "Centi-Kilomurderers" (those who killed "only" in the hundreds of thousands) and *excluding* the victims of regular ("legitimate") warfare, Rummel's grim accounting reaches a total of some 169 *million* individuals murdered by their own or other peoples' governments between 1900 and 1987, a number that is manifold higher than that of victims of violent street crime to which media reporting dedicates so much more attention (Savelsberg 2010:9). Not included here are the numbers of rape victimization and hundreds of millions of displacements that resulted from the same episodes of mass violence

Occurrences of mass violence differ in many ways, including methods of killings, the regimes under which they occur (albeit mostly authoritarian or dictatorial), their execution in times of peace versus war (albeit mostly during wars), and the number of victims. Yet, all of them involve collective action, complex social organization, including formal organization, with front-line, low-level actors who execute the dirty work as well as high-level actors whose hands remain untainted by the blood for the shedding of which they bear ultimate responsibility.

Institutional Responses and the Justice Cascade

The twentieth century also has brought remarkable change. Legal scholar Martha Minow (1998) suggests that its hallmark was not the horrendous atrocities committed in its course. Too many past centuries can compete. Instead, humanity's new inventiveness and efforts toward restricting human rights perpetration distinguish the twentieth century from previous ones. Minow lists human rights conventions, truth commissions (see also Hayner 2001), vetting procedures, compensations programs, amnesties, public memorializations, and apologies. While Minow also addresses mechanisms of criminal law and justice, political scientist Kathryn Sikkink (2011) focuses on them. She argues that the late twentieth and early twenty-first centuries are characterized by a "justice cascade," a massive increase in individual criminal accountability for grave human rights violations. And she argues that the justice cascade has beneficial consequences. It has the potential of reducing world suffering (see also Jo and Simmons 2016). Leaders of human rights movements express similar optimism (Neier 2012).

Shape and Conditions of the Justice Cascade

Sikkink's recent book (2011), recipient of the Robert F. Kennedy Center for Justice and Human Rights' 2012 Robert Kennedy Book Award, documents how prosecutions against individual human rights perpetrators in domestic, foreign and international courts increased almost exponentially in recent decades. She counts by country the number of years in which prosecutions were conducted. Values, in the single digits during much of the 1980s, rose to about 100 by the mid-1990s, to 300 a decade later, and they approached 450 by 2009 (Sikkink 2011:21).

Domestic justice systems drive this increase, partly due to the adoption of international human rights norms by a growing number of countries. Their willingness is enhanced by the complementarity principle of the 1998 Rome Statute, the foundation of the International Criminal Court (ICC): domestic courts have primary jurisdiction as long as they are able and willing to pursue cases (Article 17). As they operate "in the shadow" of the criminal court thus, nation states prosecute cases at times specifically to keep them under their own domestic jurisdiction. Simultaneously, the adoption of the Rome Statute and the establishment of the ICC in 2002, on the heels of a series of ad hoc tribunals (Yugoslavia, Rwanda, Sierra Leone, Cambodia, East Timor), document the weight of the international level of the justice cascade in its own right. And indeed, international and foreign prosecutions also increased substantially.

What were the sources of this remarkable development? Sikkink (2011) sets the stage with challenging cases that did not result from military defeat. She provides a detailed study of Greece (1975), Portugal (1976), Spain (1975–78) and Argentina (1985) to show that regional opportunity structures had developed by the 1970s that favored transitional justice proceedings. Examples for such structures are the creation of the European Court of Human Rights in 1959, and the foundation of Amnesty International in 1961, an organization that played a central role in the Darfur crisis (see chapter 3 in Savelsberg 2015).

Soon after its foundation, Amnesty International became actively engaged in Greece. Its activism coincided with a supportive international legal environment, and this situation advanced the launching of trials. The 1975 "Torture Declaration" was being prepared concurrently with the Greek torture trials and adopted by the UN General Assembly just a few months after their conclusion. And yet, at this time, trials occurred only after "ruptured" transitions from dictatorship to democracy (Greece, Portugal, Argentina) as opposed to "pacted" transitions (Spain). By the 1990s, however, conditions had changed. Ruptured transitions were no longer a prerequisite for criminal trials against human rights perpetrators as the cases of Guatemala, Chile, and Uruguay illustrate. The institutionalization of the human rights regime had progressed, and the fear of blowbacks had diminished in light of experiences from the 1970s.

Initial steps toward human rights prosecutions eventually resulted in a decentralized, interactive system of global accountability that challenged national sovereignty. Sikkink (2011:96–125) identifies two contributors, "streams" to use her metaphor. The first stream is constituted by international prosecutions, from Nuremberg and Tokyo via the International Criminal Tribunal for the former Yugoslavia (ICTY) and its equivalent for Rwanda (ICTR) and finally on to the ICC with its jurisdiction over cases of aggression, war crimes, crimes against humanity, and genocide.

The second stream consists of domestic and foreign prosecutions such as those in Greece, Portugal, and Argentina in the mid-1970s and the Pinochet case of 1998–99. In addition, a "hard law streambed" led from various conventions like the Genocide Convention (1948), Geneva Convention (1949), Apartheid Convention (1980) and Torture Convention (1987), via the Inter-American Convention on Forced Disappearances (1996) to the Rome Statute (1998). This spread of human rights initiatives, and their solidification in a system, was not simply the result of contagion. Instead, individuals, associations, trans-governmental networks, penetrated by an epistemic community of criminal law experts, and NGOs such as Human Rights Watch (HRW) and Amnesty International, achieved the progressive institutionalization of individual criminal liability, that is, *criminalization* and *individualization* of international law (see Keck and Sikkink 1998). In addition, transnational advocacy networks applied leverage politics that shamed evil doers, and accountability politics that "tricked" nations into commitments, which they might have entered into merely for symbolic and legitimacy reasons, to then hold them accountable. The 1975 Helsinki Accord is just the most famous example (Keck and Sikkink 1998).

Other analysts emphasize the weight of different types of actors in the establishment and spread of human rights norms. Hagan, for example, in his study of the International Criminal Tribunal for the former Yugoslavia (ICTY), focuses on officials within judicial institutions, specifically successive chief prosecutors, each of whom brought a new form of "capital" to bear. All of them combined innovative strategies with established legal practices: from securing international support (Richard Goldstone) to sealed indictments and surprise arrests (Louise Arbour) to Carla del Ponte's charges against former President Milosevic. Innovative strategies eventually become "doxa," Hagan argues: taken-for-granted legal standards in the emerging international criminal tribunal in The Hague.[1] Yet elsewhere, David Scheffer, former U.S. Ambassador and right hand of U.S. Secretary of State Madeleine Albright, highlights diplomats as crucial contributors in the establishment of international judicial institutions, from the ICTY to the ICC (Scheffer 2012).

No matter the relative weight of each of these types of actors, their interactions contributed to the passing of the Rome Statute in 1998 and the establishment of the International Criminal Court (ICC). The ICC entered into force in 2002 when 60 countries had ratified the Statute. By 2013 the number of ratifying countries had

[1]Once established, they diffuse in the international legal system, even if names shift, as Meierhenrich (2006) has shown for the notions of "conspiracy" (U.S. law), "criminal organization" (International Military Tribunal at Nuremberg), and "joint criminal enterprise" (ICTY).

more than doubled, and many—but not all—of those charged have made acquaintance with the imposing court building in The Hague.

An Example: Responding to Darfur in the Context of the Justice Cascade

In the year 2000, around the time of the formation of the ICC, disturbing events began to unfold in the Darfur region of Sudan. Activists against Sudan's ruling elite had issued *The Black Book: Imbalance of Power and Wealth in Sudan.* Distributed widely, especially in the surroundings of mosques after Friday prayers, the *Black Book* castigated the domination of Sudan by "only one Region (Northern Region) with just over 5% of Sudan's population" (Seekers of Truth and Justice 2003:1). A March 22, 2004 translation, signed by "Translater," informs us that "[A]s of last year (March 2003), some of the activists involved in the preparation of the Book took arms against the government" (Seekers of Truth and Justice 2004:1).

Indeed, February and March of 2003 saw the formation of the Sudan Liberation Army (SLA) and the Justice and Equality Movement (JEM), two organizations that led a violent rebellion against the government of Sudan. Their armed actions were surprisingly effective. In April of 2003 rebel groups famously attacked the Sudanese military's el Fasher air base, destroyed numerous planes of the Sudanese air force and killed almost 100 soldiers. The government of Sudan and its military, supported by Janjawiid militias, responded with brute force. A first wave of mass killings unfolded between June and September of 2003. Targets did not just include armed rebels but primarily civilian villagers, including elderly men, women, and children. A cease fire held only for a few months, and in December 2003 President al-Bashir vowed to "annihilate" the Darfur rebels.

His vow had consequences, evoking a second wave of mass killings that lasted from December of 2003 through April of 2004. Massive displacements of the civilian population were the consequence. Tens of thousands of lives were extinguished as a direct result of violence and many more during the Darfuris' flight from the violence and due to problematic conditions in displaced person camps in Sudan and refugee camps in neighboring Chad.

Much of the Western world began to take note only after the first peak of killings (summer 2003) had subsided and when the second wave (winter 2003–2004) was under way. The first public pronouncement, a "genocide alert," issued by the United States Holocaust Memorial Museum (USHMM) in January of 2004, was followed by a series of op-ed pieces in prominent American media; a speech by UN Secretary-General Kofi Annan on April 7, 2004, on the occasion of the 10th anniversary of the Rwandan genocide, before the UN General Assembly; UN Security Council (UNSC) Resolution 1564, instituting an International Commission of Inquiry on Darfur on September 18, 2004; and the UNSC's referral of the case of Darfur to the ICC on March 31, 2005. Parallel to UN interventions, a massive civil society movement evolved. In the United States, the Save Darfur movement, gathering almost 200 liberal and conservative organizations under its umbrella.

The U.S. Congress resolved that the violence in Darfur amounted to genocide. Then-Secretary of State Colin Powell initiated the famous "Atrocities Documentation Survey," a survey of more than 1000 Darfuri refugees in the camps of Eastern Chad. Based on findings from this survey, he determined, at a hearing before the Senate Foreign Relations Committee on September 9, 2004, that genocide was being committed. President George W. Bush followed suit a few weeks later.

Importantly in our context, soon after the UNSC referred the case of Darfur to the ICC on March 31, 2005, the court took action. And, after almost 2 years of investigation, on February 27, 2007, the ICC's chief prosecutor Luis Moreno-Ocampo applied for an arrest warrant against Ahmad Harun, then Sudan's Deputy Minister for the Interior and responsible for the "Darfur Security Desk," and against Ali Kushayb, a Janjawiid leader. Both were charged with crimes against humanity and war crimes. On April 27, 2007 the court issued a warrant of arrest against both actors for war crimes and crimes against humanity. It took another year until the prosecutor also applied for an arrest warrant against Sudanese President Omar al-Bashir, charging crimes against humanity, war crimes, and genocide (July 14, 2008). The judges did not initially follow this application in its entirety, but on March 4, 2009, they issued a warrant against al-Bashir for crimes against humanity and war crimes. With more than a year's delay and 5 years after the UNSC referral to the ICC, on July 12, 2010, the court followed up with a warrant against the President of Sudan for the crime of genocide.

The International Criminal Court (ICC) thus places itself at the center of the judicial field and its engagement with the mass violence in Darfur. Its interventions clearly seek to discredit potential denial of atrocities, or even glorification of those responsible for their perpetration. Reading the indictment provides a clear sense of such "degradation" (Savelsberg 2015, pp. 40–42).

The court did not just issue this warrant, but, through its press offices, it sought to communicate it to a broad public.[2] My analysis of news media from eight Western countries shows how media communicated the court's message to a world audience: the depiction of President al Bashir as a criminal perpetrator. Chances that media present crime frames to display the violence increased with several of the court's interventions (Savelsberg 2015, Chapter 10; Savelsberg and Nyseth Brehm 2015). The historical notion of leaders of violent movements as heroes (Giesen 2004) or the denial of their violence (Cohen 2001) gave way, in the case of Darfur as in some recent cases, to their depiction as criminal perpetrators, at least partially.

Importantly, the court did not act alone. An in-depth analysis of Amnesty International illustrates a supplemental NGO fight to end impunity. Interviews with Amnesty workers in eight countries show how Amnesty's narrative resembles that of the judicial field. Respondents insist that justice, once achieved, will help reach other goals such as peace (see Savelsberg 2015, Chapter 2). In addition to NGOs, the fight for criminal justice intervention is also intensely supported by some

[2] On ICC efforts to shape public opinion locally, for the case of Northern Uganda, see Golden 2013.

countries (and formally supported by many more). The United States stood out in international comparison, despite its strong opposition to the ICC, seeking to advance a criminalizing frame for Darfur and a definition of the violence as genocide. Crucial contributors were civil society groups, organized under the umbrella of the Save Darfur campaign. The George W. Bush administration followed suit, despite its opposition to the International Criminal Court (ICC), but under the pressure of civil society. Conditions for this transmission include the porousness of boundaries between civil society and the state in the United States. Media reflect the consensus between civil society and the state. They highlight the crime frame, label the violence a genocide and use dramatic bridging metaphors to shed light on the violence of Darfur by referencing past genocides, including the Holocaust (see Savelsberg 2015, Chapter 3).

In short, civil society, International Non-Governmental Organizations (INGOs), transnational advocacy networks (TANs), national governments, the UN and the ICC acted to criminalize the violence of Darfur and to initiate a legal case. Darfur thus took its rightful place in the context of the justice cascade. Driving forces are the same as those the literature has identified in other cases. But what were the consequences? What expectations are invested into the justice cascade, and how do they materialize, generally and in the case of Darfur?

Consequences of the Justice Cascade: Between Hope and Cautionary Notes

The institutions with which humankind has responded to massive human-induced suffering are historically new. Practitioners and scholars alike have invested substantial hope in their effectiveness while others have raised cautionary arguments. Evidence is still limited, but the justification of some hopes and of some objections has been the subject of scholarly exploration.

Hope and Signs of Support

Scholars as well as movement actors and practitioners anticipate consequences of the justice cascade with substantial optimism. Sikkink (2011) herself draws hope from her Transitional Trial Data Set, an impressive collection of data on a large number of transitional justice situations. Her statistical analyses suggest, cautiously worded, that prosecutions of human rights perpetrators, including high-level actors, while achieving retribution, do not systematically produce counter-productive consequences as some critics have suggested. They may in fact advance later human rights and democracy records, especially where trials are accompanied by truth commissions (Kim and Sikkink 2010).[3] Observations by practitioners such as Neier support these findings: "The fact that international humanitarian law has now been enforced through criminal sanctions that the various tribunals have imposed on hundreds of high-ranking military officials, guerilla leaders, civilian officials, and heads of government has contributed immensely to awareness of the rules for the conduct of warfare and for the seriousness with which they must be regarded" (Neier 2012:132). And, most recently, analyses by Jo and Simmons (2016) indicate, based on preliminary data, that ICC interventions indeed reduce violent victimization for which state leaders and rebel commanders are responsible.

Political scientists typically argue that the reduction of violence after judicial intervention demonstrates the deterrent effect of criminal justice. They combine a notion of political and military figures as rational actors with an understanding that an increase in the risk of prosecution and punishment from zero to at least modest levels may reduce inclinations to commit future crimes. Support, with regard less to the severity, but more to the likelihood of punishment, comes from criminological research (e.g., McCarthy 2002; Matsueda et al. 2006).

Yet, it is necessary to complement the deterrence mechanism with a cultural one. Even for deterrence to work, memories of past sanctions must be ingrained in the minds of future cohorts of political and military actors. Past sanctions must become part of the collective memory in which they share. The second argument may thus be more powerful: a cultural or socialization mechanism, not just as a precondition of deterrence, but as a force in its own right. Building on a recent line of scholarship, collective memories created by criminal proceedings against human rights offenders potentially delegitimize grave violations, thus reducing the likelihood of their recurrence. Potential violations may no longer even appear on the decision tree of rational actors.

Early on, practitioners expressed hope that criminal trials in major cases of mass violence could write history, and thus contribute to collective memories suited to delegitimize massive violations of human rights. Consider statements by Justice Robert Jackson, the American chief prosecutor at the International Military Tribunal in Nuremberg (IMT), who famously argued: "Unless we write the record of this movement with clarity and precision, we cannot blame the future if in days of peace it finds incredible the accusatory generalities uttered during the war. *We must establish incredible events by credible evidence*" (quoted in Landsman 2005:6–7; my emphasis). President Franklin Delano Roosevelt thought along similar lines. As his confidant, Judge Samuel Rosenman noted: "[Roosevelt] was determined that the question of Hitler's guilt—and the guilt of his gangsters—must not be left open to future debate. The whole nauseating matter should be spread out on a permanent record under oath by witnesses and with all the written documents" (in Landsman 2005:6).

In scholarship, expectations of criminal law's delegitimizing functions are grounded in classic writings (Mead 1918) and supported by a new line of

[3] See also, in support of these arguments, a comprehensive literature review on "The Prosecution of Human Rights Violations" (Nobels 2010).

neo-Durkheimian work in cultural sociology. Here criminal punishment is interpreted as a didactic exercise, a "speech act in which society talks to itself about its moral identity" (Smith 2008:16). The potential weight of this mechanism for our theme becomes clear if indeed the IMT in Nuremberg and the Universal Declaration of Human Rights initiated the extension of the Holocaust and psychological identification with the victims, as Jeffrey Alexander (2004) argues, for the memory of the Holocaust. Judicial events like Nuremberg, the Eichmann trial in Jerusalem, or the Frankfurt Auschwitz Trial produced cultural trauma: members of a world audience were affected by an experience to which they themselves had not been exposed.

Empirical research by historians and sociologists shows that criminal trials have the capacity of coloring not just narratives of recent events, but also the collective memory of a more distant past in the minds of subsequent generations (Savelsberg and King 2011). Once generated, delegitimizing memories – in a positive feedback loop—further promote human rights standards. This notion is supported by Daniel Levy and Natan Sznaider's insight that "[t]he global proliferation of human rights norms is driven by the public and frequently ritualistic attention to memories of their persistent violations" (Levy and Sznaider 2010:4).

The effectiveness of the criminal justice narrative is well documented, for the case of Darfur, in a media analysis of two leading newspapers, one conservative and one liberal-leaning, in each of eight Western countries. A coding of some 3400 articles and a (multivariate and multi-level) statistical analysis of the resulting data set shows that criminal justice interventions translate into a heightened depiction of the violence in Darfur as criminal violence, as crimes against humanity and as genocide (Savelsberg and Nyseth Brehm 2015).

In short, practitioners and scholars invest much hope in the new institutions world society created in response to mass violence. Some scholarship has demonstrated that such hope is not unfounded. It is supported by a mechanism of deterrence (Sikkink 2011; Jo and Simmons 2016), but also by a cultural mechanism as criminal justice interventions portray powerful and celebrated actors as criminals when they directly or indirectly initiate mass atrocities (Savelsberg 2015).

Notes of Caution: Limits of Criminal Justice Intervention

Others challenge such hope (e.g., Goldsmith and Krasner 2003; Snyder and Vinjamuri 2003/4; Pensky 2008). Most recently, Osiel (2014), while expressing sympathy with the idea of international criminal justice, pronounces that "international criminal law is unlikely to endure as anything more than an intermittent occasion for staging splashy, eye-catching degradation rituals, feel-good spectacles of good will toward men." He points at the absence of the world's largest powers (China, Russia, United States) from the Rome Statute, power politics in the United Nations Security Council (UNSC) (consider Syria in the 2010s), the risks of *coup d'états* when nations prosecute past ruling juntas or dictators, partisan case-selections in post-transitional justice proceedings, and the risk of "victors' justice."[4] Yet others highlight the risk that one-sided memories of victimization and a competition for victim status, potential outcomes of flawed transitional justice, may in fact propel cycles of violence (Barkan 2013).

All of these arguments are to be taken seriously. I here focus on two points of caution that may weaken the cultural effect of criminal justice intervention. The first is the limiting institutional logic of criminal law and the distorted memories it generates. Criminal law focuses on individual perpetrators, at the expense of larger structural and cultural forces that contribute to waves of mass violence, forces that sociologists might highlight. It is bound by a binary guilty-versus-not-guilty logic, disregarding the grey zones that social psychologists would recognize. It is bound by specific rules of evidence, more limited than those applied by historians. The story of the past told in criminal court is thus always highly selective (see Pendas 2006 on the Frankfurt Auschwitz Trial; Marrus 2008 on the Nuremberg Doctors' Trial; Savelsberg and King 2011 on the My Lai Trial).

In addition, the criminal justice narrative always has to contend with competitors, for example in the realms of humanitarian aid and diplomacy. Some illustrations for the case of Darfur must suffice. Representations of mass violence in the humanitarian aid field, examined for the case of Doctors Without Borders (MSF), differ substantially from human rights narratives. Aspects of suffering are highlighted that can be addressed by humanitarian aid programs. The Government of Sudan is treated cautiously. Long-term conditions are privileged over government actions that directly caused the violence. The humanitarian catastrophe frame is privileged over the state crime frame and actors shy away from the genocide label. The powerful position of the Government of Sudan vis-à-vis the humanitarian aid field is identified as a crucial condition for such representation. Despite a global humanitarian representation, variation of narratives in the humanitarian aid field is also noted. In addition to cross-national variation, lawyers within MSF are less divorced from the logic of the justice cascade than members of other professions, especially physicians. Conflicts between human rights and humanitarian fields may, however, give way to a division of labor when humanitarian organizations produce evidence of suffering that justice institutions use to attribute criminal responsibility (see Savelsberg 2015, Chapter 4). Humanitarian aid-oriented countries follow a similar logic (for the example of Ireland, see Savelsberg 2015, Chapter 5). Like the criminal justice field, the humanitarian field competes for acceptance in world society.

Representation of mass violence in the diplomatic field, explored through interviews, reveals a diplomatic master narrative that is similarly distinct from the delegitimizing criminal justice account (see Savelsberg 2015, Chapters 6 and 7). It

[4] Multiple contributions at conferences on "Legal Frames of Memory," held in Warsaw in fall of 2013, and on "Contested Past, Contested Present: Social Memories and Human Rights in Post-Communist Europe," held in Minneapolis in March of 2015, provided evidence (e.g., Stan 2013; Czarnota 2015).

focuses on long-term and structural causes of the conflict and avoids naming responsible actors, using the crime frame and applying the genocide label. The role of the Sudanese state in the diplomatic field is decisive as diplomats depend on active participation by its high ranking politicians. Diplomats have internalized their field's institutional logic. Analyses relativize arguments by Samantha Power (2002) for the U.S. and Karen Smith (2010) for Europe, according to which cautious language of diplomats, even in the face of genocide, is reflective of the reluctance of rational actors to get involved, attributing such caution instead to the habitus of diplomats and its rootedness in the structural conditions of their field.

Competing fields such as humanitarian aid and diplomacy thus offer representations of mass violence that compete with, and thereby reduce, the delegitimizing power of the criminal justice narrative. Simultaneously though, they pose counterweights against the limitations of that narrative. We should bear in mind, though, that analyses of world media show that the criminal justice narrative trumps these competing accounts in their respective effects on world opinion (Savelsberg 2015; Savelsberg and Nyseth Brehm 2015).

Conclusions

Much world suffering is the direct result of human action, especially mass violence. Importantly, when we consider alleviating world suffering, some actions that cause mass violence have been redefined, in the course of the late nineteenth and twentieth centuries, from heroic deeds of mighty state builders to criminal acts. War crimes, crimes against humanity, and genocide are among them. One of today's crucial questions is if such redefinitions, and the new institutions which have contributed to them, are capable of relieving world suffering. This essay has focused on one type of institution, new criminal law interventions, named the "justice cascade" (Sikkink 2011) and highlighted the mass violence of Darfur as an example (Savelsberg 2015). The evidence is fresh, and more time is needed to observe the effects of historically new institutions. Yet, initial empirical analyses indicate, despite cautionary notes, that these institutions may reduce human-induced suffering, through the deterrence effect (Jo and Simmons 2016) or through a cultural redefinition of mass violence (Savelsberg and King 2011). The hope may be utopian, that the civilizing effect and the domestic pacification that the build-up of state institutions has achieved at the level of modern nations (Elias 1978; Johnson and Monkkonen 1996), might be repeated at the world level. There is no doubt that more work toward improving new international and global institutions, including those of criminal justice, and research on their functioning, is an imperative if alleviation of world suffering is to be achieved.

References

Alexander, J. C. (2004). On the social construction of moral universals: The 'Holocaust' from war crime to trauma drama. In J. C. Alexander et al. (Eds.), *Cultural trauma and collective identity* (pp. 196–263). Berkeley: University of California Press.

Barkan, E. (2013). *Justifying atrocities: Contested victims*. Lecture at Legal Frames of Memory conference. Warsaw, Poland.

Cohen, S. (2001). *States of denial: Knowing about atrocities and suffering*. Cambridge: Polity Press.

Czarnota, A. (2015). *Law as Mnemosyne married with Lethe: Quasi-judicial institutions and collective memories*. Paper presented at Contested past, contested present: Social memories and human rights in post-communist Europe conference, Minneapolis, 2015.

Elias, N. (1978). *The civilizing process*. 1st American ed. Mole Editions. New York: Urizen Books.

Giesen, B. (2004). *Triumph or Trauma*. Boulder: Paradigm.

Golden, S. (2013). *After atrocity: Community reconstruction in Northern Uganda*. University of Minnesota, Doctoral Dissertation.

Goldsmith, J., & Krasner, S. D. (2003). The limits of idealism. *Daedalus, 132*(1), 47–63.

Hayner, P. B. (2001). *Unspeakable truths: Confronting state terror and atrocity*. New York: Routledge.

Jo, H. & Simmons, B. (2016). Can the international criminal court deter atrocity? *International Organization, 70*(3), 443–475.

Johnson, E. A., & Monkkonen, E. H. (Eds.). (1996). *The civilization of crime: Violence in town and country since the middle ages*. Urbana: University of Illinois Press.

Keck, M. E., & Sikkink, K. (1998). *Activists beyond borders: Advocacy networks in international politics*. Ithaca: Cornell University Press.

Kim, H., & Sikkink, K. (2010). Explaining the deterrence effect of human rights prosecutions for transitional countries. *International Studies Quarterly, 54*(4), 939–963.

Landsman, S. (2005). *Crimes of the holocaust: The law confronts hard cases, Pennsylvania Studies in Human Rights*. Philadelphia: University of Pennsylvania Press.

Levy, D., & Sznaider, N. (2010). *Human rights and memory, Essays on Human Rights*. University Park: Pennsylvania State University Press.

Marrus, M. (2008). The Nuremberg doctors' trial and the limitations of context. In P. Heberer & J. Matthäus (Eds.), *Atrocities on trial* (pp. 103–122). Lincoln: University of Nebraska Press.

Matsueda, R. L., Kreager, D. A., & Huizinga, D. (2006). Deterring delinquents: A rational choice model of theft and violence. *American Sociological Review, 71*(1), 95–122.

McCarthy, B. (2002). New economics of sociological criminology. *Annual Review of Sociology, 28*, 417–442.

Mead, G. H. (1918). The psychology of punitive justice. *American Journal of Sociology, 23*, 577–602.

Meierhenrich, J. (2006). Conspiracy in international law. *Annual Review of Law and Social Science, 2*(1), 341–357.

Minow, M. (1998). *Between vengeance and forgiveness: Facing history after genocide and mass violence*. Boston: Beacon Press.

Neier, A. (2012). *The international human rights movement: A history, Human Rights and Crimes against Humanity*. Princeton: Princeton University Press.

Nobels, M. (2010). The prosecution of human rights violations. *Annual Review of Political Science, 13*, 165–182.

Osiel, M. (2014). The demise of international criminal law. *Humanity Journal,* June 10, 2014 (http://www.humanityjournal.net/blog/the-demise-of-international-criminal-law/)

Pendas, D. O. (2006). *The Frankfurt Auschwitz Trial, 1963–65: Genocide, history and the limits of the law*. Cambridge/New York: Cambridge University Press.

Pensky, M. (2008). Amnesty on trial: Impunity, accountability, and the norms of international law. *Ethics & Global Politics, 1*(1–2), 1–40.

Power, S. (2002). *A problem from hell: America and the age of genocide*. New York: Perennial.
Rummel, R. J. (1994). *Death by government*. New Brunswick: Transactions Publishers.
Savelsberg, J. J. (2010). *Crime and human rights: Criminology of genocide and atrocities*. London: Sage.
Savelsberg, J. J. (2015). *Representing mass violence: Conflicting responses to human rights violations in Darfur.* Oakland: University of California Press. (An open access version of the book is available online at: http://www.luminosoa.org/site/books/detail/3/representing-mass-violence/.)
Savelsberg, J. J., & King, R. D. (2011). *American memories: Atrocities and the law*. New York: Russell Sage Foundation.
Savelsberg, J. J., & Nyseth Brehm, H. (2015). Global justice, national distinctions: Criminalizing human rights violations in Darfur. *American Journal of Sociology, 121*(2), 564–603.
Scheffer, D. (2012). *All the missing souls: A personal history of the war crimes tribunals*. Princeton: Princeton University Press.
Seekers of Truth and Justice. (2003). *The black book* (no place or publisher).
Sikkink, K. (2011). *The justice cascade: How human rights prosecutions are changing world politics*. New York: W.W. Norton.
Smith, P. (2008). *Punishment and culture*. Chicago: University of Chicago Press.
Smith, K. (2010). *Genocide and the Europeans*. Cambridge: Cambridge University Press.
Snyder, J., & Vinjamuri, L. (2003). Trials and errors: Principle and pragmatism in strategies of international justice. *International Security, 28*, 5–44.
Stan, L. (2013). Civil society and post-communist transitional justice. Paper presented at Legal Frames of Memory conference. Warsaw, Poland.

Chapter 23
The Commercial and Non-commercial Sexual Exploitation of Children in North America: Canada, Mexico and the United States

Richard J. Estes

Introduction

The sexual exploitation of children (SEC) is among the most heinous of crimes. As stated by this volume's editor, Ron Anderson, in a personal message to this author:

> It is hard to over-exaggerate the misery of children exploited for sex, especially those trafficked to totally new locations where a different language is spoken. Some children are deceived, coerced, drugged, or kidnapped before being trafficked for commercial sexual exploitation. Vulnerable young children might be trained by traffickers or pimps who pretend to have a romantic interest, but then use violence and rape to control the child. As children tend to be clueless about the prostitution trade, they do not know what is happening until they find themselves raped and forced to take clients. Some children are trafficked directly to homemade prisons, where they are held against their will, coerced, raped, and delivered by armed guards to places where clients pay for sexual services. Any of these acts of violence could be devastating for adults, so it is hard to imagine the deep, long-term suffering that children must endure." (Anderson 2015a).

This project began its focus on three main types of sexual exploitation of children: child pornography, juvenile prostitution, and the sale and trafficking of children across jurisdictional and international borders. It soon became apparent that the research could be better organized along a continuum of increasing harm to children, namely child sexual abuse, child sexual assault, and other sexual exploitation of children. The latter category produces the most harm and suffering to children, probably because it encompasses commercially driven sexual exploitation of children.

Tragically, parents, especially those living under dire circumstances in impoverished communities, may facilitate this practice and, in many cases, are actually the

R.J. Estes (✉)
School of Social Policy & Practice, University of Pennsylvania,
Philadelphia, PA 19104-6214, USA
e-mail: restes@upenn.edu

R.E. Anderson (ed.), *Alleviating World Suffering*, Social Indicators Research Series 67, DOI 10.1007/978-3-319-51391-1_23

persons who seduce vulnerable children into their eventual commercial sexual exploitation. Children may be assigned legitimate jobs such as a jockey or department store stock room worker but, in time, they, too, are pressured into commercial sex work—a phenomena known as modern day slavery, in which largely deceived and manipulated children are either owned, or mostly controlled, by adults who benefit directly from their sexual exploitation (Bales 1999; Shelly 2010; USDOS 2015a). All forms of this exploitation are associated with profound levels of human suffering for which effective solutions often prove elusive. Deception, manipulation, and coercion of children (and often their parents or other caregivers as well) are typical aspects of sexual exploitation of children in all three countries of the North American region (Anderson 2015c; USDOJ 2015a; USDOS 2015a, b).[1]

Estes and Weiner (2001, 2005), prior to the latter's death in 2009, and their research colleagues in Canada and Mexico detailed this phenomenon in considerable depth (Azaola and Estes 2003; Estes and Weiner 2001; Estes et al. 2005). The nature of these crimes against children is terrifying, and in every case leaves deep emotional scars from which children may never fully recover. Certainly their parents and extended kinship networks suffer as well, especially as the specifics of their exploitative situation become clear (Kessler et al. 2004; RAINN 2015).

The Focus of This Chapter

This chapter discusses five overlapping patterns with respect to the exploitation of children in sexual activity: (1) the nature, extent, and severity of the child sexual exploitation within the North American region[2] with a focus on all three of the region's countries; (2) identification of the major social forces that contribute to the different types of sexual exploitation of children; (3) likely scenarios regarding the containment of sexual exploitation of children; (4) a discussion of a series of interrelated recommendations designed to halt region-wide increases in the sexual exploitation of children; and (5) the prerequisites necessary to alleviate the suffering experienced by these children as they mature into adulthood. The recommendations outlined in the chapter are multidimensional and focus on the responsibilities of state and non-state actors in alleviating suffering experienced by child victims of sexual exploitation.

---

[1] The United States is one of two countries that is not a signatory member state of the United Nations' *Convention of the Rights of Children* (1989); the other country is Somalia. Thus, all laws pertaining to the protection of children from sexual exploitation, including commercial sexual exploitation, in the United States are either national or state in origin.

[2] Mexico frequently is considered as an exclusively Latin American country. Geographically, and as a member of the North American Free Trade Agreement (NAFTA), however, Mexico is included in this study as a member nation of the North American region. Another justification for doing so is the large number of Mexican nationals as well as the nationals of other Latin American nations that use Mexico as a gateway into Canada and the United States.

Research Methods

The research summarized in this chapter is the result of a multiyear, multimethod, and multidimensional approach to the study of child commercial sexual exploitation in the North American region, e.g., child pornography, juvenile prostitution, and trafficking in children for sexual purposes. The major phases involved in the research are summarized in Appendixes A and N of Estes and Weiner (2001). These methodologies included: (1) extensive literature reviews covering our understanding of the historical and contemporary nature of sexual exploitation of children in Western societies; (2) focus group meetings with persons who specialize in the issue of child sexual exploitation in specifically targeted cities in Canada [N=7], Mexico [N=8], and the United States [N=13]; (3) interviews with selected child victims of commercial sex, living either on the streets or in protective institutions [N=200]; (4) a limited number of interviews with adult customers of child sex (limited owing to the highly illegal nature and reporting requirements of the sexual crimes involved) [N=50]; (5) a limited number of interviews with cooperative adult traffickers of children for sex (again, limited owing to the highly illegal nature involved in the reporting requirements of sexual crime), [N=15]; (6) interviews with key policy- and other decision-makers responsible for planning and implementing programs designed to protect children from commercial sexual exploitation [N=40]; (7) statistical surveys of local, state, and national organizations concerned with commercial sexual exploitation of children [N=125]; (8) informal discussions with law enforcement, human service, and child advocacy groups dealing directly with the sexual exploitation of children for commercial purposes [N=70]); and (9) analyses of each country's laws and legal codes relating to this disturbing issue.

Child Sexual Exploitation in North America

Child pornography, child prostitution, and trafficking in children for sexual purposes are not new phenomena in North America (Azaola and Estes 2003; Estes 2001; Tremblay et al. 2001). Collectively, these forms of child sexual exploitation are referred to by sociologist Kevin Bales and others as manifestations of "modern-day slavery" (Bales 1999; *Frontline* 2006). Sexual slavery cuts across all social classes and income groups and occurs among the most and least educated members of communities worldwide (Moran 2015; Shelly 2010). Unfortunately, these activities historically have included adults and children, the latter frequently referred to as "street children." Indeed, historical evidence shows a long history of child sexual exploitation in the United States and in other countries of the North American region (Estes 2001; Estes and Weiner 2001, 2005). These patterns are well documented in the literature of child protection agencies, some of which are identified throughout the body of this chapter.

Considerable commercial sexual exploitation of children came after the sexual liberation movement of the 1960s in the United States, the main country of destination for many child victims of sex trafficking. International dimensions of the commercialized aspect of this phenomenon increased during the 1980s and 1990s following the collapse of the former Soviet Union, which resulted in the displacement of large numbers of young people from education and jobs. Today, tens of thousands of citizens of the recently independent republics of the former Soviet Union (especially from Moldova, Ukraine, and the Russian Federation) have made their way into Europe and, eventually, into the United States and the economically advanced nations of Europe, East Asia (Japan and South Korea) and Oceania (Australia and New Zealand). Many of these newly independent countries served as "countries of origin" of trafficked persons, whereas Western and other economically advanced societies serve as "destination countries," albeit certain countries served as both, e.g., the Russian Federation (Shelly 2010; USDOS 2015b). Trafficked persons arrived on the shores of North America from other world regions as well, e.g., from sub-Saharan Africa, Mexico, the Philippines, and others (USDOS 2015b)

Definitions of Child Sexual Abuse, Child Sexual Assault, and the Commercial Sexual Exploitation of Children

The primary definitions used to distinguish the three primary forms of child sexual exploitation are summarized in Table 23.1. All three manifestations of child sexual abuse, sexual assault, and commercial sexual exploitation exist on a continuum with each category of sexual exploitation associated with higher levels of vulnerability and suffering by the child victims, during and sometimes long after their victimization (Kessler et al. 2004; Maltz 2002; RAINN 2015; Raymond 2011).

The dynamic involved in commercial sexual exploitation of children follows a pattern. Unrelated older children or, most typically, unrelated adults in their early or mid-20s to mid-30s, recruit children specifically for the purpose of performing sexual acts that work to the advantage of the adult recruiters. The child's share of money earned from such activities (pornography, prostitution, or cross-jurisdictional sex trafficking) is usually minimal, thereby keeping children dependent on their victimizers for basic financial support.

Children are rarely able to extricate themselves from such situations without the assistance of interested adults, law enforcement, or representatives of social agencies. Families often actively search for the location of their missing child(ren), albeit the extent of the search typically depends on the situation or adult perpetrators associated with the initial sexually exploitive experience.

Table 23.1 Three major types of child sexual exploitation and their definitions[a]

Child sexual abuse	Child sexual assault	Commercial sexual exploitation of children
Child sexual abuse is any sort of non-consensual sexual contact. Sexual abuse can happen to adults as well as children of any age. Most child sexual abuse consists of adults engaging in explicit sexual contact or relations with children who have not yet reached adult age status.	Child sexual assault is any sexual act (including sexual touching) in which the recipient has not reached an adult age. The sexual assault of a child is considered more serious if the child is coerced or physically forced to engage against their will.	Sexual exploitation of children in its most egregious, and often most suffering-ridden expression of sexual exploitation, involves a commercial relationship in which monetary or non-monetary goods or services are traded for child sexual abuse, with or without assault.
	Sexual assault is a form of sexual violence, and it includes rape (such as forced vaginal, anal, or oral penetration or drug facilitated sexual assault), groping, forced kissing, or torture in a sexual manner. In brief, it is any involuntary child sexual abuse.	Sexual exploiters of children do not always use money or monetized goods. Often vulnerable children will trade sex for alcohol, drugs, popularity, personal attention, concert tickets, designer clothing, jewelry, and electronic devices. While these are informal forms of commercial transactions, they *are* nonetheless commercial exchanges.
		Children often are caught up in trafficking for the purposes of sexual slavery and may undergo coercion, brutality, and enforced pov
		erty. Children may be further subjected to violence from their adult customers or "johns."

[a]These three types of child exploitation are defined and discussed in Wikipedia (2015a, b) as well as in child sexual exploitation literature generally.

Children at Risk of Commercial Sexual Exploitation

At the outset of this project with my co-investigator, the late Neil Weiner, we had expected to find just three primary categories of children at special risk of commercial sexual exploitation: (1) child victims of pornography; (2) adolescents engaged in juvenile prostitution; and (3) domestic and international children participating in international sexual trafficking rings (Bales 1999; USDOS 2015b). Indeed, these three groups of children were confirmed to be at the greatest risk, but we also identified additional groups of children who were suffering from sexual abuse and assault. The various groups of children identified through the research (N=4) are listed in Table 23.2. Each of the four groups requires a highly specialized approach to suffering alleviation treatment tailored to the unique circumstances surrounding their recruitment and participation in sexually exploitative activities.

Table 23.2 Groups of children at the highest risk of commercial sexual exploitation

GROUP A (60%): *Sexually exploited youth not living in their own homes*
Runaways
"Thrownaways"
Homeless youth
GROUP B (20%): *Sexually exploited children living in their own homes*
General population
Public housing
GROUP C (10%): *Sexually exploited child victims of other groups*
Female gang members
Transgender street youth
GROUP D (10%): *Child victims of international dimensions of commercial sexual exploitation*
Foreign children ages 10–17 brought into the United States either legally or illegally
Unaccompanied minors entering the United States
Non-immigrant Canadian and Mexican children ages 10–17 entering the United States for sexual purposes
U.S. youth ages 13–17 living within driving distance of a tourist-type Mexican or Canadian city
Non-immigrant youth aged 13–17 trafficked from the United States to other countries

Source: Estes and Weiner (2001)

Trends and Patterns Related to Contemporary Expressions of Commercial Sexual Exploitation of Children

Many of the child vulnerability patterns that existed in America at the turn of the century remain with us today. Most of these children have run away from home or from child institutions, and others have abandoned family or institutional foster care in favor of what most perceive to be a "freer" life on the streets (USCB 2007). Many of these children survive on the streets through a combination of begging, drug sales, illegal day labor, and, yes, commercial sex work (including pornography and juvenile prostitution). Most of these children live in "squats" (abandoned or dilapidated houses or apartments) and others in low-priced motel rooms with as many as five to seven sharing the same living space. Others live temporarily in vans, station wagons, or cheap cars to have a means of transportation (Street Child Project 2015).

Though the number of commercially sexually exploited children cannot be estimated with precision, there is evidence that child victims in North America number in the tens of thousands at any moment (USDOJ 2015a; USDOS 2015a, b). Their numbers appear to shift from one period of time to the next, but the children counted always include a variety of physically abused and neglected children. Many boys over the age of 16 are forced onto the streets as "thrownaways," i.e., young people who are difficult to manage and do not conform to either family or community norms. Others are victims of domestic sexual abuse, assaults by family members, relatives, and even by various clergy members (Child Welfare Information Gateway 2015). Drug use and engagement in property crimes is rampant among these populations of children. Older adolescents also frequently function as "managers" (actually pimps) in the street community of a limited number of girls who work for them as prostitutes in exchange for protection, housing, and for regular access to street drugs (Anderson 2015b; Stegall and Mercedes 2014).

What has changed since the turn of the century in North America, however, is an increasing willingness on the part of the general public to engage in efforts to return these children to safety—to their families of origin when appropriate and, if not, to various types of foster care arrangements. The extent of the sexual exploitation of children for commercial reasons is reflected in the growing numbers of governmental and non-governmental organizations engaged in rescuing street children from such activities. The commitment also is reflected in increasingly rigorous legislation, better educated law enforcement officers, and more awareness by health care professionals (Kessler et al. 2004; Ratican 1992). Specialized child advocacy organizations also have emerged that provide street children with venues where they are welcome to shower, obtain a change of clothing, and receive nutritious meals without being compelled by the providers to change their lifestyle (although a "hand up" is almost always available for those youth who wish to leave "the life"). Alleviating the suffering of children associated with commercial sexual exploitation is particularly difficult and will involve a broad spectrum of state and non-state actors, as well as many years of "wraparound services" (housing, education, vocational training, family counseling) and individualized mental health treatment for the most seriously affected children.

Factors that Contribute to the Commercial Sexual Exploitation of Children

The psychosocial dynamics that contribute to the abandonment of children by their families of origin to the insecurities and obvious dangers associated with street life are many and varied (Lloyd 2012; Warren and Phelps 2012). A history of chronic physical or sexual abuse within the context of the family is certainly one of the main drivers of this phenomenon. For example, single parents (mostly mothers) are averse to their daughters telling them about sexual advances made by the mother's boyfriend. In Canada and Mexico, at the same time, fathers frequently cannot overcome the sense of disappointment they feel in their incorrigible sons who violate family and community norms, which brings them to the attention of law enforcement authorities. The problem is also widespread among families in the United States. Confrontations between family members and police over a child's behavior has often had a negative effect on the families, who feel admonished as inadequate parents unable to properly control their children (Finkelhor and Ormod 2001).

From our study, peer pressure is yet another major influence on the behavior of vulnerable children. For boys, the use of alcohol and drugs with peers predominated as a method of coping, whereas with girls, access on the part of their sexually active friends to more expensive clothing, jewelry, and related top-shelf purchases had the most significant impact (Van Drannen 2012). These patterns were pervasive through the population of children we interviewed; we frequently heard the same stories from caregivers in transitional housing facilities designed to serve abandoned and street children (Phelps and Larkin 2013).

Social-Psychological Dimensions of Commercial Sexual Exploitation of Children

The long-term psychological impact of suffering associated with sexual abuse, sexual assault, and commercial sexual exploitation of children has been studied extensively. All of the studies report serious challenges for these victims as they seek to assume adult roles as spouses and parents and even as employes (Ratican 1992). Many of these studies describe sexual abuse of types that foster post-traumatic stress disorder (PTSD), i.e., an illness characterized by chronic anxiety, depression, sleeplessness, reliving their abusive experiences in dreams, the inability to develop truly intimate relationships with their adult partners, and psychological distancing between themselves and others (Maltz 2002; McNew and Abell 1995). The impact of these sources on the suffering of children is devastating and leaves permanent scars on the psyche of those who have been victimized.

Social and Familial Dimensions of the Commercial Sexual Exploitation of Children

Assuming that some children have agency over their well-being, what is it about them that could, or would, motivate them to enter into the world of child commercial sexual exploitation? This question is especially relevant for children older than 13, who, in the main, are able to exercise at least some choices over the wide range of activities in which they engage, including sex work. The answers to this question are unique to the individual child and to the quality of the relationship that exists between the child and his or her own parents and other members of the child's family of origin (Raymond 2012; S., Miss 2008; Moran 2015). We also know from our field research that a substantial number of young adolescent girls are attracted to the material goods that they can purchase using sex-work money. Many of these girls are members of middle class and even more affluent families who already have been sexually active with boyfriends or others on a casual basis (Estes and Weiner 2001).

The motivations for boys engaging in commercial sex work differ from those of girls. Many of the boys we encountered were in fact thrownaway children whose incorrigible behavior at home (drug and alcohol use, theft, fighting with siblings) resulted in their parents, usually the father, telling the boy to leave home and not to return unless and until certain behavioral requirements were met. Girls, by contrast, frequently leave home to be with a boyfriend or to be with a group of slightly older girls who share the same values. The sense of humiliation that girls and boys experience when living on the streets, especially by exchanging sex for money, is frequently dulled by the frequent "highs" associated with the use of street drugs.

All aspects of this situation are complex and render intervention more difficult with older children (Estes and Weiner 2005). Neither boys nor girls engaged in sex work fully enjoy the situations in which they find themselves, as they feel trapped and unable to take the steps necessary to extricate themselves of the horrific conditions to which they are exposed (Lloyd 2012; S., Miss 2008). The failure of law enforcement authorities to take a more active role in apprehending these suffering children only adds to the mix of reasons for why these types of situations persist and new cohorts of children are added to the sexually exploited population (Gattas et al. 2012).

Child Abuse and Neglect, Including Child Sexual Exploitation

Table 23.3 identifies the number of *child abuse and neglect cases* reported to United States human service authorities between 1999 and 2005. A substantial number of these cases include suspected reports of child sexual abuse and child sexual assault. The numbers reported in the 6-year period are staggering, i.e., nearly one million of America's 74.2 million children (1.2% annually of all children). These aggregated numbers, however, mask the actual incidence of each individual type of offense included in these totals.

The number of children who were abused and neglected has fluctuated over the 7 years for which data are available from the American Humane Association, which reported the counts for the NCANDS, the National Child Abuse and Neglect Data System. It is difficult to know if the changes in the numbers of children reported year-by-year results from random fluctuations alone or partly from actual changes in abuse and neglect of children.

Table 23.3 Incidence of child abuse and neglect in the United States, 1999–2005

Year	Abused and Neglected Children
1999	829,000
2000	881,000
2001	903,000
2002	896,000
2003	906,000
2004	872,000
2005	899,000

Source: American Humane Association (2016)

Officially Reported Incidence of Child Sexual Abuse and Sexual Assault in the United States

The closest approximation of the incidence of child sexual abuse and child sexual assault are those reported annually by National Center for Victims of Crime (NCVC), the leading resource and advocacy organization for crime victims and those who serve them since 1985. The general parameters of these patterns are summarized in the bulleted list below and include data for Alaska and Puerto Rico as well as that of selected Canadian and Mexican children who have taken up illegal residency in the United States. The numbers reported in the list are quite dramatic and report that 28% of all children in the United States between the ages of 7 and 13 eventually are sexually victimized, often by members of their own families. Here are findings of the National Center for Victims of Crime (NCVC 2015): 1 in 5 girls and 1 in 20 boys is a victim of child sexual abuse:

- Self-report studies show that 20% of adult females and 5–10% of adult males recall a childhood sexual assault or sexual abuse incident;
- Over their lifetime, 28% of U.S. youth ages 14 to 17 had been sexually victimized;
- Children are most vulnerable to the abused between the ages of 7 and 13.

The Suffering Associated with Child Homelessness, Runaways, and Thrownaways

Being a single child on the streets can be a very solitary, usually devastating, experience. In addition to their youth and lack of maturity, these children have no way of supporting themselves, apart from the sale of their bodies or what children refer to as "survival sex." Homeless children, however they arrived in this situation, are profoundly lonely, feel vulnerable, and, frequently, are looking for an adult or group of older children who can accord them some measure of social protection. Such children easily fall victim to drug abuse and commercial sexual exploitation.

In the research reported in this study, the age of the youngest child identified was 9—a latency-age girl of Mexican-American origin living on the streets of Las Vegas, Nevada. This child, whom we shall refer to as "Agnes," reported that she had "been on her own" for a year prior to our encounter with her. Our research team quickly surmised that Agnes was drug intoxicated, suffering from severe depression, and made herself available for street sex by almost any adult "for whom the price was right" (a variable price that depended on the last time she had had food or a drug "fix"). Fortunately, we were able to secure Agnes's cooperation in participating with the local nongovernmental organization that specializes in serving homeless children.

After several weeks stabilizing Agnes, the agency arranged for her referral to a local psychiatric facility that also specialized in the care of acutely mentally ill children. Agnes was never reunited with her family of origin inasmuch as she cited her father as the source of the sexual abuse that caused her to run away from home. Paradoxically, her short-term actions did not take her to a place of safety, but instead to an environment in which she was repeatedly exploited over and over again.

In our all-too-brief communications with Agnes, she wanted to tell her personal story to us. Like so many other children we encountered, she wanted to share her experiences in order to reduce the risk of other children becoming victims of sexual exploitation. She was guarded about the specifics of her story, however, and we could not use it to return her to her home state or to her local community.

Even so, the presence in Las Vegas of a highly skilled agency that was prepared to work with children such as Agnes represented an exceptional situation in our several years of engaging in research with sexually exploited street children. Rarely had we been able to partner with a full-spectrum, child-serving agency that could, and would, respond comprehensively to the complex needs of children such as Agnes. Sadly, we learned of Agnes' death from a drug overdose just a year after the project concluded. She had secured the drugs from another child in the same psychiatric institution in which they were receiving treatment. From our perspective, however, the cause of death was the commercial sexual exploitation of which Agnes was a victim, and the drugs were simply instrumental in helping to alleviate the deep-seated pain that Agnes and other of her friends experienced.

Recommendations for Alleviating the Suffering of Sexually Exploited Children

The suffering experienced by child victims of sexual exploitation can be profoundly reduced, especially if responsible adults recognize the early signs of sexual exploitation. But to realize this goal, considerable effort must be made to improving our approaches to early detection and prevention. Some of these are highlighted below. Societal commitments reducing child suffering is central to each of the recommendations.

Protect the Children—A Societal Commitment

Child victims of commercial sexual exploitation rarely can protect themselves from the sexual assaults inflicted on them by adults. The situation is especially serious for those children living in homes with adult sexual predators and in situations where they expose themselves to sexual activity in exchange for money or other material things of experienced value to them. Children rarely have a sense of the long-lasting suffering to which they are exposing themselves in the process of these exchanges of sex for "things" of transient value.

Protect the Children: The Role of the Family

Families are in a unique position to intervene early in situations involving commercial sexual exploitation of their children. To do so, however, they need to be informed about the risks of such exploitation—both within their own household and among neighbors and other adults who have regular or easy contact with their children: neighbors, teachers, sports coaches, members of the clergy, adult "friends", among others. Other families, those that participate willingly in the exploitation of their children, require a broad range of legal and social service interventions—often resulting in the removal of children from their families of origin.

Protect the Children: The Role of the Schools and the Larger Community

Schools, community centers, and other places where children congregate can assume a major role in helping to reduce the incidence of children exposed to sexual exploitation, especially via their capacity "to hear" the often obscure sexual concerns expressed by children. Teachers and community center personnel, to be effective, though, need to be educated in the symptoms commonly associated with the sexual exploitation (e.g., depression, chronic somatic complaints, often faint references to abuse by parents, quiet pleas for help, and others) and be prepared to act on the cases in which these symptoms are confirmed. Such sensitivity can develop through training provided by specially prepared physicians, social service personnel, and law enforcement personnel who have extensive experience in the early detection of sexual exploitation of children (Estes, Cooper, & Giardino 2005).

The media also can play a major role in promoting the sexual safety of children, especially through the careful reporting of cases and statistics. Such exposure should focus on the societal implications of these practices. At the same time, reports can include positive actions, including hotline telephone numbers that children, parents, and others can use to reduce the incidence of future cases.

Protect the Children: The Role of Governmental and Nongovernmental Organizations

Given the cross-jurisdictional nature of most commercial sex crimes committed against children, a single lead agency at the federal level needs to be given primary responsibility for protecting children from these crimes. Currently, 14 federal agencies share this responsibility (DHHS, Customs and Postal Service, the Department of State, among others). But the sheer number of the agencies reduces the effectiveness of the public sector in responding—in a coherent way—to the many manifestations of the often difficult-to-discern cases of child commercial sexual exploitation.

Nongovernmental organizations also must maintain a proactive role in identifying child victims, but currently, the resources available to most for doing so fall far short of the services needed (Estes 2005, 2007). The result is that the level of suffering experienced by underserved children continues to be extraordinary, and resources available to help alleviate their suffering remain too few. A more creative set of private-public partnerships are needed to advance comprehensive solutions to the problem (Estes and Zhou 2015).

Target Adult Sexual Exploiters of Children for Punishment, Not the Children

Tragically, the victims of child sexual exploitation often are revictimized by the law enforcement and human services agencies created to serve them. Revictimization may take one of several different forms: (1) blaming child victims for their own exploitation, thus increasing the already high level of emotional suffering they experience; (2) treating child victims as criminals, often as felons, who require punishment rather than social care; (3) an unwarranted emphasis on the part of law enforcement in responding to child sexual exploitation when, in fact, a broader range of human services and clinical services are needed, especially in the treatment of dysfunctional families in which child sexual exploitation is all too prevalent; and (4) neglect on the part of human service funders in support of the comprehensive services required by severely impaired child victims of sexual exploitation (Estes et al. 2005; Gattas et al. 2012).

Increase Penalties Associated with the Commercial Sexual Exploitation of Children

Considerable variation exists across state and provincial lines in all three North American countries with respect to the seriousness assigned by the region's legal systems to persons convicted of child sexual exploitation. Thus, to effectively reduce the incidence of these sex crimes and to achieve some measure of alleviating the associated suffering, it is important that: (1) ages of sexual consent laws be made uniform across all state and provincial jurisdiction; (2) given the seriousness of this crime against children, penalties imposed on adult perpetrators should be increased significantly, and (3) the legal penalties should be adjusted to the differences in age between child victims and their adult exploiters (Azaola 2001; Azaola and Estes 2003).

Rigorously Enforce Existing National Laws Associated with the Commercial Sexual Exploitation of Children

A confirmed pattern of benign neglect exists in many communities regarding the enforcement of sexual crimes committed against children, including those involving child commercial sexual exploitation. To be effective in reducing child sexual exploitation, all three countries must provide more assertive national and provincial leadership in enforcing what now are already aggressive regional and national laws.

Strengthen and Expand Regional and National Task Forces Focused on Child Victims of Commercial Sexual Exploitation

Several already functioning governmental agencies focused on child sexual exploitation need to be expanded: (1) multijurisdictional task forces on child sexual exploitation, and (2) national child commercial sexual exploitation task forces. Both types of federal and regional entities have proven to be effective in working cooperatively across international and jurisdictional boundaries. Both also lend themselves readily to decentralization at the provincial, state, and local levels and, thus, within the reach of child victims of commercial sexual exploitation (ICAC 2015; USDOS 2015b).

Federally sponsored Internet Crimes Against Children (ICAC) task forces also have experienced considerable success in reducing the incidence of electronic child pornography and, in due course, juvenile prostitution. Since their inception in the United States in 1998, ICAC programs have contributed to the arrest of thousands of sexual predators and have resulted in seizing many thousand computer and electronic websites. The CyberTipline of the National Center for Missing and Exploited Children (NCMEC), the nation's central task force on child pornography and training center, needs to be further strengthened (Azaola and Estes 2003; NCMEC 2015; Tremblay et al. 2001).

Promote a Fuller Spectrum of Effective Public–Private Partnerships for Combating the Sexual Exploitation of Children

A successful regional campaign to combat child sexual exploitation requires active participation on the part of all stakeholders in child protection. These stakeholders include: (1) governmental agencies charged with leadership responsibility in combating the problem at all levels of political organization; (2) child-serving nongovernmental organizations and agencies; (3) associations and networks of children and young adults who were sexually exploited for commercial gain; (4) associations and networks of parents and guardians of runaway, thrownaway, homeless, and

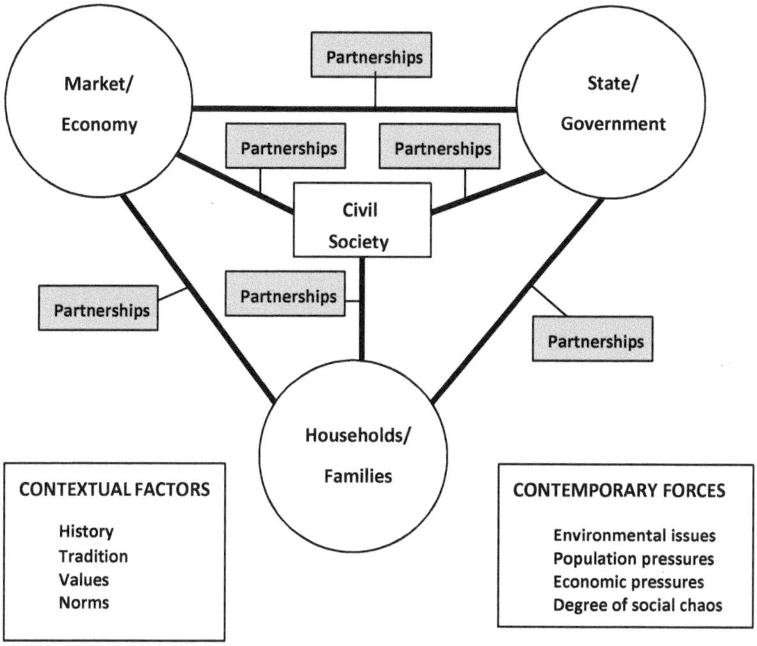

Fig. 23.1 Public-private mix of partners needed to halt child sexual exploitation (Source: Based on Estes and Zhou (2015) and reprinted with permission from the International Journal of Social Welfare and John Wiley and Sons Publisher)

otherwise missing children; and (4) nongovernmental organizations engaged in advocacy, research, and educational activities on behalf of these children and their families.

Figure 23.1 depicts the broad range of public-private partnerships designed to reduce the risk of child sexual exploitation. Developed by Estes and Zhou (2015), this figure illustrates the many possibilities that exist in all aspects of society for preventing, treating, and otherwise alleviating the suffering that child victims are exposed to through sexual exploitation (Anderson 2015b; S 2008; Shelly 2010).

Enlarge the Regional Pool of Child Sexual Exploitation Specialists

A serious shortage exists in all three of the region's countries in the number and type of specialists who deal with the sexual exploitation of children. These shortages are most apparent in the forensics area but also exist in the judicial and prosecutorial agencies at all levels of legal organization. There also remains an urgent need for more social workers, psychologists, psychiatrists, educators, physicians, lawyers, police officers, even coroners with specialized training in the diagnosis and treatment of child sexual exploitation. The central governments of each country also need to take a more active role in promoting education and training in responding to child sexual exploitation issues in all areas of their work.

Undertake More Research on Perpetrators and Victims of Child Sexual Exploitation

More needs to be understood about the nature, causes, and extent of the child sexual exploitation in North America and other regions of the world (2015b). This information is particularly needed for communities in which these children are largely hidden from public view, and thus, their personal histories of suffering are unknown and untold. The following avenues of research are needed, including dissemination of findings through the use of the public media, in pursuing multi-tiered solutions to the sexual exploitation of children. Among the most important questions to be pursued:

- Apart from the factors that we already have identified, what other forces compel children to leave the comparative safety of home for the dangers associated with street life (Azaola and Estes 2003; Estes and Weiner 2001; Moran 2015; Raymond 2012)?
- What is the precise nature of functions performed by major market actors in supporting child sexual exploitation, especially those roles played by hotels, bus companies, airlines, and others that profit directly from the commercial exploitation of children?
- Why is it that some children engage in survival sex including those involved in commercial sex work for varying periods of time (Warren and Phelps 2012)?
- For those children who are able to exit "the life" more successfully than others, what are the underlying dynamics that contribute to their exit from commercial sex work? What type of support and treatment services do they need? And, in extreme cases, what actions should be taken against their adult exploiters, including recruiters, enforcement personnel and, yes—customers?
- Homosexual and transgender children engage in commercial sex work for longer time periods than children who self-identify as heterosexual. Why is this, and more fundamentally, what special efforts need to be undertaken to protect sexual minority children from years of recurrent suffering associated with commercial sex work? The approaches taken to respond effectively to the needs of sexual minority children appear to differ appreciably from those needed for sexual majority children, including access to a much fuller range of outreach and protective services (Azaola 2001; Feinauer et al. 1996; Kessler et al. 2004; Lloyd 2012; Maltz 2002; McNew and Abell 1995; Phelps and Larkin 2013; Warren and Phelps 2012).
- Far more needs to be known about the adults who perpetuate sexual victimization and exploitation of children. Who are they, and how did they become

involved in this activity? What proportion of the adult perpetrators of sexual exploitation against children were, themselves, victims of sex abuse as children (Estes 2001, 2007; NCMEC 2015; RAINN 2015; Tremblay et al. 2001)? What is the nature and extent of child sexual exploitation by adult perpetrators?
- Considerable effort must be undertaken to coordinate the efforts of local, provincial, state, national, and regional authorities in solving the underlying causes of child sexual exploitation. These efforts must be carefully coordinated with judicial authorities and, in turn, with probationary personnel who will be charged with responsibility of supervising adult sexual exploiters of children over the long term (Estes et al. 2005; NCMEC 2015).

Given the nature of the sex crimes committed against children, none of the research agendas outlined above will be easy to implement. To achieve this goal will require active partnerships, based on cooperative endeavors with the U.S. Department of Justice, other regional and national law enforcement agencies, and major research-oriented charitable foundations focused on children. Such approaches to second generation research must be pursued vigorously if we are to alleviate the profound levels of suffering experienced by sexually exploited children, their families, and even the communities in which these crimes take place.

Conclusions

Protecting North America's children from sexual exploitation is a complex and difficult challenge. Each year the number of children exposed to this form of exploitation affects tens of thousands of vulnerable children in the North American region's three countries and subjects them to unparalleled levels of human suffering (Bales 1999; Shelly 2010; USDOS 2015b). Alleviation of the suffering associated with these experiences is difficult to achieve because of their covert character.

Despite the difficulties involved, considerable progress has been made recently in combating the sexual exploitation of children throughout North America. Certainly clinicians have become more skilled in the early identification and intervention into suspected cases of sexual abuse. Similarly, law enforcement and human service professionals are increasingly more sensitive to the pervasive nature of child pornography and juvenile prostitution including the long-term consequences of child sexual exploitation. Increasingly, parents and others around the world have begun to understand that sexual exploitation of children is a problem that afflicts not only impoverished nations but *all* nations.

These important advances in recognizing the existence of the sexual exploitation of children contribute to a growing worldwide intolerance of such practices. As a result, global strategies to combat this victimization have been developed, regional compacts that seek to prevent such exploitation have emerged, and new and more comprehensive national and local laws designed to protect children have been passed. Teachers, physicians, social workers, child advocates, and others are now actively working with police, judges, and other law enforcement officials to weave more secure social safety nets designed to protect children from sexual exploitation.

Children themselves have joined in the effort, including "experiential youth" (youth actively involved in the sex trade) and other former child victims of sexual exploitation. But more partners and more steps are urgently needed to alleviate the suffering associated with commercial sex work and other sexual exploitation imposed on children.

The kind of suffering experienced by children who are victims of this ugly practice is not short-lived. Along with the fear, confusion and trauma suffered by the victims in the early stages of sexual abuse or assault is the further, and possibly longer-lasting impact: disease and sickness, mental illness, poverty, and even—as in the case of young Agnes—death. Without a determined effort to address and alleviate, if not solve, the problems and suffering that result from this exploitation, society as a whole will suffer if its youngest members are not safely allowed to become healthy, contributing, confident adults.

References

American Humane Association. (2016). *Child abuse and neglect statistics*. http://www.american-humane.org/children/stop-child-abuse/fact-sheets/child-abuse-and-neglect-statistics.html. Accessed 06 Jan 2016.

Anderson, R. (2015a). Personal communication to the author, 09 December 2015.

Anderson, R. (2015b). *Global suffering on the rise*. World suffering and compassionate relief of suffering (April 15). http://worldsuffering.org/global-suffering-on-the-rise/. Accessed 08 Dec 2015.

Anderson, R. (2015c). *World suffering and quality of life*. Dordrecht: Springer.

Azaola, E. (2001). *Child sexual exploitation in Mexico—A national report*. Mexico City: CIEASAS & Siglo XXI Veintiuno Editores.

Azaola, E., & Estes, R. J. (2003). *La infancia como mercancia sexual: México, Canadá y Estados Unidos*. Mexico City: CIEASAS & Siglo XXI Veintiuno Editores.

Bales, K. (1999). *Disposable people: New slavery in the global economy*. Los Angeles: University of California Press.

Child Welfare Information Gateway. (2015). *Perpetrators of child sexual abuse*. https://www.childwelfare.gov/topics/can/perpetrators/perp-sexabuse/. Accessed 15 Nov 2014.

Estes, R, J. (2001). The sexual exploitation of children: A working guide to the empirical literature. Philadelphia: University of Pennsylvania School of Social Work.

Estes, R. J. (2005). *Medical, legal & social science aspects of child sexual exploitation: A comprehensive review of child pornography, child prostitution, and internet crimes against children*. St. Louis: G.W. Medical Publishing.

Estes, R. J. (2007). *Child sexual exploitation: Quick reference for healthcare, social services, and law enforcement professionals*. St. Louis: G.W. Medical Publishing.

Estes, R. J., & Weiner, N. A. (2001). *The commercial sexual exploitation of children in the United States*. Philadelphia: University of Pennsylvania School of Social Work.

Estes, R. J., & Weiner, N. A. (2005). The commercial sexual exploitation of children in the United States. In S. W. Cooper, R. J. Estes, A. P. Giardino, N. D. Kellogg, & V. I. Vieth (Eds.), *Medical, legal, & social science aspects of child sexual exploitation: A comprehensive review of pornog-*

raphy, prostitution, & internet crimes (pp. 95–128). St. Louis: G.W. Medical Publishing, Chapter 5.

Estes, R. J., & Zhou, H. M. (2015). A conceptual approach to the creation of public–Private partnerships in social welfare. *International Journal of Social Welfare, 24*(4), 348–363.

Estes, R. J., Azaola, E., & Ives, N. (2005). The commercial sexual exploitation of children in North America. In S. W. Cooper, R. J. Estes, A. P. Giardino, N. D. Kellogg, & V. I. Vieth (Eds.), *Medical, legal, & social science aspects of child sexual exploitation: A comprehensive review of pornography, prostitution, & internet crimes* (pp. 297–335). St. Louis: G.W. Medical Publishing, Chapter 15.

Feinauer, L., Callahan, E., & Hilton, H. G. (1996). Positive intimate relationships decrease depression in sexually abused women. *American Journal of Family Therapy, 24*(2), 99–106.

Finkelhor, D., & Ormod, R. (2001). *Child abuse reports to the police.* Washington, DC: U.S. Department of Justice and Delinquency Prevention. https://www.ncjrs.gov/pdffiles1/ojjdp/187238.pdf. Accessed 01 Dec 2015.

Frontline. (2006). PBS: Sexual Slaves (aired February 7). http://www.pbs.org/wgbh/pages/frontline/slaves/. Washington, DC: Public Broadcasting Service. Accessed 15 Oct 2015.

Gattas, G. J. F., Figaro-Garcia, C., Landini, T. S., & Estes, R. J. (2012). Commercial sexual exploitation and missing kids in the coastal region of Sao Paulo State, Brazil. *Journal of Applied Research on Children, 3*(2).

Internet Crimes Against Children (ICAC). (2015). *Multijurisdictional task forces.* https://www.icactaskforce.org/Pages/Home.aspx. Accessed 06 Nov 2015.

Kessler, M. R. H., Nelson, B., Jurich, A., & White, M. (2004). Clinical decision-making strategies of marriage and family therapists in the treatment of adult childhood sexual abuse survivors. *American Journal of Family Therapy, 32*(1), 1–10.

Lloyd, R. (2012). *Girls like us: Fighting for a world where girls are not for sale—A memoir.* New York: Harper Perennial Books.

Maltz, W. (2002). Treating the sexual intimacy concerns of sexual abuse survivors. *Sexual and Relationship Therapy, 17*(4), 321–327.

McNew, J., & Abell, N. (1995). Posttraumatic stress symptomatology: Similarities and differences between Vietnam veterans and adult survivors of childhood sexual abuse. *Social Work, 40*(1), 115–126.

Moran, R. (2015). *Paid for: My journey as a prostitute.* New York: N. N. Norton and Co..

National Center for Missing and Exploited Children (NCMEC). (2015). *CyberTipline.* http://www.missingkids.com/cybertipline/. Accessed 06 Nov 2015.

National Center for Victims of Crime (2015). *Child sexual abuse statistics.* http://www.victimsofcrime.org/media/reporting-on-child-sexual-abuse/child-sexual-abuse-statistics. Accessed 06 Nov 2015.

Phelps, C., & Larkin, W. (2013). *Runaway girl: Escaping life on the streets.* New York: Penguin.

Rape, Abuse, & Incest National Network (RAINN). (2015). *Adult survivors of childhood sexual abuse.*https://rainn.org/get-info/effects-of-sexual-assault/adult-survivors-of-childhood-sexual--abuse. Accessed 06 Nov 2015.

Ratican, K. (1992). Sexual abuse survivors: Identifying symptoms and special treatment considerations. *Journal of Counseling & Development, 71*(1), 33–38.

Raymond, J. (2011). Effects of sexual abuse last for decades. *NBC News* (30 June). http://www.nbcnews.com/id/43594639/ns/health-health_care/t/effects-sexual-abuse-last-decades-study-finds/#.VmG0NDZdGP8. Accessed 15 Nov 2015.

Raymond, J. B. (2012). *Not a choice, not a job: Exposing the myth about prostitution and global sex work.* Washington, DC: Potomac Books.

S., Miss. (2008). *Confessions of a working girl.* Chicago: Sourcebooks.

Shelly, L. (2010). *Human trafficking: A global perspective.* Cambridge: Cambridge University Press.

Stegall, A., & Mercedes, C. (2014). 3 juveniles recovered, 16 pimps, 75 prostitutes arrested in sex trafficking operation. *Fox 19 Now* (June 23). http://www.fox19.com/story/25847987/3-

juveniles-recovered-16-pimps-75-prostitutes-arrested-in-sex-trafficking-operation. Accessed 04 Dec 2014.
Street Child Project. (2015). *Advocate*: Research. http://www.thestreetchildproject.org/causes-effects/. Accessed 15 Oct 2015.
Tremblay, P., et al. (2001). *Child sexual exploitation in Canada: Child sexual network among jailed Canadian inmates*. Montreal: University of Montreal Centre for Criminology.
U.S. Department of Health & Human Services, Administration on Children, Youth, & Families (USCB). (2007). *Child maltreatment 2005*. Washington, DC: U.S. Government Printing Office.
U.S. Department of State (USDOS). (2015a). *What is modern slavery?* http://www.state.gov/j/tip/what/index.htm. Accessed 08 Nov 2015.
U.S. Department of State (USDOS). (2015b). *Trafficking in persons annual report, 2015*. Washington, DC: Superintendent of Documents.
United States Department of Justice (USDOJ). (2015a). *Child exploitation and obscenity division*. http://www.justice.gov/criminal-ceos. Accessed 05 Nov 2015.
United States Department of Justice (USDOJ). (2015b). *National drug intelligence center*. http://www.justice.gov/archive/ndic/about.htm. Accessed 05 Nov 2015.
Van Drannen, W. (2012). *Runaway*. New York: Emer Books of Random House.
Warren, L., & Phelps, C. (2012). *Runaway girl: Escaping life on the streets*. New York: Viking Books.
Wikipedia. (2015a). *Sexual assault*. https://en.wikipedia.org/wiki/Sexual_assault. Accessed 09 Nov 2015.
Wikipedia. (2015b). *Commercial sexual exploitation of children*. https://en.wikipedia.org/wiki/Commercial_sexual_exploitation_of_children. Accessed 03 Dec 2015.

Part V
Preventing Future Suffering

Chapter 24
Socializing Students in Higher Education to Alleviate Human Suffering Among the Homeless

Meg Wilkes Karraker

Introduction

The state of being without a home necessarily varies by culture, and given the large number of nomadic communities, the prevalence of world homelessness eludes rigorous estimation. However, a 2005 study by the United Nations claimed there were 100 million homeless around the world, which is about 2% of adults (United Nations 2008). Homeless persons typically are highly visible in any large city around the world including the United States, where shelters for the homeless may increasingly serve women and children as well as men. Yet U.S. Census studies have rarely found more than a half million homeless on any given day. A study by Link and associates in 1990 concluded that 13.5 million (7.4% of adults) were "lifetime homeless," those who had ever slept in shelters, abandoned buildings, etc. (Link et al. 1995).

In the state of Minnesota, where this study was conducted, the average winter temperature ranges from 16° F in the southern part of the state to 6° F in the north, discouraging many from homeless from remaining in the state. Nevertheless, during any given year, an estimated 40,000 adults, youth, and children (almost 1% of the total state population) lack shelter (Owen and Gerard 2013).

Suffering remains a constant companion for most homeless persons, especially the weak, the sick or the mentally ill. While homelessness may seem mostly a matter of inconvenience and stress, those caught in in its grip find themselves suffering from hunger and poverty, nutrition, lack of healthcare, greatly increased crime victimization, deprivation from job markets and embarrassingly visible marginality within society (Lee et al. 2010). Not surprisingly, the homeless have greater risk of addiction, suicide and many mental health disorders. Also, lack of safety and other risk factors lead to shorter life expectancies.

M.W. Karraker (✉)
University of St. Thomas, St. Paul, MN, USA
e-mail: mwkarraker@stthomas.edu

R.E. Anderson (ed.), *Alleviating World Suffering*, Social Indicators Research Series 67, DOI 10.1007/978-3-319-51391-1_24

The costs of providing emergency and inpatient medical services, police and correctional systems, and other public resources are exorbitantly expensive. Speaking on *The Daily Show*, Shaun Donovan, U.S. Secretary of Housing and Urban Development said, "Because, at the end of the day… between shelters and emergency rooms and jails, it costs about $40,000 a year for a homeless person to be on the streets" (Moorhead 2012). These costs provide practical incentives to the humanitarian pressures to reduce homelessness and its embedded suffering.

The causes of homelessness are not mysterious. Morse (1992: 4) and others have carefully dissected the diverse paths by which individuals and populations come to be homeless – "extreme poverty, low job skills, high unemployment rates, high rates of personal-social adjustment problems (e.g., mental disorders, alcoholism, criminality), low levels of social support, high levels of life crisis." The Wilder Foundation identified five key reasons why people are homeless in Minnesota. (1) People living on the margins are the last to recover from downturns in the economy such as the recent Great Recession. (2) Insufficient housing results from an "affordability gap" between rent and mortgage costs and personal income. (3) Barriers to living independently include cognitive, mental or physical issues, experience with domestic abuse and other violence, and cumulative adverse life events that inhibit skills and networks for a stable life course. (4) Youth who experience childhood trauma and health issues are more likely to experience homelessness. (5) Persistent racial disparities around home ownership, health, educational achievement, and other issues compound the risk of homelessness for people of color, especially African Americans and Native Americans (Owen and Gerard 2013). Ironically, the causes of suffering often function as the negative consequences of homelessness. In summary, Lee et al. (2010) concluded that the "emerging consensus in the sociological research community is that homelessness is, fundamentally, a structural problem rooted in the larger political economy." In other words, too many poor people compete for too few low-income housing units.

The depth of individual human suffering associated with homelessness is almost unfathomable. The transient living circumstances associated with homelessness strain social relationships, contribute to stress and depression, and inhibit access to health care (Garcia-Rea and LePage 2010). Children and young adults are at particular risk of homelessness, suffering a range of consequences, including physical, cognitive, emotional, and social well-being, debits that have lifelong consequences for quality of life. Unaccompanied homeless youth have physical and mental health challenges, including histories of abuse and other trauma (Amherst H. Wilder Foundation 2013). Compared to other children, homeless children are twice as likely to experience hunger and twice as likely to have a learning disability, repeat a grade, or be suspended from school (American Psychological Association 2015).

In religious institutions and workplaces; among children, youth, adults, and senior citizens; from elementary schools through postgraduate programs, volunteering to serve communities is widespread. When asked in a Gallup World Poll (2011) in 2010 "have you volunteered your time to an organization in the last month," 43% of Americans polled answered "yes." While the United States ranked second behind Sri Lanka, quite a few of the other very civically engaged countries were developing nations. Empirical studies of civic engagement among youth and young adults worldwide are of particular interest. (See for example de los Angeles Torres et al. (2013) on Chicago, Mexico City, and Rio de Janeiro and Zhang and Lin (2008) on China).

How then to mobilize people to do something about the human suffering associated with homelessness in their communities? Can experience engaging one-on-one with people living homeless change citizens' attitudes and future behaviors toward alleviating this scourge? And most relevant for this chapter, does higher education have a responsibility in this regard?

As any director of a center that shelters homeless people will tell you, their guests include the occasional person enrolled in college. Nonetheless, few college or university students in developed countries have personal experience with homelessness. Service learning (also referred to as civic engagement, community engagement, community-based learning, or simply service sociology (Treviño 2012)) has become a mainstay in American higher education.

In 1986, Campus Compact, a national organization that aims to advance civic and social responsibility among college and university students, had 76 members; today members number 1100 (Campus Compact 2014). In 2006 the Carnegie Foundation for the Advancement of Teaching selected 76 U.S. colleges and universities to receive its first Community Engagement Classification (Driscoll 2009). Less than a decade later, in 2015, that number had more than tripled, to 240 U.S. colleges. In collaboration with the U.S. Community Population Survey, the Corporation for National and Community Service (a federal agency that promotes civic engagement) estimates that in 2012, 3.1 million college and university students volunteered more than 118 million hours of service valued at \$2.5 billion (Corporation for National and Community Service 2013).

Classes that use service learning often tie learning objectives to substantive outcomes. For example, in my introductory sociology course at the University of St. Thomas (one of those 240 institutions), I invite students to engage the sociological perspective in their service at a center that provides shelter and services for men and women living homeless. I ask them to consider Berger's (1963: 23) admonition that "things are not what they seem." However (whether they admit it or not) one of the primary objectives among many instructors who use service learning is often to raise the consciousness of the learner about the suffering of others. In sociology, we teach George Herbert Mead's (1934) concept of taking the role of the other, sometimes relating it to the development of empathy.

A report on the 2015 We Day Minnesota, a yearlong, school-based educational service program, reported that youth engagement in service programs grew an astonishing 204% from 2013–2014 to 2014–2015 (*Star Tribune* 2015). Yet in spite of the popularity of service learning in education, knowledge of the effects of that pedagogy is incomplete. One web survey of alumni who have participated in the Wilder Foundation's Youth Leadership program reported positive outcomes in personal growth, including self-confidence and becoming more aware of personal strengths, as well as pride in own culture and cultural understanding of others. The same survey also found ongoing civic engagement (voting in the most recent national election and volunteering in the past year) at higher rates than other young adults in Minnesota (Valorose 2015).

Following a brief review of the literature, this chapter offers insights from data from a survey of undergraduate students, before and after they had engaged in a service learning experience at a center providing services for men and women living homeless in the Twin Cities of St. Paul/Minneapolis, Minnesota.

This paper assesses progress on two co-curricular objectives as students move beyond familiar comfort zones, immersing themselves in a new environment and interacting with people out of their ordinary social sphere. I hypothesized that after completing the service learning experience, students would express:

H1: More accurate knowledge and fewer stereotypes regarding homeless people and homelessness.

H2: Greater affirmation of principles of social justice.

Effects of Community Engagement on Attitudes and Behaviors

Research on the effects of service learning on student achievement is inconclusive. This is not surprising, given the diverse qualities of service learning practices and the paucity of controlled, longitudinal studies. However, some research has found that students who participate in service learning have changes in attitudes about social problems and social justice. For example, Mobley (2007) found that upper division undergraduate students who partnered with advocates and homeless clients had significant changes in a positive direction in their perceptions of individuals who are homeless and some small changes in attitudes about social justice. Likewise, Okpala et al. (2009) found that participation in service learning is associated with gains around students' social justice values such as support for diversity, fairness, patience, and work ethic.

To contribute to the ongoing need to assess attitudinal and behavioral outcomes of service-learning, I offer findings from a short-term longitudinal sample of undergraduate students in Introduction to Sociology classes at the University of St. Thomas, a private university in the upper Midwestern United States. My findings may surprise those who have been skeptical about, and those who have been long-time enthusiasts of, service learning as part of the undergraduate curriculum.

Engaging Undergraduate Students

In Introduction to Sociology (SOCI 100), I require that students in their first semester at the University of St. Thomas complete three three-hour sessions at Catholic Charities of St. Paul and Minneapolis Dorothy Day Center. The Dorothy Day Center (Catholic Charities of St. Paul and Minneapolis 2015) was built in downtown Saint Paul, Minnesota, in 1981. Intended to be only a short-term, daytime drop-in facility, on the first day, the Center served 50 people coffee and rolls. In 2014, the Center sheltered approximately 250 people each night, providing some cots but mostly mats for men and women to sleep on the floor. The Dorothy Day Center also offers a variety of services to clients experiencing homelessness, including hot meals to hundreds of people every day, a special shelter program for 40 women, shower facilities, counseling, and a computer lab.

Students' tasks at Dorothy Day included checking guests in at the start of the evening (including administering sobriety tests), distributing bed linens, laundering bed linens, setting out mats for sleeping, serving the evening meal, distributing hygiene supplies, and monitoring shower times. Students also had opportunities to engage in informal conversation with the clients and the staff, while observing interactions among the same.

The sociology class was not exclusively focused on homelessness, but over the course of the semester, the topic was integrated into the course as follows:

- During the first week of the semester, students engaged in a 30-min observation of homelessness in St. Paul's twin city of Minneapolis.
- Also during the first week, students studied a series of frescoes depicting seven virtues often associated with religious social teaching (faith, justice, prudence, hope, temperance, fortitude, charity), relating them to social responses to homelessness.
- In the first month of the semester, the program director for the Dorothy Day Center visited the class to provide orientation to the center and to answer questions about student service learning at the Center.
- Also in the first month of the semester, the community education and leadership manager for the Office of Social Justice for Catholic Charities of St. Paul and Minneapolis visited the class to provide an overview of homelessness in the context of social justice.
- During the semester, students had access to published resources on homelessness that were posted by the sociology instructor on the course Blackboard site.
- Students were required to compose a three-page paper with two scholarly references on homelessness for the sociology course, integrating their observations at the center.

Following students' completion of their hours of service, the director and the manager at Catholic Charities conducted a semi-structured focus group with the class. The primary purpose of the focus group was to solicit students' comments regarding their experience serving, while giving them an opportunity to process that experience. (The course instructor left the room for the portion of the discussion relating to the value of the service-learning experience for the sociology course.)

Research Methods and Analysis

An ongoing assessment to examine changes in students' attitudes was approved by the University of St. Thomas Institutional Review Board as IRB #470953-1. Student participation was voluntary and responses were confidential. At no time after identification numbers had been assigned were students' names linked to their responses. Furthermore, to reduce concerns that students might be placed at risk for their responses, data were not analyzed until after each course had ended and final grades had been submitted.

She study uses a questionnaire administered at an academic advising session prior to the first day of class and again after the students had completed the last of three three-hour service learning sessions and the debriefing session conducted by the director and the manager from Catholic Charities. The questionnaire was developed in consultation with Marty Roers (community education and leadership manager for the Office of Social Justice for Catholic Charities of St. Paul and Minneapolis), who has extensive experience directing and assessing service learning. With the instructor's permission, the questionnaire used in this study included questions administered to students in an upper division undergraduate sociology course at Clemson University on Policy and Social Change.

The questionnaire included a set of demographic questions, followed by three sections: (1) knowledge and attitudes toward homeless people, (2) attitudes toward social justice, and (3) expressions of self-efficacy. Each attitudinal item was measured on a 5-point Likert-type scale (1 = Strongly Agree to 5 = Strongly Disagree).

Population and Sample

This project studied students enrolled in a first-semester, first-year program at the University of St. Thomas that assigns students to courses that meet core requirements in the university curriculum. All the students in this sample were enrolled in Introduction to Sociology. Students did not have a choice in the courses in which they are enrolled, although they could (and some in this sample did) drop the course for a variety of reasons (e.g., conflicts with courses later added, desire to take fewer credits). Hence, when asked to identify their reason(s) for taking the course, they all indicated they were doing so "for the credits" and "for the day/time the course was offered."

Although 23 students were enrolled in the course, the final number of valid cases for the sample was 16. The lower number reflects net loss from (1) students who did not complete the entire pre-test or post-test and (2) students who dropped the course and who therefore did not complete the post-test. Also, one student added the course late and so completed only the post-test, so that student was also not counted in the sample.

For the most part, the section was a virtual snapshot of the first-year class entering in 2013 at the University of St. Thomas. All of the students were 18 years old on their last birthday. Two students self-identified as a race or ethnicity other than white. All but one student reported being a member of a church, synagogue, temple, or other religious group and 60% of those identified as Catholic. (The University of St. Thomas is a part of the Catholic Archdiocese of St. Paul and Minneapolis.) All but two students indicated at least one intended major and those majors ranged across the colleges of arts and sciences, business, education, and engineering. At 56%, women were slightly over-represented in comparison to men at the University of St. Thomas.

Findings

I assessed changes in attitudes in the first-year Introduction to Sociology course after completion of service learning and associated pedagogy in two co-curricular areas: (1) knowledge and stereotypes regarding homelessness and (2) principles of social justice.

Knowledge and Stereotypes Regarding Homeless People and Homelessness

Prior to participating in service learning, students held attitudes toward homeless people that could, for the most part, be described as centered between agreement and disagreement, with means ranging from 2.5 to 3.7 on the 5-point scale, which ranged from strongly agree at "1" to strongly disagree at "5." Student attitudes tended to persist between the pre- and post-tests, with small to moderate changes in the direction of less negative stereotypes and more accurate knowledge following the service learning experience. Paired sample tests of differences between pre- and post-test means yielded t-tests that were significant at $p \leq .05$ for all the items listed in Table 24.1.

Table 24.1 Opinion questions on which the students studied significantly improved

Attitude items	Pre-	Post-	Initial opinion	Change in opinion
1. Most homeless people are unclean	2.7	3.8	Mixed	Much greater disagreement
2. Most homeless people are white	3.4	3.8	Disagreement	Greater disagreement
3. Public assistance (welfare) provides people with sufficient funds on which to live	3.1	3.9	Disagreement	Greater disagreement
4. Homeless people often move from shelters to permanent housing	3.6	3	Disagreement	Less disagreement
5. There is little that can be done for homeless people, except to address their immediate needs for shelter and a meal	3.5	3.9	Disagreement	Greater disagreement
6. I would feel comfortable having a conversation with a homeless person	2.5	1.9	Mixed	Greater disagreement

The first four items in the table all express negative or inaccurate stereotypes of homeless communities: that homeless are unclean; predominately nonwhite; have enough funds to live on; and often get permanent housing. As shown in Table 24.1, the students shifted significantly on all four items toward greater accuracy in their perceptions.

Social Justice Orientation

Social justice is the typical philosophical and moral underpinning in the discipline of sociology as well as Catholic social teaching principles embedded in Catholic education and social service (Catholic Charities 2016). While there may be disagreement on the nature of specific principles of social justice, service learning's value is generally stated in terms of enhancing principles of social justice, especially in the context of principles of Catholic social teaching (Catholic Charities of St. Paul and Minneapolis 2016). Therefore, several opinion items were included on commitment to social justice.

Prior to participating in service learning, students expressed strong support for certain social justice issues. For example, students tended to agree with "I am compassionate toward the homeless" (mean = 1.94) and "I believe that, in working with others, I can help solve society's problems" (mean = 1.94). The only social justice items that changed significantly over the course of the semester were items 5 and 6 in Table 24.1. Item 5 says: "There is little that can be done for homeless people, except to address their immediate needs for shelter and a meal." This item expressed the essence of the "option for the poor" as stated in many documents on the principles of Catholic social justice. The students expressed stronger disagreement with this statement (implying support for the principle) after their service learning experience.

In addition, following their service learning experience, students were more likely to agree with the statement "I would feel comfortable having a conversation with a homeless person," which indicates an improvement in positive feelings for the homeless and acceptance of them generally. While this expresses an attitude of increased inclusiveness for homeless people, this principle is also framed in terms of "solidarity" with all peoples. This indicates that social justice learning took place as a result of the service-learning experience of these students.

Implications

The sample on which this study is based is admittedly small and limited. However, what the sample lacks in size, it makes up in control of extraneous variables such as age and stage in the undergraduate career. Further, as service-learning projects go, this one was neither as extensive in hours nor curricular-content as some might be.

Even so, this study suggests what can be done in terms of outcomes with even a short-term service-learning experience.

The University of St. Thomas is a Catholic college of the Archdiocese of St. Paul and Minneapolis that has a mission that states:

> *Inspired by Catholic intellectual tradition, the University of St. Thomas educates students to be morally responsible leaders who think critically, act wisely, and work skillfully to advance the common good.*

Students at the University of St. Thomas encounter the Catholic part of the mission frequently, even if they are not well-schooled in principles of Catholic social teaching. The extent to which undergraduates actively endorse that mission could be the subject of another study, but my conversations with students suggest that the number of 17-year-olds who choose institutions like the University of St. Thomas on the basis of such lofty institutional missions (versus career, friendship, geographical, or other agendas) is probably very small.

This modest project contributes to our understanding of the attitudinal and intended behavioral changes that can occur when undergraduate students engage in service learning around a pressing social issue like homelessness. Some findings may surprise faculty who have been skeptical about service learning. Specifically, students who engage in service learning with homeless people as part of an undergraduate course may become:

- Less stereotyping of some characteristics of homeless people and more knowledgeable about homelessness in their community.
- Less pessimistic that something can be done for homeless people beyond meeting immediate needs.
- More comfortable interacting with a homeless person.

Marty Roers, community education and leadership manager of Catholic Charities of St. Paul and Minneapolis' Office of Social Justice, debriefed each class after their experience serving at the Dorothy Day Center. He reported complementary observations. Speaking in the class setting, students in each class shared their sense of dignity and respect for those experiencing homelessness, as well as a sense of "accompaniment," i.e., seeing, meeting, and actually talking with people living homeless. (Roers has noted that students frequently referred to people living homeless as "them.")

Other findings may disappoint those who are long-time enthusiasts of service learning. Students who engage in service learning as part of an undergraduate course may not make enormous leaps regarding either their attitudes toward social justice. However, we must keep in mind this study involved 18- and 19-year olds in the first semester of their college experience. Developmental change and personal agency do not move that quickly. However, Roers also reported that, especially students in the sociology classes (compared to the philosophy and theology classes) would ask questions like "What else can I do?" and "What systems can be put in place to help or prevent homelessness."

Also (as students are quick to remind anyone who assumes otherwise), American students do not arrive at college as novices when it comes to service learning around pressing social problems. Most if not all of these students report having been previously engaged in community service with their families, schools, religious communities, and other voluntary organizations. For example, some students described their positive experiences with Feed My Starving Children, a non-profit Christian organization that packages and ships food around the world. However, anecdotal evidence suggests that much of the previous service has been of that nature, not face-to-face with human suffering.

Implications for Future Research

Service learning is often what some may call a "feel good" pedagogy. Whether tutoring educationally at-risk children in the Twin Cities of Minneapolis and St. Paul or working with economically-challenged families along the Mexican-U.S. border, undergraduate students at the University of St. Thomas often report that community-based learning, particularly in service to disadvantaged populations, is among their favorite part of any class. While students often report feeling troubled by the depth and breadth of the social problems they observe, they also report that they came away from helping others with very positive feelings and, as this research suggests, a greater sense of efficacy.

But, from a pedagogical perspective, good vibes are not enough. Given the high investments required on the parts of students, faculty members, and institutions for effective service learning, we really need to know more about the outcomes of that experience. Specifically, how do undergraduate students change across their life course after participating in service-learning experiences?

A follow-up with students in these panels as they approach graduation or at a period of time after graduation would be useful to determine the stability of effects observed in this study. Certainly more research is needed to explicate the link between service-learning experiences among young adults with later adult volunteering. Of critical importance, given that suffering on such a scale as homelessness can only be addressed through strenuous, concerted efforts in civil society, what is the prospect of these changed undergraduates moving forward with broader civic efforts to alleviate human suffering?

At least one panel study has found that religion and religiosity increase volunteerism over the adult life course (Johnston 2013). Given the religious affiliation of the university from which this sample is drawn and the religious identification of the students, as well as the Catholic affiliation of the service-learning site, the intersections of religious identification and religious engagement with service learning are of interest. Samples drawn from other populations (e.g., state-supported colleges or universities; colleges or universities representing other faith traditions) might give deeper insight into the extent to which religion or religiosity shapes the experience of service learning.

Conclusions

Midway through data collection for this chapter, Catholic Charities of St. Paul and Minneapolis, in partnership with the city of St. Paul, announced plans for expansion into new facilities (Melo 2014) for the social problem that, three decades ago, was considered a temporary issue. Financial resources are tight and the need for social service and civic action continues to grow in areas such as homelessness.

Organizations like Dorothy Day depend on committed, reliable volunteers for basic human capital. At the same time, these organizations have a strong, vested interest in determining just how much benefit they can reap from the considerable resources they must invest in recruiting, selecting, training, and supervising volunteers. While the students in this study not only washed the laundry, laid out mats, and served food, they also offered a measure of respectful interpersonal interaction. That considerable social asset is not lost on either the professional staff or, most importantly, the people living homeless. And, as this research reveals, these young adults came away with increased comfort in speaking to someone who is more disadvantaged than them.

Organizations with long-term investments in their communities hope to socialize long-term commitments to service and pay off in the form of citizens who understand and support organizational missions. Will the greater comfort and confidence experienced by undergraduate service learners translate into their feeling more empowered to do something beyond meet immediate needs, beyond "putting a bandage on" a social problem? Those organizations (and professors) hope they are helping to socialize a new generation of citizens committed to action for the common good. Such appears to be the case for at least some of the undergraduates in this study. Snyder and Dwyer (2012: 482) remind us that regardless of whether collective prosocial behavior (including volunteerism) is motivated by self- or other-oriented (altruistic) concerns, prosocial efforts, "the volunteers, their recipients, and society stand to gain more as a result of those actions."

From his debriefings with sociology classes, Roers reported that students had approached him to ask if they might return to serve at the Dorothy Day Center after the course ends. Others have asked if they might bring their student club to serve. Many follow through, serving on their own, with a friend, or with groups. After each semester, at least one student has contacted me to inquire about additional service. And they follow through as volunteers and with even more ambitious efforts. For example, in 2015, students at the University of St. Thomas organized a fund-raiser for the Dorothy Day Center and worked with the university's food service to put in place an ambitious food recovery network between the university and Dorothy Day.

Service learning could be a highly commendable means to the goal of fostering civic engagement among undergraduates. As such, it serves as an exemplar of Burawoy's (2004) public sociology, extending the promise of sociology's tools and knowledge beyond the academy and spanning boundaries from the academy to the community (Nyden 2014). Organizations like Academics Without Borders and the International Professors Project exemplify civic engagement opportunities for faculty members who seek to put conscience into civic action, perhaps modeling those commitments for our students. Beyond setting the stage to address social problems, I agree with Keyes (2014: 19) that civic engagement is "also about helping our students develop a suite of skills that will allow each of them to pursue a better life."

Not surprisingly, students involved in comprehensive programs that formally integrate service learning with academic coursework show greater increases in civic responsibility than either students involved in service not formally integrated with coursework or students not involved in service (Myers-Lipton 1998). Service-learning pedagogy can be a labor-intensive (and, if things do not proceed as planned) risky endeavor for the faculty member. Research on the effects of service learning in terms of teaching and learning, in particular around the variables like knowledge and stereotyping and social justice that directly affect later civic engagement, would provide incentive to faculty members to make the effort.

Civic-minded professors who embrace service learning hope we are extending the socialization of students in the liberal arts to include growing commitments to alleviating suffering in this world through efforts for the common good. The Association of American Colleges and Universities (2014) maintains:

> *It is the unique and historical responsibility of higher education in a democratic society to be the provider of intentional opportunity for broad and deep civic learning and civic action. No other institution provides that.*

Anderson (2012) has even developed pedagogical tools to move students studying research methods to consider questions about the meaning of life "and perhaps to become intrinsically motivated to help others."

This chapter describes how one local, community-based education program may promote attitudes conducive to relieving suffering. Would that we knew more about how such experiences translate into attitudes that grow behaviors toward the common good not only in face-to-face engagement, but regarding institutionalizing efforts through social policy as well as global initiatives.

We have reason to be hopeful regarding higher education as an agent of socialization to alleviate human suffering. Speaking shortly before his death in 1995 to a meeting of the American Academy of Arts and Sciences, Ernest Boyer (1996, p. 18) reflected on the place of higher education in American society:

> *[O]ur outstanding universities and colleges remain, in my opinion, among the greatest sources of hope for intellectual and civic progress in this country ... in the search for answers to our most pressing social, civic, economic, and moral problems.*

Acknowledgements Thanks to then-undergraduate sociologists Darek Albertson, Olamide Fadahunsi, and Kylee Joosten for data assistance. Kelly Sardon-Garrity, program panager, Office of Civic Engagement, University of St. Thomas, provided useful information on community engagement. Finally, as always, Ron Anderson exemplifies that which is the collegial best in an editor.

References

American Psychological Association. (2015). *Effects of poverty, hunger, and homelessness on children and youth*. http://www.apa.org/pi/families/poverty.aspx/. Accessed 15 Aug 2015.

Amherst H. Wilder Foundation. (2013). *Homelessness in Minnesota: 2012 results*. http://www.wilder.org/Wilder-Research/Publications/Studies/Homelessness%20in%20Minnesota%202012%20Study/Homelessness%20in%20Minnesota%20%20Findings%20from%20the%202012%20Statewide%20Homeless%20Study.pdf. Accessed 16 Aug 2015.

Anderson, R. (2012). *Generation X students reflect on the meaning of life*. Paper presented at The Future of Social Science Research Methods Conference and Babbie Center Dedication, Chapman University, 21 March.

Association of American Colleges and Universities. (2014). *Bringing theory to practice, civic series teaser*. Online video. http://www.aacu.org/bringing_theory/CivicSeries.cfm#CS. Accessed 16 Jan 2014.

Berger, P. (1963). *Invitation to sociology. A humanistic perspective*. Garden City: Doubleday.

Boyer, E. L. (1990). The scholarship of engagement. *Bulletin of the American Academy of Arts and Sciences, 49*(7), 18–33.

Burawoy, M. (2004). 2004 presidential address: For public sociology. *American Sociological Review, 70*(1), 4–28.

Campus Compact. (2014). Campus Compact membership survey 2014: Three decades of institutionalizing change, 2014. Boston: Campus Compact. http://kdp0l43vw6z2dlw631ififc5.wpengine.netdna-cdn.com/wp-content/uploads/2015/05/2014-CC-Member-Survey.pdf. Accessed 18 Aug 2015.

Carnegie Foundation for the Advancement of Teaching. (2015). *Carnegie selects colleges and universities for 2015 community engagement classification*. http://www.carnegiefoundation.org/newsroom/news-releases/carnegie-selects-colleges-universities-2015-community-engagement-classification/. Accessed 15 Aug 2015.

Catholic Charities of St. Paul and Minneapolis. (2015). Dorothy Day Center. http://cctwincities.org/DorothyDayCenter. Accessed 16 Aug 2015.

Catholic Charities of St. Paul and Minneapolis. (2016). *Major encyclical, conciliar and key teaching documents*. https://www.cctwincities.org/education-advocacy/catholic-social-teaching/major-documents/. Accessed 8 Feb 2016.

Corporation for National and Community Service. (2013). Volunteering in civic life in America. http://2013.volunteeringinamerica.gov/. Accessed 18 Aug 2015.

de los Angeles Torres, M., Rizzini, I., & del Rio, N. (2013). *Citizens in the present: Youth civic engagement in the Americas*. Urbana: University of Illinois Press.

Driscoll, A. (2009). Carnegie's new community engagement classification: Affirming higher education's role in community. *New Directions for Higher Education, 147*(1), 5–12.

Gallup World Poll. (2015). *Civic engagement highest in developed countries*. http://www.gallup.com/poll/145589/civic-engagement-highest-developed-countries.aspx. Accessed 3 Jan 2016.

Garcia-Rea, E. A., & LePage, J. P. (2010). Reliability and validity of the World Health Organization quality of life: Brief version (WHOQOL-BREF) in a homeless substance dependent population. *Social Indicators Research, 99*(2), 333–340.

Johnston, J. B. (2013). Religion and volunteering over the adult life course. *Journal for the Scientific Study of Religion, 52*(4), 733–752.

Keyes, C. (2014). The eudeamonic and the civic. In D. W. Howard (Ed.), *Civic Provocations* (pp. 19–22). Washington, DC: American Association of Colleges and Universities Bringing Theory to Practice.

Lee, B. A., Tyler, K. A., & Wright, J. D. (2010). The new homelessness revisited. *Annual Review of Sociology, 36*, 501–521.

Link, B. G., Phelan, J., Bresnahan, M., Stueve, A., Moore, R. E., & Susser, E. (1995). Lifetime and five-year prevalence of homelessness in the United States: New evidence on an old debate. *The American Journal of Orthopsychiatry, 65*, 347–354.

Mead, G. H. (1934). *Mind, self, & society from the standpoint of a social behaviorist*. Chicago: University of Chicago Press.
Melo, F. (2014). St. Paul eyes higher ground as it seeks to upgrade homeless shelter. *St. Paul Pioneer Press,* January 4. http://www.twincities.com/localnews/ci_24878509/st-paul-eyes-homeless-shelter-replace-crowded-dorothy. Accessed 29 Jan 2016.
Minnesota Department of Natural Resources. (2015). *Climate*. http://www.dnr.state.mn.us/faq/mnfacts/climate.html. Accessed Aug 14 2015.
Mobley, C. (2007). Breaking ground: Engaging undergraduates in social change through service learning. *Teaching Sociology, 35*(2), 125–137.
Moore, E. W., Warta, S., & Erichsen, K. (2014). College students' volunteering: Factors related to current volunteering, volunteer settings, and motives for volunteering. *College Student Journal, 48*(3), 386–396.
Moorhead, M.. (2012). HUD secretary says a homeless person costs taxpayers $40,000 a year. *The Daily Show,* March 12. http://www.politifact.com/truth-o-meter/statements/2012/mar/12/shaun-donovan/hud-secretary-says-homeless-person-costs-taxpayers/. Accessed 15 Aug 2015.
Morse, G. A. (1992). Causes of homelessness. In M. J. Robertson & M. Greenblat (Eds.), *Homelessness: A national perspective* (pp. 3–17). New York: Springer.
Myers-Lipton, S. J. (1998). Effect of a comprehensive service-learning program on college students' civic responsibility. *Teaching Sociology, 26*(4), 243–258.
Nyden, P. (2014). Public sociology, engaged research, and civic education. In P. Levine & K. E. Soltan (Eds.), *Civic studies: Approaches to the emerging field* (pp. 103–113). Washington, DC: American Association of Colleges and Universities.
Okpala, C. O., Sturdivant, L., & Hopson, L. (2009). Assessment of the impact of service learning on academic growth of college students. *Journal of College Teaching & Learning, 6*(4), 65–68.
Owen, G., Gerard, M.D. (2013.) Survey shows: 5 key reasons people are homeless in Minnesota. Amherst G. Wilder Foundation. *Community Matters* Blog. http://www.wilder.org/Blog/Lists/Posts/Post.aspx?ID=63. Accessed 14 Aug 2015.
Snyder, M., & Dwyer, P. C. (2012). Altruism and prosocial behavior. In I. B. Weiner (Ed.), *Handbook of psychology* (2nd ed., pp. 467–485). Hoboken: Wiley.
Star Tribune. (2015). *Welcome, We Day, and thanks, students*. November 3. http://www.startribune.com/welcome-we-day-and-thanks-to-minnesota-students/339642951/. Accessed 6 Nov 2015.
Treviño, A. J. (2012). The challenge of service sociology [Presidential addresss]. *Social Problems, 59*(1), 2–20.
United Nations. (2008). *UN-HABITAT unveils state of the world's cities report*. London: UN-HABITAT.
U.S. Census Bureau. (2015). State and county QuickFacts: Minnesota. http://quickfacts.census.gov/qfd/states/27000.html. Accessed 16 Aug 2015.
Valorose, J. (2015). Instilling the value of civic engagement in youth. Amherst H. Wilder Foundation. *Community Matters*. http://www.wilder.org/Blog/Lists/Posts/Post.aspx?ID=147. Accessed 22 Dec 2015.
Zhang, Y., & Lin, J. (2008). Vounteerism in China: National policies, student responses, and two case studies of self-organized volunteer programs. *Chinese Education and Society, 41*(3), 3–13.

Chapter 25
Existential Suffering in the Social Context of Cancer Risk

Lea Hagoel

Introduction

Cancer, a fatal, overwhelming group of diseases, known to patients and physicians for centuries, constitutes an immense global burden of suffering and loss, spreading from the more developed countries to the less developed ones. This is not the known viral or bacterial infectious diseases that spread in populations. Rather, it is the case of social-cultural norms which are adopted and spread, causing health-related life styles associated with certain cancers. For example, breast cancer was shown to be associated with mothers having their first child at an older age than in traditional societies, with having fewer children, and with avoiding breast-feeding: all these are currently more frequent in developed countries, yet are being adopted in other parts of the world as well.

Much effort has been devoted to helping cancer patients in all age groups, providing them with treatment to alleviate their suffering, and in some cases, a cure. Using statistical data and personal experience reports, this chapter surveys the burden of cancer-related suffering, particularly, that of existential suffering. Such suffering emerges in asymptomatic individuals, defined as *being at-risk* to develop cancer; they are invited for medical tests intended to identify disease development in its early stages.

Beck's "risk-society" provides a sociological context of relevant epidemiological and public health constructs. These constructs are translated here, including the medical rationale behind population programs for the early detection of cancer in

L. Hagoel (✉)
The Department of Community Medicine and Epidemioogy, Carmel Medical Center and the Faculty of Medicine, Technion, Haifa, Israel
e-mail: mdlea@technion.ac.il

R.E. Anderson (ed.), *Alleviating World Suffering*, Social Indicators Research Series 67, DOI 10.1007/978-3-319-51391-1_25

Table 25.1 Cancer incidence and mortality

World wide	No. of new cases	No. of deaths
Total (All disease sites)	12,677,900	7,671,500
Colorectal Cancer	1,233,000	608,000
Breast[*] Cancer	1,383,000	458,000
North America	No. of New Cases	No. of Deaths
Total (All disease sites)	1,603,900	638,400
Colorectal Cancer	177,100	58,400
Breast[a] Cancer	205,500	45,600

U.S. Census Bureau (2008)
[a] Only women

at-risk target populations. Early detection of cancer offers patients relatively simple treatment, and is expected to alleviate their suffering and that of their families.

However, implementing the idea of cancer screening carries unexpected, unintended consequences. Similar to the pain associated with medical procedures, intended to lead to a cure, the very definition of large groups in the population as *being at-risk* to develop cancer, produces worries, difficulties, and stress. Attention is drawn to the existential suffering involved in cancer risk assessment for otherwise healthy individuals, resulting from the change in the actual definition of individual health. Viktor Frankl's contribution to coping strategies for existential suffering concludes the chapter with a promising perspective on the complexities involved.

Worldwide estimates of the cancer burden entail considerable suffering (Table 25.1, based on (Ferlay et al. 2010)). It is estimated that in 2008 alone, 12.7 million new cancer cases were diagnosed and 7.6 million cancer deaths occurred, worldwide (p. 2902). These authors note that the world's population continues to grow and to age, which means that 'the burden of cancer will continue to increase… if rates remained unchanged' (p.2916). In North America, 1.2 million new cancer cases were diagnosed in 2008 and 0.6 million deaths occurred. Breast and colorectal cancer (CRC) are cancer diseases to which the highest morbidity and mortality rates are attributed in many countries, with commensurate personal, medical, social and economic burdens. In 2008, breast and CRC contributed equally, accounting together for one fifth of the global cancer burden, (Table 25.1), as well as for the high rates of morbidity and mortality from cancer in North America.

Others (Are et al. 2013) agree that, 'The global cancer burden is expected to rise significantly and will disproportionately affect the less developed world' (p. 221), predicting further cancer-related human suffering. For each diagnosed patient, relatives share the painful situation, as do friends, colleagues, and neighbors. There is grim picture of endless disease-related suffering, physical pain, harsh medical treatments, temporary or permanent disability, loss of work-time or even work places, economic difficulties and, grief, which is no less obvious.

"Cancer" is a popular lay term for many cancer diseases, differing from each other (among others) in frequency, etiology, developmental paths, risk factors, treatment options, and survival rates. Clearly, prevention of all diseases is preferable to needing a cure, but scientifically established cancer-control preventive measures exist for only a few cancer-diseases thus far; disease detection in its early developmental stages is the next best to prevention. In such cases, screening is offered to individuals in population target-groups, according to medical criteria. Screening tests are intended to single out individuals who may be developing a disease but are as yet asymptomatic. In the case of cancer, risk is assigned to individuals by pre-defined criteria (e.g., age and/or gender). They may be, then, invited to undergo specific tests, and if diagnosed, offered appropriate treatment. The medical rationale is based on the relatively simple treatment in early stages of cancer, compared to diagnosis and treatment in later stages of the disease.

Expert epidemiologists agree that, from a public-health perspective, it is justified to offer population-level screening for two of the three leading cancer diseases worldwide: *breast and CRC*. Such an intervention program would aim at diagnosing and treating patients at *average risk* (who are defined not personally, but rather by group-level criteria, such as age/gender) for these diseases in the early stages of disease development. For most cancer diseases, screening is not recommended by official health-policy authorities. The reason is that several important, specific parameters combined are required in order to establish a professional consensus. In the case of breast and CRC, these factors have been established and they include, among others: the natural history of the diseases, similar in both cases in that detection in early (pre-symptomatic) stages is possible; the availability of medical modalities considered safe, effective, and acceptable to the public; extant epidemiological evidence (based on large Randomized Clinical Trials, RCTs) that routine, systematic screening (using specific test modalities) contributes to a decrease in disease morbidity and mortality (Faivre et al. 1999; Roder et al. 2008); *and* the availability/accessibility of treatment options which are preferable to those used in later stages of disease diagnosis, to assist patients and improve medically-assessed outcomes.

The Predicament

In a context such as outlined above, the existence of "cancer-control prevention measures" means that population-level screening programs could make a significant difference to the cancer burden: many more patients would be diagnosed in the early stages of the disease (rather than in later stages, as many are diagnosed following symptom presentation); they would receive relatively simpler treatments; and, have higher recovery and longer survival rates. For this to occur, they would need to participate routinely, repeatedly (annually for CRC, once every 2 years for breast cancer), between the ages 50 to74, in the recommended screening tests for *average-risk* populations, as defined in epidemiological screening criteria for such populations: mammography, for breast cancer, and Fecal Occult Blood Test (FOBT) for CRC. A consensus supporting these recommendations exists in countries where organized screening programs for average-risk populations are offered (International cancer screening network 2009). Individuals who have a first-degree relative diagnosed with either breast or CRC are considered to be at *high-risk* for these diseases. In such cases, follow-up recommendations are made *individually,* according to different criteria than the ones used for population screening, and will not be discussed here for lack of space.

In 2008, the population at *average-risk* for breast and CRC in the US included some 74,125,000 women and men between the ages 50–74 (US census report for 2008). This population-size reflects the proportions of the immense existing global cancer burden, and adds a significant 'cluster' of vulnerable individuals, in harm's way merely because they were assigned to the average-risk group for breast and/or CRC pursued (relatively) new risk assignment and its meaning for them. The target populations for (breast and CRC) screening include these individuals. It should be noted that cancer screening was a medical innovation 2–3 decades ago; this innovation has spread among medical professionals of various specialties, and is now being passed on slowly to the general (lay) public.

The discussion turns now to the context of being assigned a cancer risk, its personal and social effects, and to some coping strategies. The issues addressed in this chapter are embedded in Ulrich Beck's notion of a risk society: his global-, macro-, and individual-level analysis of what he termed "risk society" provides a comprehensive sociological context for the epidemiological practice of population and individual risk-assessment. Beck explains risk society as a stage of modernity characterized by man-made risks. Risk itself is the outcome of human decisions, but is beyond our control. A significant part of the difficulty experienced when living with risk is the helpless anticipation of the risked event to occur. The possibility of being diagnosed with cancer is threatening and tragic. This means living with the anticipated *future* of disaster, as well as with the constant *present* attempts to avoid it. The danger is present, agitating, charged with uncertainty, and unbalancing. The implementation of cancer screening as a form of preventive medicine turns cancer risk-assessment into an individual experience. Cancer screening of eligible individuals in defined target populations has become the focus of population intervention programs in many countries (Klabunde et al. 2015). Individuals are personally invited for specific tests (often free of charge), at a pre-determined frequency, to identify (as early as possible, in the natural history of the disease) those who may be developing cancer.

What does it feel like, being in this position? What are the reactions of healthy, asymptomatic people in the community, who are invited to undergo (breast and CRC) screening? The answer is in individual accounts. Authentic quotes were collected over two-decades by this author who served on the team of the National Programs for breast and CRC screening, established in the 1990s by Clalit Health Services, the largest Health Maintenance Organization in Israel. These programs initiate the mailing of screening invitations to everyone in the target population at average risk for breast and CRC. The multidisciplinary medical team is responsible for planning, administration of free-of-charge tests and process/outcome monitoring (through to the final stages of the process, including diagnosis and treatment), and evaluation research. As a medical service, daily interactions take place with insured members in the target population for biannual mammograms and/or annual FOBT.

Insured members call the program offices to react to the invitation, to ask questions, or share their thoughts regarding the initiatives, which in the early years of the programs were innovative, even unanticipated, for many of the invitation addresses; some of their statements are quoted in this chapter. Additional quotes which appear below were expressed in focus group research and in interviews with individual laypersons.

Risk-assessment for cancer may cause perplexity or anxiety. A person ceases to be 'healthy' by virtue of having been invited to be tested. Not yet diagnosed with a disease, they hope for confirmation that they are healthy: *'Doc, what do you mean, I'm at risk for CRC?'* (Hagoel and Feder-Bubis 2016); they may go on to say: *'I feel OK, why undergo a medical test?'*, or *'I performed the test last year'*, as their own risk perception lags behind their (medical) risk group assignment and its medical implications. Women offered a mammography test following a screening indication reply, *'Right after I discover a lump…, I will see my doctor; immediately, that morning.'* As the 'lump' may be a symptom, this would, evidently, not constitute breast cancer early detection. In other cases individuals might ask, *'What do you know about my family that's behind this screening test invitation?'*, or *'Who decides [the screening test criteria]?'*

Some prefer to postpone: *"I've got a [test-] kit at home. I have read the instructions and left the envelope closed, until I am ready to perform the test;"* they may be worried, preferring avoidance rather than taking action in advance: *"I refuse to hear the [bad] news; thinking about a bad result raises fears,"* or rationalizing: *"the fear inhibits rational thinking, thus causing avoidance of the test, but fear is always present when we approach a [medical] test situation. And I have so many other issues in my life… why introduce this too?"; "the very thought of undergoing any medical test is so stressful;" "I understand very little about medicine and believe you should act according to how you feel… if I'm sick, I'll agree to testing…if I'm happy, why introduce trouble into my life? It's a 'Pandora's box' ."* Finally, a general comment is frequently heard: *"I'm really anxious about every test [referring to FOBT]… even the preventive ones…waiting for the results I constantly think about this…every year I debate again, within myself, whether I should skip the test or not… it's too stressful!"*

Professional teams in organized cancer screening programs see some of the invitees accepting the invitation, with others remaining reluctant. "Barriers" to participation are not the main concern here; the issue is the position in which invited individuals are placed, by their very definition of "being at (*average/high*) risk".

Patients are referred for testing using a *diagnostic indication,* following a complaint presented to the physician. A *screening indication* for testing is not obvious (although, this is changing, with the diffusion of health literacy). "Asymptomatic", means in laypersons' language – "healthy", as symptoms are central to motivating help-seeking. To the observer, medical procedures used are similar in both screening and diagnostic situations. Thus, their medical and social meanings overlap, adding to the confusion. In Beck's words: "Non-knowing permeates and transforms human conditions of life and suffering;" this is when "individuals are robbed of their power of judgement… the inability-to-know has become an ineradicable part of their lamentable condition" (Beck 1992, p. 115–116).

Furthermore, there is no direct bridge between the (epidemiologically) known percentages of population-risks, to the unknown future of each individual in this population. It is very difficult to cope with this insurmountable gap. Individuals ask: *"What does it mean that I have 28% risk for developing cancer?"* Even with careful consideration of information provided, ethical criteria observed, and individual autonomy recognized, some suffering is bound to result. The established *population-level benefits* co-exist with the *price 'paid' at the individual level*, to which we turn next.

Beyond the medically based social categories of 'healthy' and 'ill (acute/chronic)', a new medical category has been inadvertently created: 'individuals-at-risk', or 'in the target population for early detection' of cancer. The 'at-risk' status places one in limbo, between 'healthy' and 'diagnosed with-'. Based on an aggregated statistical approach, the new medical category, 'invited for screening', is applied to health system users. 'Well' and 'ill' are the opposite ends of a continuum to which the new, intermediate status option – 'at risk' – has been added. It is applied to individuals who cease to be 'healthy' by virtue of their having been invited to undergo a screening test. Not yet diagnosed with a disease, they hope for the (uncertain) re-confirmation of their own self-assessment as healthy. This cryptic socio-medical status, in itself, and the constant awareness of one's vulnerability, is often experienced as stressful, doubt-ridden and ambiguous.

"Cancer candidacy" (Macdonald et al. 2013), or being a *potential* cancer victim, causes an awareness that many tend to be rejected immediately, intuitively. The experience of fear is an effective motivator for rejecting the 'at risk' label, but more than fear is involved.

A series of fundamental, intricate questions emerges in the mind of the person-at-risk, which are not trivial, or mundane, but are existential. People ponder their lives, how they have led them thus far, life's purpose, what the future holds, what can and cannot be done about health, achievements, relationships; this becomes an encompassing ever-present experience, stretching from the past into the future – such is existential suffering (Best et al. 2015), which impairs these individuals' quality of life.

Existential Suffering and the Search for Meaning

Being assigned to the population sub-group at *average* risk for CRC, by merely having reached the age of 50, is a notification individuals take personally, seriously, thoughtfully. Knowing about this personal status has an effect on a person's entire life, on their self-management, their plans, and their desires. This depends, among others, on the risk communication techniques used; while this has an important role in the process, even more so in high cancer-risk families, it is not discussed here for space limitations. Questions arise, such as, "Did I do what I wanted to in this life? Who am I? Where do I want to go from here?" Insufficient answers lead to despair, to a strong sense of helplessness, of hopelessness. This experience can be categorized as "distress resulting from threat or damage to one's body or self-identity" (Anderson p.10). It is existential suffering.

Suffering appears in a variety of forms (physical pain, mental, or social suffering) and contexts (produced internally or externally by nature, by other persons/groups or institutions, even societies). Existential suffering is mental suffering produced externally; for example, as medical information delivered by professionals that assigns an individual to a category predicting their risk for developing a cancer disease. This is a form of suffering caused by the news that someone is at risk for developing cancer.

Suffering, particularly existential suffering is related in the literature mainly to diagnosed cancer patients (Best et al. 2015), with some researchers referring to the excruciating meaning of the *average* or *high* "at risk" label. Best et al. (2015) found it is important to acknowledge such suffering reported by individuals, as this future threat enters their lives. Hallowell (2006) notes that living with ovarian cancer risk carries, "the responses of an emotional and relational self" (p. 9), while Rubin et al. (2014) point to practical aspects of such suffering in terms of parenthood planning for BRCA1/2 mutation carriers. The problem of suffering due to risk and its consequences is encountered world-wide, as exemplified by research from Cuba, Greece, Germany (Gibbon et al. 2010), and Australia (Gibson et al. 2015; Ward et al. 2015).

Existential suffering consists of the absence or loss of meaning that is exhibited by indications of hopelessness, negative self-worth, loss of meaning, and spiritual or moral confusion (Williams 2004). Suffering may be the result of struggles with the meaning of one's existence, perhaps even in confronting one's potential death. With many optional synonyms, Beck defines the range of possible reactions to this state: *between prudent concern, crippling fear and hysteria.* Victor Frankl, a psychiatrist and Holocaust survivor, focuses on the meaning of one's life as the perspective of coping with suffering, including existential suffering. With little control over what caused the suffering, one can still *reframe* the situation in a beneficial way. Some individuals have this stance as a "built-in" part of their outlook on life. They may be spiritually inclined, or lean on religious beliefs as sources of meaning, strength, and a balanced, harmonious inner existence. They may use meditation or other techniques to relieve themselves from harsh life experiences. Others need to be inspired in such moments; the following paragraphs provide examples.

Frankl's initial axiom is that the meaning of life is central to human existence (Frankl 1985). He notes that the search for meaning involves a choice, between disregard for meaning, a [unclear to what this refers] deep layer of life, and contemplating what life presents us with and how to approach, appreciate, and consider these options. This choice is "second best", some say, to that of being able to choose what will actually happen in our lives, sadly beyond our reach. Nevertheless, how we accept reality can still change our experience of this reality. For Frankl, human beings are in search of a meaning to assign to their lives, which transcends the actual conditions of this life.

The cliché about life's immeasurable value is old, yet human beings often aspire for more. The purpose of life, an enigma philosophers have tried to resolve for millennia, is addressed now and again by individuals in search of their own version of this purpose, to avoid an *existential vacuum* manifesting itself in a state of boredom. Accepting a purpose is a source of strength for individuals: "…being human always points… to something, or someone, other than oneself – be it a meaning to fulfill or another human being to encounter. The more one forgets himself – by giving himself to a cause to serve or another person to love – the more human he is and the more he actualizes himself" (Frankl 1985; p. 133). The meaning of life is constantly changing and can be revealed in action, in a worthwhile experience, or in suffering.

Drawing on his personal experience and observations of the extreme conditions forced on concentration camp prisoners, Frankl notes: "… man does have a choice of action… man can preserve a vestige of spiritual freedom, of independence of mind, even in such terrible conditions of psychic and physical stress… everything can be taken from a man but one thing: the last of human freedoms – to choose one's attitude in any given set of circumstances, to choose one's own way" (p. 86). This noble purpose, to live by one's beliefs, gives one strength. In the worst of circumstances, "the way they [some prisoners] bore their suffering was a genuine inner achievement. It is this spiritual freedom – which cannot be taken away – that makes life meaningful and purposeful" (id, p. 87). In other words, beyond the concentration camp experience, "Everywhere man is confronted with fate, with the chance of achieving something through his own suffering" (id, p. 89); creativity and enjoyment are sources of meaning, but so is suffering, as the sufferer can choose, if not the situation, then to move through it with dignity and morality, turning it into a human achievement.

Frankl suggests a technique to cope with the unavoidable suffering discussed in this chapter: "if … one cannot change a situation that causes his suffering, he can still chose his attitude" (id, p.172), and "[to] master a hard lot with [the] head held high" (id, p.173). This is a fresh perspective which offers one to move beyond struggle and despair to choose one's own reaction, to recruit courage from within, to pick a humanly honorable stand in spite of what one is experiencing. Frankl's examples are extraordinary and yet they can be applied to the risk situation. This is a path for living life to the fullest, acknowledging its multiple layers.

Inspiration is provided by a group of six women interviewed by this author in the waiting room of a mammography clinic. They had scheduled their screening mammography tests at the same time that morning, and had arrived and waited together. They said it was their decision to treat this bi-annual event as if it was one of their weekly coffee get-togethers. As close friends they supported each other in the stressful days before, as well as after the test (until the arrival of the results). Their explanation was simple: *"Fear? Of course we are afraid; and worried. But you know what? We are together in this, and we 'bring the fear along' to the clinic. Still, we do what we think is right. That helps: being together, the situation becomes bearable."* The insight of assigning a new, positive meaning to the situation is an example of how Frankl's approach can be helpful. On the rational level, these women accepted the medical recommendation, took responsibility, and supported each other with the power of their friendship and love of life. They were thus able to undergo the difficult situation.

The Alleviation of Existential Suffering

Coping with this situation involves its recognition, expressed compassion, verbal articulation, and legitimacy; suffering is an incremental attribute. This, along with the added existential dilemma of being at risk, stigmatizes, frightens, and overburdens the individual in need of the medical team's attention, to alleviate the resulting distress (Beck 1992; Balmer et al. 2014). Resistance to screening invitations may reflect (among other reasons) individuals' strong resistance to contemplating the meaning of the 'at-risk' label, of the threat to their emotional well-being. Thus, even if the objective situation cannot be changed, quality of life can be improved, with relief from existential suffering. A few solutions were noted above; each, if adopted, can lead to alleviation: religious beliefs, meditation techniques, and generally an acceptance of the *human condition* and the maintenance of inner balance.

This is made possible by the *choice-element* which might seem irrelevant, and yet could make a difference in the sufferers' lives. In Victor Frankl's work on logotherapy, his analysis of the human search for meaning, particularly assigns meaning to uncontrollable negative events, and urges mental flexibility (reflexivity). This can enhance feelings of courage, endurance, achievement and dignity. Disease-risk information is often theoretical, far from our concrete daily lives, and yet we allow it to overpower us; but we can choose to reject negativity. The understanding of a threat to one's life is not really news for an open-minded person who recognizes that immortality is not an option. Suffering, real as it may be, stems from our subjective view of its underlying causes. Friends and family may often be counted on for direct personal support. Alleviation of existential suffering is available through medical services and interventions, counseling, educational as well as therapeutic psychological support.

Another valuable avenue for coping with the existential suffering discussed in this chapter is through the normalization of cancer control and its establishment as part of routine health maintenance. The medical innovation of the 'at-risk for cancer' status will, eventually, become a regular part of preventive medicine, for laypersons and for medical professionals alike. While medical teams need to be aware of patients' fears, including the threat of stigma, moving towards a proportional view of the (often theoretical) threat could alleviate suffering in this situation. It could also contribute to public health, in that resistance to valuable follow-up recommendations and tests would decline.

Adopting a new health habit requires effort, which eventually is understood and accepted: *"Taking preventive action is of no interest to people… I'm sorry I don't do more in this regard;" "how is it possible, that rational people don't take care of themselves? Are they really such cowards?;" "if you really care about your health, then – there are things you need to do: to be healthy is to undergo periodical tests... one has got to be systematic about this;" "I appreciated the HMO's sending FOBT kits in the mail, paying attention to the public as a whole, this is right.... and it's not only this test, also the flu vaccinations; it's not an economic issue, the HMO care about us;" "I've been doing it for years but missed the last one. Still, for years we underwent the tests;" "We take our health for granted, but if we don't have it, all the rest becomes impossible."*

The family physician is often a significant source of support: *"From age 50 people get sick more, so tests are important, but the authority of my doctor telling me to do it [undergo FOBT] is compelling;" "When I turned 50, Dr. B. [participant's family physician]called me on the telephone and said, 'Natalia, it's time for screening tests'. Everything she told me – I actually did."*

Individuals vary in terms of the pace by which they adopt an innovation. Some are more open and 'adventurous', others are slow and hesitant. They observe people who embrace change; this is how innovations diffuse. Here is what a few 'early adopters' had to say about introducing behavioral components of a healthier, recommended life-style: *"Perhaps if they do it gradually, people will get used to the routine of taking care of their health;" "In our home, let me tell you, my wife bakes. She used to use a lot of margarine. I'm not sure even why this is produced, it's so bad for you... so I told my wife, 'fatty is tasty but we don't really need to have so much of it; less fried, getting used to more healthy stuff... I'm for it'. I mean, really fresh food, we do need to take care of our health, eat right, be active, walk...[as well as undergoing recommended medical tests]"; "the model of a healthy routine: my neighbors, both husband and wife, regularly, every morning, summer and winter, walk from their home to the sea shore... they swim and then return home. And... they live on the 8th floor, and never take the elevator. They always take the stairs;" "undergoing basic tests will gain mental peace; routine FOBT is one such test."* This acceptance is even more remarkable in women's acceptance of screening mammography: *"I undergo mammography routinely...."* says one. Another replies: *"me too, regularly"; "I do this for my daughters,"* adds the third.

Conclusion/Implications

This chapter has focused on millions of asymptomatic individuals worldwide who are labeled to be "at average risk" for breast or colorectal cancer, adding to the cancer burden of the many patients already diagnosed with the disease. By virtue of being members of the population age and/or gender groups, individuals are assigned "at risk" status as derived from epidemiological criteria for (breast and CRC) screening. The meaning of this status has been shown to affect a person's socio-medical status, particularly as it is often accompanied by an invitation for action: participating in a routine medical follow-up, or undergoing screening tests for the early detection of cancer as recommended by public health experts.

This unique status has direct implications for the wellbeing of the individuals involved. This routine preventive example of medical risk-management is unexpected from the patients' point of view. The experts who initiate it see the *population-level benefits* of cancer screening intervention programs, as do individual patients who benefit from early-stage cancer diagnosis in terms of recovery and survival. Just as a screening-test is unexpected by the invitees, the price paid on the *individual level* for this public health action in terms of the impaired quality of life, and the ensuing existential suffering, are invisible to medical teams. This gap is illustrated by the rare-to-non-existent discussion, in main-stream medical literature, of cancer risk assignment as problematic on the individual level. The limbo, in which individuals find themselves, is the place where helplessness and hopelessness thrive.

A persons' bio-social status is an important aspect of one's life, but there are aspects on which one can concentrate to reduce anxiety. Risk is ubiquitous and yet we ignore it and go on about our business. For medical professionals, when life is at stake, action to save it is not assessed in ordinary terms. When resuscitation is performed, a patient's shirt may be torn off to conduct immediate life-saving actions. At the population-level, in order to save lives and to enhance quality of life for (future) patients, and under strict screening criteria, medical professionals have deemed it worthy to screen entire population groups to identify the ones in need of medical attention. By now, for many, in countries where organized cancer screening is offered, this has become routine. Solbjør et al. (2015) say, "screening has become a routine part of ordinary life" (p. 558), which might help to bring individuals back from *hysteria* to *prudent concern*, turning cancer-related existential suffering to another one of life's difficulties we have come to accept and cope with. Though it is beyond the scope of this chapter to suggest a new research agenda, these concluding remarks offer a direction such research could take.

References

Are, C., Rajaram, S., Are, M., et al. (2013). A review of global cancer burden: Trends, challenges, strategies, and a role for surgeons. *Journal of Surgical Oncology, 107*, 221–226. doi:10.1002/jso.23248.

Balmer, C., Griffiths, F., & Dunn, J. (2014). A qualitative systematic review exploring lay understanding of cancer by adults without a cancer diagnosis. *Journal of Advanced Nursing, 70*, 1688–1701. doi:10.1111/jan.12342.

Beck U (1992) *Risk society: Towards a new modernity* (Published in association with Theory, Culture & Society). Sage.

Best, M., Aldridge, L., Butow, P., et al. (2015). Conceptual analysis of suffering in cancer: A systematic review. *Psychooncology, 24*, 977–986. doi:10.1002/pon.3795.

Faivre, J., Tazi, M. A., ElMrini, T., et al. (1999). Faecal occult blood screening and reduction of colorectal cancer mortality: A case-control study. *British Journal of Cancer, 79*, 680–683. doi:10.1038/sj.bjc.6690107.

Ferlay, J., Shin, H.-R., Bray, F., et al. (2010). Estimates of worldwide burden of cancer in 2008: GLOBOCAN 2008. *International Journal of Cancer, 127*, 2893–2917. doi:10.1002/ijc.25516.

Frankl, V. E. (1985). *Man's search for meaning*. New York: Pocket books.

Gibbon, S., Kampriani, E., & Nieden, A. z. (2010). BRCA patients in Cuba, Greece and Germany: Comparative perspectives on public health, the state and the partial reproduction of "neoliberal" subjects. *BioSocieties, 5*, 440–466. doi:10.1057/biosoc.2010.28.

Gibson, A. F., Lee, C., & Crabb, S. (2015). "Take ownership of your condition": Australian women's health and risk talk in relation to their experiences of breast cancer. *Health, Risk and Society, 17*, 132–148. doi:10.1080/13698575.2015.1032215.

Hagoel, L., & Feder-Bubis, P. (2016). Mind the cancer screening gap between medical rationale and laypersons' reasoning. *Journal of Internal Medicine, 279*, 563–565. doi:10.1111/joim.12472.

Hallowell, N. (2006). Varieties of suffering: Living with the risk of ovarian cancer. *Health, Risk and Society, 8*, 9–26. doi:10.1080/13698570500532322.

International cancer screening network. (2009) *Colorectal cancer screening activities in ICSN countries*. http://appliedresearch.cancer.gov/icsn/colorectal/screening.html. Accessed 7 Jul 2013

Klabunde, C., Blom, J., Bulliard, J.-L., et al. (2015). Participation rates for organized colorectal cancer screening programmes: An international comparison. *Journal of Medical Screening*. doi:10.1177/0969141315584694.

Macdonald, S., Watt, G., & Macleod, U. (2013). In search of the cancer candidate: Can lay epidemiology help? *Sociology of Health & Illness, 35*, 575–591. doi:10.1111/j.1467-9566.2012.01513.x.

Roder, D., Houssami, N., Farshid, G., et al. (2008). Population screening and intensity of screening are associated with reduced breast cancer mortality: Evidence of efficacy of mammography screening in Australia. *Breast Cancer Research and Treatment, 108*, 409–416. doi:10.1007/s10549-007-9609-5.

Rubin, L. R., Werner-Lin, A., Sagi, M., et al. (2014). "The BRCA clock is ticking!": Negotiating medical concerns and reproductive goals in preimplantation genetic diagnosis. *Human Fertility, 17*, 159–164. doi:10.3109/14647273.2014.940003.

Solbjør, M., Skolbekken, J.-A., Østerlie, W., & Forsmo, S. (2015). Women's experiences with mammography screening through 6 years of participation—A longitudinal qualitative study. *Health Care for Women International, 36*, 558–576. doi:10.1080/07399332.2014.989438.

U.S. Census Bureau. 2008. *Current population survey*, Annual Social and Economic Supplement.

Ward, P. R., Coffey, C., & Meyer, S. (2015). Trust, choice and obligation: A qualitative study of enablers of colorectal cancer screening in South Australia. *Sociology of Health & Illness, 37*, 988–1006. doi:10.1111/1467-9566.12280.

Williams, B. R. (2004). Dying young, dying poor: A sociological examination of existential suffering among low-socioeconomic status patients. *Journal of Palliative Medicine, 7*, 27–37. doi:10.1089/109662104322737223.

Chapter 26
Exploring Caring Economies and Alleviating Suffering

Mehmet Kocaoğlu and Rhonda Phillips

Introduction

Market-based economic models generally presume self-interest to be a given. Market models for the most part tend to ignore community welfare and non-economic, human well- being. There is no certainty that if market-based approaches fail to translate into improved quality of life for the majority of community members, there will be a correction. In other words, current economic approaches may be considered "uncaring" in the sense that the emphasis is on monetary outcomes, not necessarily improvement in well-being and quality of life, even though that has been the result in many situations throughout modern history. Here is one example: Kuwait and France have the same levels of per capita Gross Domestic Product (GDP), yet indicators of quality of life vary drastically; France's higher gender equality is surely one of the factors helping to lift the overall quality of life in this comparison (Eisler 2007).

It cannot be denied that people gain access to many opportunities with each passing day under market conditions based on values of power, hierarchy, and sometimes, greed. Improvements in many dimensions of life have been made like no other time in history, with more people having access to wealth and all that it conveys. On the other hand, suffering caused by problems brought by market-based economic approaches has increased over the past few decades, especially in regard to access and equity issues, and the imbalance of wealth distribution in many

M. Kocaoğlu
Department of Political Science, Purdue University, Beering Hall of Liberal Arts and Education, Room 2216J, West Lafayette, IN 47907-2098, USA
e-mail: mkocaog@purdue.edu

R. Phillips (✉)
Purdue University, Windsor Halls, Duhme Room134,
West Lafayette, IN 47906-4238, USA
e-mail: RPhillips@purdue.edu

R.E. Anderson (ed.), *Alleviating World Suffering*, Social Indicators Research Series 67, DOI 10.1007/978-3-319-51391-1_26

countries of the world. For example, suffering caused by market-based economics may consist of one or more of the three types of suffering: physical, mental, or social suffering in Anderson's classification (2014: 3, 2015: 3–6).

In contrast to market-based economics, "caring economics," as defined by Eisler (2007: 8) is a system that supports policies and rules based on the value of caring for ourselves, others, and nature. The ideas around caring for ourselves and our environment, and caregiving to others, are instrumental to the underlying ethos of caring economics. Eisler (2007:9) also remarked that, "It's not realistic to expect changes in uncaring economic policies and practices unless caring and caregiving are given greater value."

Basic assumptions of market-based economics can lead to a variety of problems, especially in situations where issues of inequity or unequal access permeate: loss of sense of caring for others, alienation to his/her own work, anxiety, addictions, prevalence of diseases resulting from insecurity and stress, work-family conflict, and gender inequality. These problems may cause additional physical, mental and social suffering in both the personal and working lives of human beings. In this chapter, we explore how ideas around caring economics can help alleviate suffering. Based on values such as caring, altruism, compassion, partnership, and solidarity, caring economics may represent an important alternative to reducing suffering produced by market-based economic models.

Is a Different Understanding Possible?

Research recently conducted on human nature has shown that a different understanding of human nature is possible (Singer 2015b). In particular, research in neuroscience and psychology has revealed that the belief in humans' nature of self-interest is not a rigid or permanent reality. Empirical results obtained from these studies show that humans have a nature that includes altruistic behavior, caring, relationships and relational goods, and partnerships. In light of these findings, might suffering caused by current economic models be reduced if dominant values such as power, hierarchy, competition, egoism, and greed are augmented with other values like empathy, compassion, caring, and partnership?

The assumption that humans act merely with the motivation of self-interest mostly leads to neglect of the feelings enabling humans to adopt altruistic motivations. It is necessary to accept that humans would have motivations other than merely self-interest. From the very beginnings of modern market-based economics, Adam Smith (2002:11) points out that humans have enjoyment in the happiness of others despite their own self-interested nature. Singer (2015a:30–31) in particular argues that there is a natural and inevitable relationship among people in regards to feeling each other's pain rather than merely acting on self-interest. According to experiments in neuroscience, Singer claims that people act with the motivation of empathy and compassion felt for each other's pain.

To explore this, experiments were conducted on couples by using the brain imaging techniques (fMRI) in neuroscience. Each of the partners received pain through the electrodes attached to their fingertips. Both partners could see on a screen which of them was suffering. In this case, brain responses of one of the partners were recorded while she/he was witnessing the other partner's suffering. Although the neural network is activated during suffering by oneself, it was often seen during the experiment that the network is also activated in the case of suffering by another. The finding that humans give similar neural responses as they witness others' suffering is an evidence that, as suggested by Singer, we each have a bond to another. In the context of experiments based on monetary exchange, Singer (2015a: 34–35) also found that women feel deeper empathy for others who are exposed to injustice or suffering than men. Similar laboratory work also revealed that people feel more empathy for individuals within their group when compared to individuals outside their group.

According to one of the basic assumptions of market-based economic theory, it is natural that humans act on the motivation of self-interest. But there are numerous studies proving that humans also naturally act in an altruistic way when faced by suffering of others. Research in neuroscience demonstrates that individuals who grew up in a culture emphasizing the importance of self-interest motivation could adopt the actions of altruistic behavior about reducing the suffering of others after a short training (Davidson 2015: 52, Singer and Klimecki 2014: 877). Davidson (2015: 52–56) conducted experiments finding that participants show more altruistic behaviors in making economic decisions after participating in training sessions over a two-week period. In the experiment, the participants were divided into two groups. In one group, some of the participants were given training on compassion and loving kindness. The remaining participants were trained on how to find positive ways to respond in adverse situations on the basis of cognitive therapy. As a result, it was seen that those receiving training on compassion showed more altruism in making economic decisions.

Singer (2015b) promotes that empathy and compassion, while natural capacities, need to be developed and require training. In the ReSource project, conducted at the Max Planck Institute for Human Cognitive and Brain Sciences, efforts were made to answer the question as to whether humans can learn to be more compassionate. The year-long study found that mental training in compassion led to significant increases in helping, trust, and donation behaviors. This study points to the idea that "such training can change selfish preferences into the more altruistic and prosocial ones that are needed to subserve global cooperation" (Singer 2015b).

The significance of these findings holds much relevance for the topic of this chapter. It does appear we can learn to change motivations and behaviors in such a way as to help build more cooperative, sustainable societies. Singer further explains that "a lack of compassion is arguably the cause of so many of humankind's biggest failures. Certainly, we will not successfully tackle our greatest challenges without developing these attributes and fostering what is perhaps a rather old-fashioned ethical notion—that of the Common Good." (Singer 2015b).

Along a similar line, Ricard (2015: 60) states that altruism, defined as sensitivity to others' suffering, can be taught. This was found to be especially true if children, who tend to engage in altruistic behavior based on compassion, go through training at an early age about the importance of compassion, empathy, and caring. We support the idea that teaching about altruistic tendency is important to help reduce the pain of others. The behavior of self-interest admired by current economic philosophy displaces the altruistic behavior, and can contribute to people remaining indifferent to the suffering of the others, increasing the number of individuals seeking self-interest.

Widely embraced within the notion of community, altruistic behavior is an important foundation on which to reduce suffering by others and ensure cooperation. Research has revealed that relationships and cooperation between people without proximity between them cannot be explained with self-interest motivation only. Henrich et al. (2005) found out that individuals show altruistic behaviors to people who are not relatives across spectrums of communities, from small to large. Andreoni and Rao (2011: 513) also found that altruistic behavior increases as communication is established between people, allowing for self-interest to be overcome. They found that in the condition where there is only one-way communication and only the allocator could speak, 6% of the endowment is donated. But when the recipient talks, 24% of the endowment is donated. When both parties talk, 30% of the endowment is shared. Thus socialization and altruistic behavior correlate strongly. In particular, communication increases the allocator's level of empathy and allows for the establishment of a relationship on altruistic grounds.

Although altruistic behavior is widely expected of the wealthy, it is observed among people of all income groups. Moreover, recent research (Piff et al. 2010; Harbaugh 2015) shows that people in lower income groups unexpectedly show more altruistic behaviors. Generally,, individuals belonging to the lower-income group are expected to be more worried about meeting their own basic needs. But this does not necessarily restrict altruistic behaviors of people in lower-income groups. Studies in the United States reveal people with lower incomes give more to charity than the rich. In a study (Piff et al. 2010: 775–776) carried out with a trust game, lower income people were reported to have a tendency to give out 43% of what is provided for them. According to Piff et al. (2010: 772), those in the lower-income groups act with motivation that existing suffering and difficulties will be overcome with social engagement and altruistic behavior.

These studies in economic behavior, psychology, and neuroscience indicate that human beings are capable of acting on altruistic motivation containing empathy and compassion. The "homo economicus" (the notion that we act rationally on our own wishes and selfishness to maximize our own utility) may yet be able to evolve and predominate.

The Role of Partnership in Alleviating Suffering

As mentioned earlier in the chapter, Eisler started the caring economy way of thinking movement. Later, it came to be called the "Caring Economy Campaign," as a project of the Center for Partnership Studies. This campaign designed and developed the Social Wealth Economic Indicators (SWEIs) to aid policy-makers in crafting economic systems that consider unpaid or underpaid labor, overall health and well-being, and the general welfare of the population (Center for Partnership Studies 2016). Partnership in this context is to help identify systems that can help the greater good of society by providing tangible tools to help assess current situations and gauge progress toward goals. Synonyms for partnership include: connection, association, alliance, affiliation, and cooperation. It is meaningful in that it implies that rather positive things can be achieved with partnerships.

The idea of partnerships as cooperatives has evolved, or re-emerged, over the last few decades, perhaps in response to concern with market-based economic systems. In earlier parts of the twentieth century, the idea of cooperative enterprises was popular. But the history of cooperatives as a means to gain economic advantages dates much further back than the last century. Throughout history, "cooperatives have flourished where the costs to individuals (and their families) of maintaining their standard of living have been too high to bear alone. As far back as the thirteenth century, skilled craftsmen formed guilds as a way to insure their livelihood in a world of considerable social and economic risk" (Gonzales and Phillips 2013: 1).

Cooperatives fell out of style in the United States for several decades; however, a recent resurgence of interest has emerged in their legitimacy and effectiveness as partnership-based structures (Burneli & Phillips 2015). They have the potential to harness economic productivity for those involved in the cooperative structure, allowing for more control over the sources of power. Inherently, cooperatives are more equitable for their members, and decision-making is shared versus other models of businesses. They are considered alternative development approaches and can be quite effective in creating shared wealth and skill attainment. Cooperative endeavors can serve as means to connect social and economic justice movements to public policy responses and to issues around social marginalization, and differences and disparities in unequal wealth distribution (Birchall 2001; Rothschild 2009).

The case of the Mondragon Corporation, probably the most recognized cooperative in the world, is worth exploring in the context of partnerships, alleviating suffering, and caring economies. It is notable that the company motto is "Humanity at Work." It is the largest business enterprise in the Basque region of Spain, and the tenth largest in the entire country. Its guiding principles clearly imply caring and concern for the member partners:

- Open admission
- Democratic organization
- Sovereignty of labor
- Instrumental and subordinate nature of capital
- Partipatory management
- Payment solidarity
- Inter-cooperation
- Social transformation
- Universality
- Education (Mondragon Corp. 2016)

For example, ideas about participatory management provide pathways for workers to express their viewpoints and work together toward improvements for enhancing the cooperative. Even more fundamental is the idea of open admission, where all can seek opportunity to join, participate, and work.

The corporation operates its own university and multiple training programs, enhancing the skills and capabilities of the members, and their region. The ability to self-organize and manage around economic opportunity (and responding to need, such as was the case in the Basque region when the cooperative efforts began) is crucial to success. Partnering with others with similar goals of addressing inequities, finding opportunities, and enhancing skills sets can be highly effective. This type of economic self-management "is a means of creating connection with community, it can be considered a form of social organization, holding much potential for impact beyond the initial impetus for cooperation (Phillips 2012: 191).

Alternative ways of thinking about economic and social well-being in terms of economic activities continue to emerge. Some are reflected in social or community-based business practices, with benefits accruing in environments where "social, natural, and cultural dimensions are important and recognized by the private sector as well as the civic sector" (Phillips 2015: 25). There are several forms of enterprise that focus on doing good while making money, including wide-spread interest in corporate social responsibility and social enterprise. There are many variations on these themes in corporations' approaches to social responsibility and sustainability. For social enterprise, there are also many variations. Typically, these entrepreneurs and their organizations are at the cross roads among the public, private, and civic (non-profit) sectors. They are seeking innovative solutions to effect positive change. Descriptions of social enterprise include:

1. The convergence of organizations toward a new landscape—a critical mass of organizations within the three sectors (private, public, and civic/non-profit) has been evolving, or converging, toward a fundamentally new organizational landscape that integrates social purposes with business methods.
2. The emergence of hybrid organizations—pioneering organizations have emerged with new models for addressing societal challenges that blend attributes and strategies from all sectors (Sabeti 2009: 2).

An interesting result is that social enterprises are often not driven primarily by profit maximization. This opens up avenues for addressing issues around inequities and other aspects of suffering from economic consequences.

Further, workplace environment can directly affect well-being and suffering. Much suffering seems to be grounded in the jobs and wages of companies that do not pay well enough or provide the caring services that alleviate suffering in the lives of workers and their families. Those companies and organizations that operate with a sense of "higher purpose" may find that happier employees are more productive, benefitting all involved. Chapman and Sisodia (2015) found that companies oriented this way exhibit determination to create multiple kinds of value for all of their stakeholders, have leaders who care about their purpose and their people, and have cultures built upon trust and authenticity and genuine caring for human beings.

The authors, who include a CEO of a large corporation, explain that with goals including profit motivation and expanding beyond, they seek to give people the power and freedom to care for each other, to trust that people want to do well and be good. This translates into creating value for everyone involved. Values are created using foundational approaches such as establishing a shared long-term vision, fostering a people-centric culture, developing leaders from within, and sending people home fulfilled. It is heartening to have the authors explain that, "the most powerful force in the universe and thus human beings and organizations is caring" (2015: 244).

There is also much interest in localization. This has been defined as, "adjustment of economic focus from the global to the local; rebuilding local economies around the meeting of local needs" (Hopkins 2011: 51). Again, approaches vary widely although some commonalities exist around ideas of building social capital, core (or nonmarket) economy activities, co-production, time banking, community-owned businesses, and locally focused community-led development initiatives (Burnell and Phillips 2015). All of these efforts include the idea of working together and increasing capacity to achieve positive outcomes for community residents. Again, the idea of partnering with others and caring for others serves as the underlying foundation of these approaches. Via these partnerships, suffering can be addressed and alleviated for community members.

Conclusion and Implications for Alleviation of Suffering

Caring economics represents a way to help alleviate suffering, by expanding emphasis from beyond economic self-interest to one that is more inclusive of compassionate actions. Market-based economic systems tend to focus on self-interest, yet reflections on "caring" could help overcome some of the negative outcomes.

Studies from neuroscience and psychology point to findings that compassionate behaviors as well as increasing altruism and trust can be increased. Using training, behaviors can be modified and compassion reinforced or acquired. The implications for alleviating suffering could be significant if more people learned about compassion, and how to be more compassionate to others, including those outside their groups. Communications play a role in enhancing compassion as an element in economic systems too, and ideas around increasing communications may help others act on feelings of empathy. Further, partnerships can be directly linked to the outcome of creating a more caring economy. More innovative, inclusive approaches to integrating a spectrum of considerations for people in relation to economic systems hold potential to directly affect outcomes. We conclude that if economies can integrate more caring attributes, perhaps not replacing existing market-based economic systems but rather expanding dimensions to be more equitable and just, there is hope that some suffering can be mitigated. After all, we created the current system; surely improvements and adjustments can be made to help alleviate suffering.

References

Anderson, R. E. (2014). *Human suffering and quality of life*. Dordrecht: Springer.
Anderson, R. E. (2015). Implication of world suffering for human progress. In R. E. Anderson (Ed.), *World suffering and quality of life* (pp. 3–31). Dordrecht: Springer.
Andreoni, J., & Rao, J. M. (2011). The power of asking: How communication affects selfishness, empathy and altruism. *Journal of Public Economics, 95*, 513–520.
Birchall, J. (2001). *The new mutualism in public policy*. London: Routledge.
Burnell, J., & Phillips, R. (2015). The "New" local. In R. Phillips & R. Pittman (Eds.), *Introduction to community development* (2nd ed.). London: Routledge.
Center for Partnership Studies. (2016). *About*. Accessed 31 July at http://centerforpartnership.org/
Chapman, B., & Sisodia, R. (2015). *Everybody matters: The extraordinary power of caring for your people like family*. New York: Penguin Publishing Group.
Davidson, R. (2015). The neural bases of compassion. In T. Singer & M. Richard (Eds.), *Caring economics: Conservations on altruism and compassion between scientist, economists, and the dalai lama* (pp. 45–57). New York: Picador.
Eisler, R. (2007). *The real wealth of nations: Creating a caring economics*. San Francisco: Berrett-Koehler Publishers, Inc..
Gonzales, V., & Phillips, R. (2013). *Cooperatives and community development*. London: Routledge.
Harbaugh, W. (2015). Why people give to charity. In T. Singer, & M. Richard (Eds.), *Caring economics: Conservations on altruism and compassion between scientist, economists, and Dalai Lama* (pp. 97–115). New York: Picador.
Henrich, J., Boyd, R., Bowles, S., Camerer, C., Fehr, E., Gintis, H., McElreath, R., Alvard, M., Barr, A., Ensminger, N. S., Hill, K., Gil-White, F., Gurven, M., Marlowe, F. W., Patton, J. Q., & Tracer, D. (2005). Economic man in cross-cultural perspective: Behavioral experiments in 15 small-scale societies. *Behavioral and Brain Sciences, 28*, 795–855.
Hopkins, R. (2011). *The transition companion: Making your community more resillient in uncertain times*. Vermont: Chelsea Green.
Mondragon Corporation. (2016). *Our principles*. http://www.mondragon-corporation.com/eng/co-operative-experience/our-principles/.
Phillips, R. (2012). Food cooperatives as community-level self-help and development. *International Journal of Self-Help & Self-Care, 6*(2), 189–203.
Phillips, R. (2015). Building community well-being across sectors with "For Benefit" community business. In S. J. Lee, Y. Kim, & R. Phillips (Eds.), *Community well-being and community development, conceptions and applications*. Dordrecht: Springer.
Piff, P. K., Kraus, M. W., Kote, S., Cheng, H., & Keltner, D. (2010). Having less, giving more: The influence of social class on prosocial behavior. *Journal of Personality and Social Psychology, 99*(5), 771–784.
Ricard, M. (2015). A buddhist perspective for survival: Altruism. In T. Singer & M. Ricard (Eds.), *Caring economics: Conservations on altruism and compassion between scientist, economists, and the dalai lama* (pp. 45–57). New York: Picador.
Rothschild, J. (2009). Workers' cooperatives and social enterprise. *American Behavioral Scientist, 52*(7), 1023–1041.
Sabeti, H. (2009). *The emerging fourth sector*. Washington, DC: The Aspen Institute.
Singer, T. (2015a). Empathy and the interoceptive cortex. In T. Singer & M. Richard (Eds.), *Caring economics: Conservations on altruism and compassion between scientist, economists, and the dalai lama* (pp. 27–45). New York: Picador.
Singer, T. (2015b). *How to build a caring economy*. Accessed 1 Aug at: https://www.weforum.org/agenda/2015/01/how-to-build-a-caring-economy
Singer, T., & Klimecki, O. M. (2014). Empathy and compassion. *Current Biology, 24*, 875–878.
Smith, A. (2002). In K. Haakonssen (Ed.), *The theory of moral sentiments*. Cambridge, UK: Cambridge University Press.

Chapter 27
Well-Being, Future Generations, and Prevention of Suffering from Climate Change

Ronald E. Anderson

Quality of Life, Sustainability and Future Generations

The research literature on "quality of life" (QOL) and well-being has grown exponentially during the lifetimes of those reading this chapter. Our research methods make it possible to investigate this family of topics in the past using historical methods and in the present using both qualitative and quantitative measurement. The future as a research context is much more problematic. Economists and others have built methods for forecasting but these instruments require extensive resources, cover a short time period, and their conclusions lack the certainty that can often accompany findings from studies of the past and present.

The Well-Being of Future Generations

An important political development occurred in 2015 when the state of Wales, UK, passed the *Well-being of Future Generations Act.* This Act of the National Assembly for Wales requires public bodies to do things "in pursuit of the economic, social, environmental and cultural well-being of Wales in a way that accords with the sustainable development principle." Not only did this legislation designate future generations as the beneficiary of government and civil society activity, but it suggested that the most effective way to enact such benefits would be to use sustainability as the guiding principle or goal. As sustainable development is explicitly mentioned, there was no question that the decision-makers chief concern was environmental integrity and the intended beneficiaries of concern were present and future generations.

R.E. Anderson (✉)
Faculty of Sociology, Department of Sociology, University of Minnesota,
Minneapolis, MN 55455, USA
e-mail: rea@umn.edu

R.E. Anderson (ed.), *Alleviating World Suffering*, Social Indicators Research
Series 67, DOI 10.1007/978-3-319-51391-1_27

Importantly, at the same time the *Well-being of Future Generations Act* was enacted in Wales, the United Nations was winding up its nearly final draft of the Sustainable Development Goals (SDG) after years of deliberation involving 193 countries (United Nations 2015). The SDGs consist of 17 goals with 169 sub-goals called targets and 304 indicators to show compliance. Several chapters in this volume, most notably those by Speidel as well as by Lagon and Kaminski, discussed the significance of these goals. Not all international leaders and scholars agree on the importance of these goals and indicators, as can be seen in the chapter by Jason Hickel.

Foundations for the Prevention of Future Suffering

Given the difficulty in targeting the future as a context for well-being research, it is useful to review the justification for concern for the well-being of future generations. Those with a moral commitment to humanity are theoretically concerned for the well-being of all known people from the present forward through time, because of the implicit commitment to future generations—which are rarely mentioned in any policy documents.

Commitment to present and future generations also depends upon one's moral principles, particularly those that promote justice, compassion and community (Wrigley 2012). Communitarianism enhances loyalty to such principles and reinforces social solidarity as well.

Intergenerational ethics commit us most powerfully to future generations. These ethics arise not only from a morality of caring or neighborliness but from future generations as extensions of oneself through interpersonal networks, "blood ties," and family genes. The notion and social practice of inheritance and family beneficiaries implement these values. Traditional moral arguments minimize obligations toward future generations. For example, some argue that our obligations disappear as our knowledge, understanding, and ability to control the relevant situations diminish (Visser 't Hooft 1985). Also compelling might be the argument that our future obligations are very different from present ones.

Future generations have no official advocate. Proposals have been made for all major democratic institutions to establish a committee of ombudsmen or a commission representing the interests of future generations (Meyer 2016), but so far no action has been taken. At a minimum, people should be encouraged to feel both solidarity with future generations and a sense of social responsibility for their well-being on ethical or religious grounds (Tanner 2010).

Addressing the needs of future generations is ethically problematic if the suffering of the present day poor or powerless is not concurrently addressed as well. Hopefully policy actions can address both populations, especially because disasters occurring in a future time-frame are likely to produce greater suffering among the poor than the non-poor (Tanner 2010). Perhaps the best succinct conclusion to the current controversy is that we should act toward the future so as not to knowingly violate the human rights of all present and future generations (Caney 2010).

Extinction, the Ultimate Failure to Prevent Suffering

Human extinction probably is the most catastrophic future event imaginable, which may account for why we rarely discuss it. A major exception is the recent *Global Catastrophic Risks* report from the Global Challenges Foundation (2016). This carefully done study defined global catastrophic risk (GCR) as an event leading to the deaths of at least 10% of the world population.

Though such a disaster would seem to be so remote as to be nearly impossible, the report claims that "the average American is more than five times likelier to die during a human-extinction event than in a car crash" (Global Challenges Foundation 2016). The report states that the most likely global catastrophes over which we have some control are nuclear war, pandemics, and catastrophic climate change. Catastrophes over which we have almost no control include asteroid impact and super-volcanic eruption.

In this chapter, catastrophic climate change will be used to illustrate and represent global catastrophes because it is the one extinction threat over which people have some influence, as opposed to a handful of decision makers. By reducing carbon emissions, we reduce a tiny slice of global warming. Climate change is used to not only discuss the prevention of suffering but to remind us of the threat of extinction.

Jamail (2013) reported his interviews of several eminent climate scientists, several of whom expressed very real concerns about possible global catastrophic events with human extinction possible from climate change. Especially of concern to them were the effects of methane gases released into the atmosphere from the ocean after the polar ice has melted. Other indicators of global warming are becoming so extreme that science cannot yet help predict the outcome of related catastrophic events.

This quote by Stoknes (2015) is typical of the expert opinions of some of the most respected climate scientists: "When the Arctic multiyear ice is soon fully gone, we may see a meltdown of methane hydrates in permafrost and seabeds. This could unleash enormous burps of methane from below, tipping the climate for … well, in human-time scales, pretty much forever" (Stoknes 2015).

Next we will review how unsustainability and climate change not only vary across time and generations of people but how they contribute to world poverty and global violence as well.

The Production of Suffering from Climate Change Disasters

Scientists and most other investigators of the impact of global warming have been forecasting chaos and loss, especially for those with few resources. (Brainard et al. 2009; Ellwood 2014; Parenti 2011; (WHO 2014) Worldwatch Institute 2015). Put simply, the argument is that climate change has begun to expand its enormous environmental disasters around the world, including searing drought in desert regions and devastating flooding of seacoast communities (Rahmstorf 2014). Although these disasters will substantially increase world suffering, that consequence of global warming is rarely made explicit, perhaps because many people worry more about comfort in the present. This is the context in which Lakoff (2014) wrote, "Global warming is the greatest moral issue facing our generation." As world suffering escalates, the moral dimension of climate catastrophes will become more and more compelling.

Baseline Trends in Climate-Related Catastrophes

The World Meteorological Organization (WMO) compiles global data on climate-related disasters, in which a disaster is defined as a destructive event meeting one of these two conditions: 10 or more people killed, 100 or more people affected (injured, infected, evacuated or homeless.) Of the 7416 climate-related disasters from 1981 to 2010, over 90% were storms, floods, and droughts. The trend in disasters has been steadily moving upward as shown by Fig. 27.1. The figure reveals how sharply the rise in major disasters has been accelerating, even during the past two decades.

Climate Change and the Alleviation of World Suffering

Over the past 150 years, but mostly the past 50 years, several major global changes have occurred. Perhaps of greatest concern is the rise in atmospheric carbon dioxide from 280 ppm to more than 400 ppm. While this might not seem like much, it is entirely caused by humans and is primarily due to the burning of fossil fuels and secondarily to deforestation. This seemingly modest rise in carbon dioxide could be catastrophic, because it leads directly to rising temperatures of the earth's oceans as well as its landmass. Both of these temperature rises lead to glacier and polar ice melting, which results in the rise of sea levels and devastating flooding of land near ocean fronts. The loss of ice sheets is particularly devastating because of the unknown methane gas reserves potentially hidden underneath and because of the many millennia that will be required to recover the ice.

Other physical impact and risks from warming include ocean acidification and loss of all types of species: ocean life, land dwellers, birds and a huge variety of

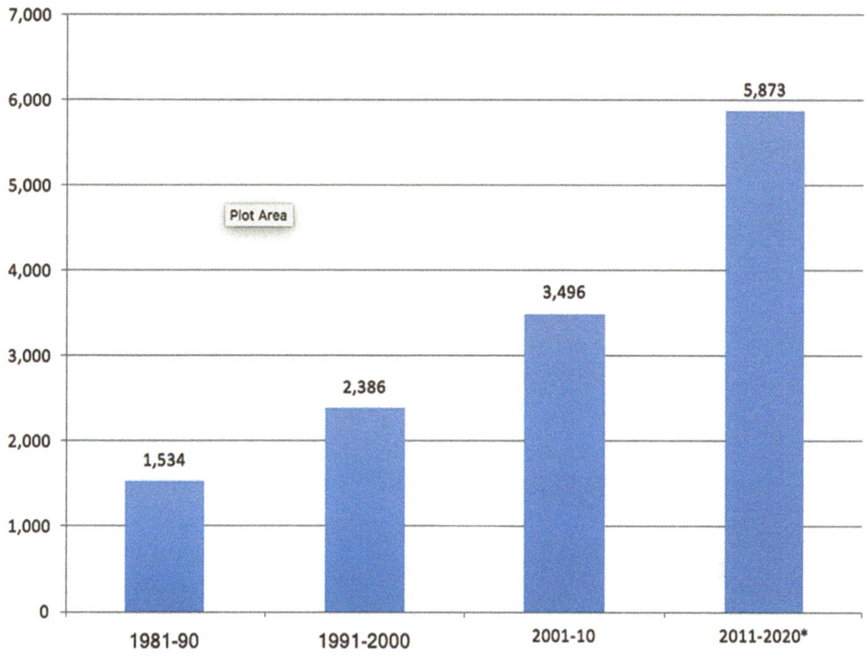

Fig. 27.1 Global climate-related disaster count rising data (Source: WMO 2016)

plants. Many species will be at risk because ecosystems will be disrupted. These changes will also disrupt food supplies even though growing seasons may expand. Perhaps the greatest threat to food supplies comes from water shortages and weather extremes.

While this major disruption of climate-related processes necessarily has created havoc and destruction during major weather events, for any given storm, draught, or disruptive event, the attribution of cause by global warming or climate change requires considerable analysis of huge amounts of data (McGuire 2012). Because of the complexity of attributing causation for any given weather event, many "climate skeptics" and "climate deniers" have emerged and some even believe that it is a hoax.

The evidence of negative effects of global warming from climate and other ecosystems has become so compelling that almost all scientists, and a majority of most national publics, agree that people-created global warming has become a serious threat. What is less well known is that global-warming catastrophes have major secondary effects, in particular, greater poverty and violence. The poverty outcome will be discussed in the next section, but here the outcome of violence will be summarized.

In a meta-analysis of 55 research studies on the impact of climate change on violence, Burke et al. (2015) concluded that, "In an ever-warming world, expect more wars, civil unrest, and strife and also more violent crime in general." They concluded that for every Celsius degree of warming in Africa there could be a 20% increase in civil conflict in Africa.

In a more concrete case, consider Syria's severe drought beginning in 2011. Farmers lost all their crops and flocked to the cities. Food and jobs were scarce, and then a civil war began with many groups trying to topple the ruling regime. At about that time Syria became burdened with crowds of refugees fleeing from Iraq. Then Syria's Arab Spring began, but soon turned into a bloody, chaotic war. Syria's climate catastrophe became an even more catastrophic war. The Syrian war has claimed a half-million lives, wounded 2 million people, generated 4.8 million refugees, and displaced 7 million within Syria (Mansharamani 2016). Of course, climate was not the only precipitating force behind the war, but the war might have been avoided had such factors not created major unrest within Syria.

Modeling the Effects of World Climate Change on Poverty from 2015 to 2030

The World Bank Group recently released a major report entitled, "Shock Waves: Managing the Impacts of Climate Change on Poverty" (Hallegatte, et al. 2016). The report is significant because it undermines the credibility of those who deny that climate change is a serious threat, especially to large numbers of people without the means to survive such disasters. It is also important because it measures many direct links between climate disasters and human poverty, both of which generate suffering, especially in the more impoverished regions of the world. The report was based upon a very large project using leading-edge econometric and microsimulation techniques to analyze available data and forecast trends to 2030.

While the United Nations in its Millennium Development Goals (MDG) project had been estimating the downward evolution of extreme global poverty, the World Bank, as already mentioned, was estimating the growth in climate-related disasters and their interaction with and impact on poverty (Hallegatte, et al. 2016).

Three types of global poverty indicators can be seen in Fig. 27.2. The top trend line is what has been called the "Ethical Poverty Line," because it is more realistic about income needs than the traditional global poverty lines. The ethical line is based upon an income of \$5/day (or 60 cents an hour), whereas the poverty line used by the MDG project and most other UN projects is represented by the bottom lines, defined by \$1.25/day income or less. The UN sometimes will report the middle line as well, which graphs the number of people living on \$2.00/day or less. The bottom lines showing \$1.25/day also depict a fork in the line, the top branch of the fork represents a worst case scenario projection and the bottom branch a best case scenario. The data for these best and worst case projections were generated by the Shock Wave report (Hallegatte, et al. 2016).

The data for the top two poverty lines were obtained from the chapter by Jason Hickel in this volume. The fact that these two lines are so flat compared to the \$1.25/

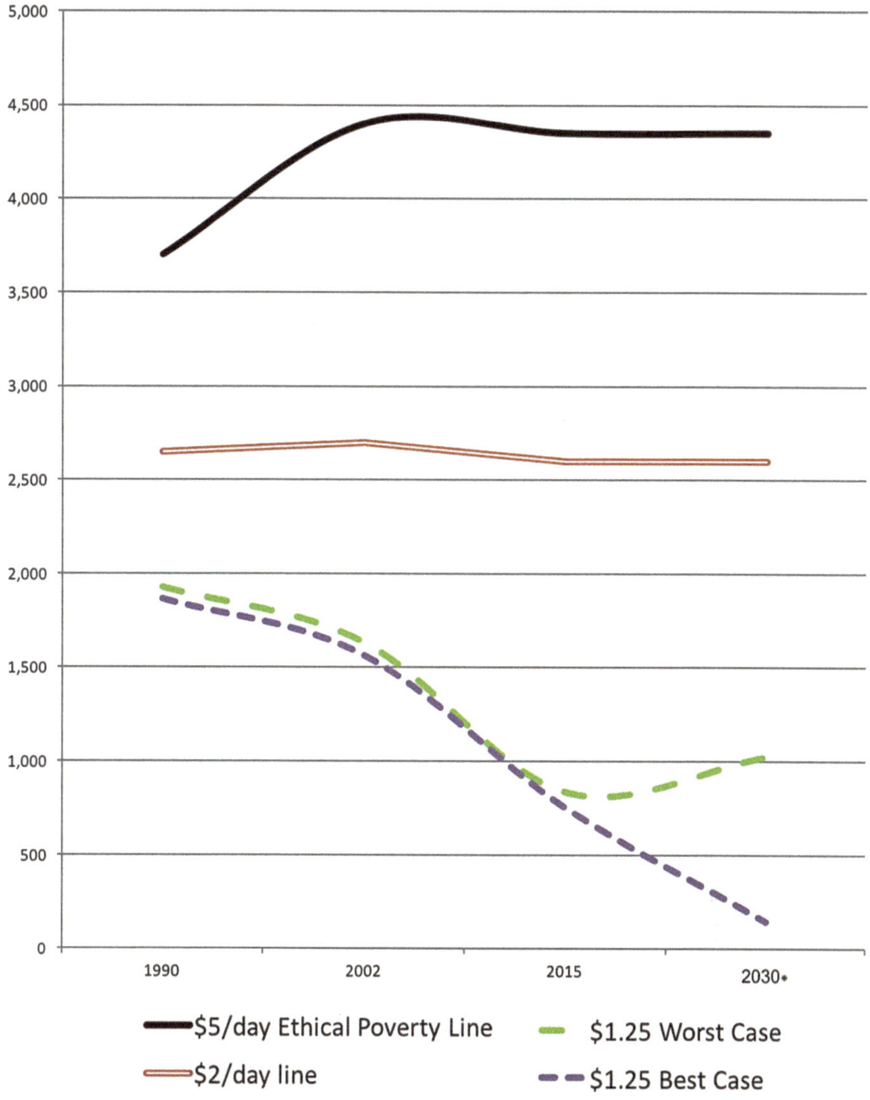

Fig. 27.2 Indicators of poverty with best and worst case scenario forecasts from the World Bank report

day poverty line, indicates that recent claims to poverty reduction around the world are not very robust. Looking literally between the lines, you can see from the chart that for the 2 million people earning only $1.25/day, almost all of them gained only a few pennies per day of income and almost none of them rose 75 cents or more to $2.00/day.

The UN uses the share of adults living on less than $1.25 per day as their indicator of extreme poverty, and by that measure, poverty has declined sharply in the past

Table 27.1 Sources of impact of climate change on poverty

Sources of impact	Percent of impact
Food/Agriculture	73%
Problem Health	27
Poor Labor Productivity	19
Disaster direct effects	5

25 years as can be seen in Fig. 27.2. For the year 2030, their worst-case scenario leaves extreme poverty at one billion, but their best-case scenario estimates it as less than 200 million.

The difference between the best and worst cases is determined by three factors: (1) existing economic, international development policies; (2) economic damage from climate disasters; and (3) the indirect and joint effects of climate change and poverty. The Shockwave report makes the following conclusions:

- As many as 100 million people could slide into extreme poverty because of rising temperatures.
- Efforts to stabilize climate change should be combined with anti-poverty activities; otherwise, they will be less efficient.
- Without proper efforts to stabilize the impact of climate change, global warming can undo decades of progress in lifting people out of extreme poverty.

There are several ways that climate will produce the predicted impact on extreme poverty. The Shockwave report estimates that these sources of impact will have the relative magnitudes as shown in Table 27.1.

The World Bank's report, Shockwave, urges closely coordinating climate and development policies, which makes sense. However, the World Bank's notion of effective development has been questioned and denounced by some experts on international development such as Banerjee & Duflo (2011), Black (2015), Darnton (2011), Easterly (2006), Munk (2013) and Moyo (2010). Given these questions, it is quite possible that the effects of climate disaster on impoverished people may be much greater than estimated by the report (Brewer 2014). If so, the likely effect of climate change disasters on world suffering will be far greater than that forecasted by the Shockwave report.

Framing Projects to Help those with Minimal Resources

Given our history of global colonialism and neocolonialism, it should not be surprising when Western nations behave paternalistically in dealing with developing nations. International development, whether organized by global institutions (e.g., the UN, the World Bank or the IMF), or national governments, or the private sector, tends to champion markets, technological innovation, and economic growth,

Table 27.2 Frame comparisons of the international development frame with the local partnership frame

Project attributes	International development frames	Local partnership frames
Mission	Finding and spending charitable aid	Resolving structural causes of poverty
Major goal	Economic growth	Livelihood maintenance
Economic engines	Markets	Cooperative organization
Leadership	Paternalistic and hierarchical leadership	Joint partners leadership
Role of Debt	Dependence on debt	Avoidance of debt creation
Investors	Reliance on Multi-Nationals	Reliance on local Eco-Systems
Community	Largely Omitted	Major, leadership role
Leadership	Novel, recent	Indigenous, experienced
Who are the main funding recipients?	Governments & intermediaries, e.g., NGOs	Participants

neglecting the wisdom of local knowledge and the power of community partnerships (Darnton & Kirk 2011). International scholars tend to frame their analyses in terms of traditional development and its institutions (cf. Sachs 2005, 2015) or local values, networks, and customs (cf. Easterly 2006).

These two different perspectives in how to achieve social progress are contrasted in Table 27.2, which suggests project attributes depending upon the frame used for the project: international development or local partnership.

When development institutions put their philosophies into practice, they often find themselves working at cross-purposes to local norms and customs. Many of these incompatibilities can be avoided if sufficient time and effort are devoted to an understanding of these local norms, customs and values, as well as their logic. Listening to indigenous wisdom is critical to successful merging of global and local values and concerns.

The mission of international development has too often been to solicit charitable funding rather than understand the role of economic and gender inequality, injustice, and aggression in maintaining poverty and stagnation. This becomes evident with examples such as giving farmers tractors. Often the machinery sits unused and rusting away because no training was given in skills to operate it and/or there was no money given for spare parts or repairs.

The Ecovillage Movement

One of the most successful development programs around the world is the Ecovillage movement. Developed from the "local upward" rather than the top down, Ecovillages have been devoted to ecological integrity on one hand and community on the other (Anderson 2017).

The Ecovillage movement is several decades old and is described in a recent book by Jobert & Dregger (2015). Most of these communities promote not only environmental sustainability but also social sustainability. Most remain active and committed to their mission. Ecovillages are spread across each of five world regions: Europe, Africa, Latin America, North America, and Asia.

All Ecovillages express commitment to sustainable and localized agriculture and food production. However, about two-thirds of the projects define peace, love, or trust as an explicit mission of the project. Some stress the importance of relationships; others, the importance of learning social responsibility or the skills to work together in groups. Thus, the high priority given to social well-being seems to have arisen from experience. Many of the Ecovillages adopt *permaculture*, the philosophy of working with, rather than against, nature, including thorough observation of natural and social systems before committing to thoughtless labor. Some believe that permaculture provides the most meaningful and effective vision that leads to both ecological and social sustainability. It has also become an inspirational vision for those who give up on development projects that drain away precious natural resources.

Though Ecovillages rarely use the terminology of well-being, many appear to have discovered the secret to infusing it into their communities. Although most Ecovillages were launched to implement environmental change, community social change became a second major direction, in part because of their commitment to building caring capital and maintaining sustainable well-being. Caring capital emerges from a variety of other-centered actions and relationships that are mutually helpful. Communities with considerable caring capital are likely to have sustainable well-being as a side benefit. Whatever the path to success as communities, Ecovillages have become models of strategies for reversing the adverse effects of unbridled development and destruction of natural resources and the ecosystem.

International Development

Moyo (2010) concluded that food and monetary aid both created corrupt institutions in Africa. And as if that were not enough damage, she shows how funds for "international development" aid contributed to horrific civil war in Africa. The aid system produces negative effects from those intended, because the aid very often is guided by political agendas and blocked by powerful but corrupt intermediaries. Moyo, an economist, tends not to look to local partnerships alone as the solution but to changes in foreign policies and reforms in aid distribution as well.

One of the policies supported by Moyo is the "conditional cash transfer program" promoted by Ferguson (2015) for South Africa. Because the cash transfers are conditional upon behavioral contributions, such as schooling or work, and because these programs are less prone to corruption, Moyo and others support them. In addition, the preliminary results for South Africa appear promising.

Tragic stories from Bolivia (Shultz & Draper 2009) unearth the harm produced by international institutions like the IMF and multinational corporations, which are managed by a few persons under the guise of democratic freedom. Struggle after struggle make it clear that what the local people need is indirect aid going to local partnership projects that function as reform movements to ensure true, local sustainability rather than sham sustainability managed by corrupt decision-makers often at national levels.

These concerns are shared by Parenti (2011), who tends to focus upon the direct link between climate change and the rise of violence of all types. A live example of Parenti's concern can be found in Somalia, where in 2011 women and children fled to Kenya to escape a severe drought laced with violence, only to be faced with rape at the border. Those who resisted were all too often killed or tortured.

Sustainable Development Goals (SDGs)

While the United Nations has been working on outlining sustainable development goals for decades, not until 2015 did they become an official project. The Millennium Development Goals (MDGs) project provided a model and the SDGs include many goals, such as reducing extreme poverty, that were central to the MDGs.

The Millennium Development Goals project emerged from the United Nations in 2000 at a convention of leaders representing most world nations interested in working together toward common development in the new millennium. Most significantly, the MDGs evolved into a global partnership for poverty reduction. While this became one of the largest development projects ever and produced improvements in many countries, expectations for its success became so unrealistic that the MDGs project also has been called the "world's biggest un-met promise." (Darrow 2012).

The Millennium Development Goals report (United Nations 2015) encompasses eight goals: eradicate extreme poverty and hunger, achieve universal primary education, promote gender equality, reduce child mortality, improve maternal health, combat diseases, ensure environmental sustainability, and develop a global partnership for development.

As the MDGs project ended, a new project, the Sustainable Development Goals (SDGs) was launched in 2015 with 193 participating countries. As already noted, the SDGs have 17 goals, 169 proposed targets for these goals and 304 proposed indicators to show compliance. One goal of the SDGs is to "end poverty in all its forms everywhere." Another goal is to "ensure healthy lives and promote well-being for all at all ages," a step forward beyond MDGs, which did not mention well-being.

The first and most visible goal of the MDGs project was to eradicate world poverty and hunger. However, the project picked such an extremely low standard for poverty—to live on $1.25 or less a day— that the project could easily claim that it exceeded its goal. In addition to this technical weakness, the MDGs had substantive problems. The MDG, with its major emphasis on poverty reduction, like most development strategies fails to recognize that the end goal should be sustainable human well-being and quality of life, rather than economic progress or even poverty reduction. Broad human progress builds upon unleashing human capabilities and respecting human rights, especially the alleviation of suffering. Poverty blocks such progress, but its relief is secondary to human well-being and quality of life. The Sustainable Development Goals project gives lip service to well-being (SDG goal 3) but it remains to be seen how much attention it will be given.

According to the Millennium Development Goals Report (United Nations 2015), poverty has gone down sharply in the past 25 years. The MDG reports evidence for world poverty reduction is that millions of daily earnings have risen from less than $1.25 per day to more than $1.25. However, many daily earnings may not have increased to more than $1.50 per day. An increment of 25 cents per day is roughly equivalent to an hourly wage increase from 15 cents per hour to 19 cents per hour, thus the rise in earnings for many may not have improved access to adequate healthcare or improved well-being in other ways.

According to the MDG's report (UN 2015), from 2006 to 2013 extreme poverty (as measured by living on less than $1.25/day) went from about 27% of adults worldwide to 18%. This was a relatively steep decline of extreme poverty of 9% of the adult world population, which possibly was due to an MDG project effect.

The so-called reduction in extreme poverty was probably misnamed, as the gain in wages may well have been only a few pennies per hour. To be confident that a perceptive reduction in poverty occurred, we need to know more about the actual distribution of poverty reductions, and we need to know whether the wage earners felt any noticeable change in their lives. This analysis points to the importance of collecting indicators of well-being in the large natural experiments like MDG and SDG.

While it would seem that the concept of sustainable development would have much to do with climate change and its mitigation, only three out of 17 SDGs directly address climate change or ecosystem issues. These three goals are: (13) take urgent action to combat climate change, (14) conserve use of oceans and marine resources, and (15) protect ecosystems and halt biodiversity loss. While sustainable development is much broader than climate change mitigation, the SDGs as a whole reflect an economic development notion of sustainable development compared to the original meaning of the phrase: conservation management. Unfortunately, this hints of capitulation to those who believe in growth at almost any cost, and rejection of those who would substitute general well-being for economic well-being in future development.

Recent Disasters that Beg for Climate Action and Improved Humanitarian Relief

Here are three recent disasters almost certainly caused in part by climate change that reveal how the effects of climate-assisted natural disasters discriminate against the poor and disadvantaged and consequently remain unjust.

Typhoon Haiyan in 2013

Typhoon Haiyan in 2013 was the strongest tropical cyclone to make landfall in history. The key drivers for typhoons include high sea surface temperatures, rising ocean levels, and heavy rains that loosen potentially active earthquakes (McGuire 2012, 2016). While the greatest destruction occurred in the Philippines, also struck were South China, Vietnam, and Micronesia. Overall, 7500 were killed or missing, at least 700,000 people displaced, and the lives of 11.3 million people upended in some way (Milman 2015). Haiyan, also known as Super Storm Yolanda, illustrates how climate-related catastrophes selectively harm the poor, especially the extreme poor. This is true for those living in poverty within both rural and urban areas. Disadvantaged groups simply do not have the resources to cope with disruptive forces such as floods and extreme temperatures, which can totally change one's life. On the other hand, the wealthy typically have access to transportation, water, and medications. Displacement and disease are two common consequences, which require additional resources from either the victims or from civil institutions. The poorer the nation, the less likely it is to have social institutions that provide transportation for evacuation, temporary housing and other social and health services.

East Africa, 2010–2016

East Africa, 2010–2016, marks a devastating drought beginning with Somalia and spreading to neighboring Ethiopia and Eritrea as well. Below-average rainfall over several planting seasons caused crop failures and death of large numbers of livestock in Ethiopia, ruining the livelihood of farmers. Ethiopia's government estimated in October 2015 that 8.2 million people needed food assistance and as many as 350,000 children already suffered from severe malnutrition. Another 700,000 moderately malnourished children and pregnant and breastfeeding mothers needed supplemental nutrition in early 2016 (*The Telegraph* 2016).

Nearly 260,000 people died during the famine from 2010 to 2012. Half of them were children under the age of 5. The crisis was caused by a severe drought, but worsened by conflict between rival groups fighting for power. While the lack of rainfall cannot be attributed to climate change, global warming and increased solar radiation, which are climate-related, have been found to be contributors (McDonnell 2015). This huge climate-related disaster illustrates the dreadful power of inequality. Specifically, farmers with small farms feel the effects of climate change much more than those with large farms. Small farms have difficulty competing with large farms because they have less flexibility over land, crops, and farming options. Chances are that the owner of a small farm cannot afford the major changes in farming practice that a large-farm owner might not have difficulty implementing (Byrd 2014).

Not only does a small farmer have a disadvantage, but so do other vulnerable groups, such as the elderly, women, and children. In many African countries, it is the responsibility of the women to carry firewood very long distances to market in order to pay for meager supplies. With heat waves and drought, such long distance carrying may become extremely difficult if not impossible, leaving the family without money to buy nutritious food and other necessities (Byrd 2014). In times of climate-based stress, children and the elderly become more vulnerable because they and their families have less money to pay for healthcare and remaining healthy.

The Small Island Developing States (SIDS)

The Small Island Developing States (SIDS) share sea level flooding and banded together under UN auspices. SIDS includes islands in the Caribbean, Pacific Ocean, and the Greater Indian Ocean region (UNEP 2014). Climate-induced sea-level rise among the world's 57 Small Island Developing States (SIDS) continues to be one of the most pressing threats to global ecosystems. These nations, home to more than 62 million people, emit less than 1% of global greenhouse gases, yet they suffer disproportionately from the climate change that global emissions cause. Typical of the SIDS challenges was the 2012 Fiji Island floods. Unprecedented flooding and landslides left eight dead and 3500 displaced in the aftermath of tropical storms.

Haiti, another SIDS nation, has experienced legendary disasters. In 2010, an earthquake killed more than 200,000 people and injured another 300,000. In addition, 1.5 million were left homeless. In October, 2016, Hurricane Matthew hit Haiti with storm surges up to 10 feet. At least 1350 people died in the storm.

As the sea level is rising at the rate of about a half-inch per year (which is several times higher than the sea rise in most other regions) not only are the islands at risk of flooding but the people are vulnerable to ground water contamination. Further, the loss of usable land threatens the populations of these small island nations. Together these climate-based changes produce annual losses in the trillions of dollars due to increased vulnerability. While the rising sea levels and temperatures threaten habitats, the global net loss of the coral reef cover will cost the international economy an estimated US $11.9 trillion, with Small Island Developing States especially affected by the loss. The huge cost results from aquatic species loss, which in turn destroys food sources.

The SIDS also are threatened by coastal land capacity, invasive alien species and threats from chemicals and waste. As most of the land disappearing under rising sea levels is owned by relatively low- income people, generally the problem is resolved by moving individuals and villages to higher elevations. Not only does this forced migration place people in undesirable locations, it also destroys culture, community, and ways of life that may have existed for centuries (UNEP 2014).

Choosing Priorities for Relieving Suffering

These three climate-induced disaster case studies reveal that physical and social destruction already occur in the present. And the extent of destruction is not trivial. Even though we can expect five to ten times (or more) greater destruction in the near future, it is logical to invest in a concerted, initial effort to minimize the loss that is forthcoming from the interaction of socio-demographic factors that magnify the effect of climate processes on the natural environment.

Both for the present and future, the negative impact of climate change is concentrated in Central America, Central South America, the Arabian Peninsula, Southeast Asia, and much of Africa (Samson et al. 2011). Yet it is the more industrialized regions of the world that produce most of the gasses that produce the vulnerability in these developing regions (UNFCCC 2007). Samson et al. (2011) argue that this situation creates a moral hazard for Western countries and others that do not compensate vulnerable countries in proportion to the harm done.

In terms of priority-setting for present as opposed to future action, another argument can be made for paying more attention to the present than the future. The present is here and now; the future can only be predicted based on what is happening in the present.

Consistent with relieving the suffering of the populations most vulnerable to climate change disasters, now and in the future, compensatory action to assist these populations with such projects as sea walls is recommended. Additional projects should assist small farmers with irrigation, storm water systems, and other water projects that make conflict-free survival possible. Another important action would be to greatly boost funding for technical assistance to countries vulnerable to climate-based disasters.

Finally, and most importantly, funding should be provided to local community projects in these more vulnerable countries to help them meet the challenges of global warming. Community projects like those of the Ecovillage network have the best chance of implementing innovative projects tailored to local challenges.

Conclusions

Hardship and suffering exist in many configurations in most corners of the world. William Vollmann (2005), after living with extremely poor people in both New York City and Nairobi slums, concluded he would rather reside in Kenya's filthy shanties than in New York's tenements because even though New York had more material goods and public utilities, Kenyans cared more about each other's well-being. Vollmann thus discovered that communities with a culture of caring help alleviate the deep suffering of those struggling under great adversity.

Policy that harnesses the energy of local ties has far more potential than policy that applies only to independent individuals. This helps explain why traditional international development often fails whereas local partnerships succeed.

Any project to alleviate suffering can be grounded in one or more time frames: past, present, or future. Humanitarian relief is delivered in the present for disasters rooted in the past. International development projects build capacities and prevention mechanisms in the present that will function as resiliencies in the future.

Climate mitigation advocacy and suffering prevention prepare us to better prepare for both the present and the future. Increasingly the present is filled with victims of chaos that had been predicted for the future. We have failed at suffering prevention from such disasters as climate-produced catastrophes.

This final chapter has argued for attentiveness to the present in order to anticipate future needs. Specifically, we seek to alleviate the suffering of vulnerable populations such as the poor and the disabled in order to address the injustices of existing policies and practices of relevant institutions.

Another undercurrent of this chapter has been that victims of climate disasters should not be viewed just as unlucky people, but as likely victims of inaction and failure to sacrifice for the well-being of present or future generations. People suffer from climate change, inequality, poverty, lack of health care, and other human-produced structural deficits. The language we use should not hide these realities. By working toward alleviating the suffering of currently victimized groups, we not only relieve their hurt but point toward the cruel injustice of failing to mitigate climate change, help recover from disasters, and alleviate large-scale, severe suffering.

Tragically, suffering in climate disaster zones is not generally a single, discrete event, but a series of linked experiences of extreme physical, mental, and social pain embedded in conflict. Recovery from such experiences, particularly among children, may not only be difficult but perhaps impossible for many who suffer as victims or observers—or both. Sometimes death may seem to be the least traumatic outcome; all too often, the victimized are left to a lifetime of intractable pain and shame-producing disabilities.

Furthermore, the poor and neglected tend to be those who suffer the most. Giving them our greatest attention at this point in history might benefit them in the future, were we in the meantime to awaken to the untenable moral "hazard" in which we have placed ourselves as de facto decision-makers.

References

Anderson, R. (2017). Community functioning that fosters sustainable social well-being. In R. Phillips & C. Wong (Eds.), *Handbook of community well-being*. New York: Springer.

Banerjee, A., & Duflo, E. (2011). *Poor economics: A radical rethinking of the way to fight global poverty*. New York: Public Affairs Press.

Black, M. (2015). *International development* (4th ed.). Oxford: New Internationalist Publications.

Brainard, L., Jones, A., & Purvis, N. (Eds.). (2009). *Climate change and global poverty: A billion lives in the balance?* Washington, DC: Brookings Institution.

Brewer, J. (2014). *An impoverished view of poverty–linguistic analysis of gates foundation annual letter*. http://www.slideshare.net/jamesdnorth/a-linguistic-analysis-of-the-gates-foundation-2014-annual-letter Accessed on 11 Jan 2016.
Burke, M., Hsiang, S. M., & Miguel, E. (2015). Climate and conflict. *Annual Review of Economics, 7*(1), 577–617.
Byrd, R. (2014). *5 reasons why climate change is a social issue, not just an environmental one*. Huffington Post Green. Accessed on 8 Feb 2016 at http://www.huffingtonpost.com/rosaly-byrd/climate-change-is-a-socia_b_5939186.html
Caney, S. (2010). Climate change, human rights and moral thresholds. In S. Humphreys (Ed.), *Human rights and climate change*. Cambridge, UK: Cambridge University Press.
Darnton, A. (2011, March 28) Aid: Why are we still stuck in 1985? *The Guardian*. http://www.theguardian.com/global-development/poverty-matters/2011/mar/28/aid-public-perceptions. Accessed 11 Jan 2016.
Darnton, A. & Kirk, M (2011). *Finding frames: New ways to engage the UK public in global poverty*. http://www.findingframes.org/report.htm. Accessed 12 Jan 2016.
Darrow, M. (2012). The millennium development goals: Milestones or millstones? Human rights priorities for the post-2015 development. *Yale Human Rights and Development Journal, 15*(1), 55–127.
Easterly, W. (2006). *The white man's burden: Why the west's efforts to aid the rest have done so much ill and so little*. New York: Penguin Books.
Ellwood, W. (2014). *The no-nonsense guide to degrowth and sustainability*. Oxford: New Internationalist.
Ferguson, J. (2015). *Give a man a fish: Reflections on the new politics of distribution*. Durham: Duke University Press.
Global Challenges Foundation. (2016). *Global catastrophic risks*. Stockholm: Global Challenges Foundation.
Hallegatte, S., Bangalore, M., Bonzanigo, L., Fay, M., Kane, T., Narloch, U., Rozenberg, J., Treguer, D. & Vogt-Schilb, A. (2016). *Shock waves: Managing the impacts of climate change on poverty*. Washington, DC: World Bank. Accessed 2016 at https://openknowledge.worldbank.org/handle/10986/22787
Jamail, D. (2013). What these climate scientists said about earth's future will terrify you. *Mother Jones*. http://www.motherjones.com/environment/2013/12/climate-scientist-environment-apocalypse-human-extinction. Accessed on 21 Oct 2016.
Jobert, K., & Dregger, L. (Eds.). (2015). *ECOVILLAGE: 1001 ways to heal the planet*. Devon: Triarchy Press.
Lakoff, G. (2014). *The all new don't think of an elephant: Know your values and frame the debate*. White River Junction: Chelsea Green Publishing.
Mansharamani, V. (2016). A major contributor to the Syrian conflict? Climate change. *PBS NewsHour*. http://www.pbs.org/newshour/making-sense/a-major-contributor-to-the-syrian-conflict-climate-change/ Accessed on 22 Oct 2016.
McDonnell, T. (2015). Scientists have figured out which natural disasters we can blame on climate change. *New Republic*. https://newrepublic.com/article/123361/scientists-know-which-natural-disasters-blame-climate-change. Accessed on 22 Oct 2016.
McGuire, B. (2012). *Waking the giant: How a changing climate triggers earthquakes, tsunamis, and volcanoes*. Oxford: Oxford University Press.
McGuire, B. (2016). How climate change triggers earthquakes, tsunamis and volcanoes. *The Guardian*. https://www.theguardian.com/world/2016/oct/16/climate-change-triggers-earthquakes-tsunamis-volcanoes. Accessed on 22 Oct 2016.
Meyer, R. (2016, April 29). Human extinction isn't that unlikely. *The Atlantic*. http://www.theatlantic.com/technology/archive/2016/04/a-humanextinction-isnt-that-unlikely/480444/. Accessed 11 Jan 2016.
Milman, O. (2015, March 25) Life in the Philippines: Preparing for the next typhoon Haiyan. *The Guardian*. Accessed on 8 Feb 2016 at http://www.theguardian.com/environment/2015/mar/25/life-in-the-philippines-preparing-for-the-next-typhoon-haiyan

Moyo, D. (2010). *Dead aid–why aid is not working and how there is a better way for africa.* New York: Macmillan, Farrar, Straus and Giroux Publishers.

Munk, N. (2013). *The idealist: Jeffrey sachs and the quest to end poverty.* New York: Knopf Doubleday Publishing Group.

Parenti, C. (2011). *Tropic of chaos: Climate change and the new geography of violence.* New York: Nation Books.

Rahmstorf, S. (2014). *Climate change–State of the science.* Accessed on 19 Oct 2016 at http://www.pik-potsdam.de/~stefan/warmingfacts.pdf

Sachs, J. D. (2005). *To heal a fractured world—The ethics of responsibility.* New York: Schocken Books.

Sachs, J. D. (2015). *The age of sustainable development.* New York: Columbia University Press.

Samson, J., Berteaux, D., McGill, B. J., & Humphries, M. M. (2011). Geographic disparities add moral hazards in the predicted impacts of climate change on human populations. *Global Ecology and Biogeography, 20*(4), 532–544.

Shultz, J., & Crane, M. (Eds.). (2009). *Dignity and defiance: Stories from bolivia's challenge to globalization.* Berkeley: University of California Press.

Stoknes, P. E. (2015). *What we think about when we try not to think about global warming: Toward a new psychology of climate action.* White River Junction: Chelsea Green Publishing.

Tanner, K. (2010). *Our responsibility to the future.* Reflections. Yale Divinity School. http://reflections.yale.edu/article/money-and-morals-after-crash/our-responsibility-future. Accessed 21 Oct 2016.

The Telegraph. (2016). *Horn of Africa famine: Somalia, Ethiopia and Kenya suffer worst drought in 60 years.* Accessed on 8 Feb 2016 at http://www.telegraph.co.uk/news/picturegalleries/worldnews/8630255/Horn-of-Africa-famine-Somalia-Ethiopia-and-Kenya-suffer-worst-drought-in-60-years.html

UNFCCC. (2007). *Climate change: Impacts, vulnerabilities and adaptation in developing countries.* United Nations Framework Convention on Climate Change. Accessing on 8 Feb 2016 at http://www.preventionweb.net/publications/view/2759

United Nations. (2015). Indicators and a monitoring framework for the sustainable development goals. New York: United Nations. Accessed on 18 Oct 2016 at https://sustainabledevelopment.un.org/index.php?page=view&type=400&nr=2013&menu=35

United Nations Environment Programme (UNEP). (2014). *Sea-level rise in small island nations-up to four times the global average – To cost US$ trillions in annual economic loss and impede future development: Shift to green policies and investment critical.* Accessed on 8 Jan 2016 at http://www.unep.org/newscentre/default.aspx?DocumentID=2791&ArticleID=10879#sthash.32Q2knCR.mdyX1oK8.dpuf

Visser't Hooft, H. (1985) *Obligations to future generations: A short essay on the ethics of sustainability.* Accessed on 18 Oct 2016 at http://www.jaysquare.com/resources/growthdocs/grow11.htm#Introduction

Vollmann, W. T. (2005). *Poor people.* New York: HarperCollins.

WHO. (2014). *Quantitative risk assessment of the effects of climate change on selected causes of death, 2030s and 2050s.* Geneva: World Health Organization.

WMO. (2016). *Disasters by decade.* Geneva, Switzerland: World Meteorological Organization. http://www.wmo.int/pages/prog/drr/ Accessed 29 Oct 2016.

Worldwatch Institute. (2015). *State of the world 2015: Confronting hidden threats to sustainability.* Washington, DC: Island Press.

Wrigley, A. (2012). Harm to future persons: Non-Identity problems and counterpart solutions. *Ethical Theory and Moral Practice, 15*, 175–190.